Emotion, Psychotherapy, and Change

Emotion, Psychotherapy, and Change

Edited by

JEREMY D. SAFRAN
The Derner Institute
Adelphi University

LESLIE S. GREENBERG
York University

THE GUILFORD PRESS
New York   London

© 1991 The Guilford Press
A Division of Guilford Publications, Inc.
72 Spring Street, New York, NY 10012

Printed in the United States of America

This book is printed on acid-free paper.

Last digit is print number: 9 8 7 6 5 4 3 2

Library of Congress Cataloging-in-Publication Data

Emotion, psychotherapy, and change / edited by Jeremy D. Safran,
  Leslie S. Greenberg.
        p.   cm.
    Includes bibliographical references and index.
    ISBN 0-89862-556-4
    1. Emotions.   2. Psychotherapy.   I. Safran, Jeremy D.
  II. Greenberg, Leslie S.
    [DNLM: 1. Emotions.   2. Psychotherapy.   WM 420 E535]
  RC489.E45E46   1991
  616.89′14—dc20
  DNLM/DLC
  for Library of Congress   90-14130
                                                                      CIP

Contributors

LARRY E. BEUTLER, PhD, Graduate School of Education, University of California at Santa Barbara, Santa Barbara, California

STEPHEN F. BUTLER, PhD, Department of Psychology, Brookside Hospital, Nashua, New Hampshire

HARTVIG DAHL, MD, Department of Psychiatry, State University of New York Health Science Center at Brooklyn, Brooklyn, New York

ROGER J. DALDRUP, PhD, Division of Educational and Professional Studies, School of Family and Consumer Resources, University of Arizona, Tucson, Arizona

DAVID ENGLE, PhD, Department of Psychiatry, College of Medicine, University of Arizona, Tucson, Arizona

EDNA B. FOA, PhD, Center for the Treatment and Study of Anxiety, Department of Psychiatry, Medical College of Pennsylvania, Philadelphia, Pennsylvania

EUGENE T. GENDLIN, PhD, Department of Psychology, University of Chicago, Chicago, Illinois

LESLIE S. GREENBERG, PhD, Department of Psychology, York University, North York, Ontario, Canada

VITTORIO F. GUIDANO, MD, Center for Cognitive Therapy, Rome, Italy

CARROLL E. IZARD, PhD, Department of Psychology, University of Delaware, Newark, Delaware

MICHAEL J. KOZAK, PhD, Center for the Treatment and Study of Anxiety, Department of Psychiatry, Medical College of Pennsylvania, Philadelphia, Pennsylvania

RICHARD S. LAZARUS, PhD, Department of Psychology, University of California at Berkeley, Berkeley, California

KATHLEEN N. McGUIRE, PhD, The Focusing Community, Eugene, Oregon

JUAN PASCUAL-LEONE, MD, PhD, Department of Psychology, York University, North York, Ontario, Canada

LAURA N. RICE, PhD, Department of Psychology, York University, North York, Ontario, Canada

JEREMY D. SAFRAN, PhD, The Derner Institute, Adelphi University, Garden City, New York

HAROLD SAMPSON, PhD, Department of Psychiatry, Mount Zion Hospital, University of California Medical Center, San Francisco, California

GEORGE SILBERSCHATZ, PhD, Department of Psychiatry, Mount Zion Hospital, University of California Medical Center, San Francisco, California

HANS H. STRUPP, PhD, Department of Psychology, Vanderbilt University, Nashville, Tennessee

Preface

The heart has its reasons, of which reason knows nothing.
—Blaise Pascal

All our so-called consciousness is a more or less fantastic commentary upon an unknown text, one that is perhaps unknowable but still felt.
—Friedrich Nietzsche

The human body is the best picture of the soul.
—Ludwig Wittgenstein

In contemporary Western culture the mind is conventionally located in the head. This has not, however, been the case in all cultures. The ancient Hebrews located the mind in the heart. Traditional Japanese culture emphasizes the importance of a type of intuitive knowing, which is localized in the abdomen. Traditional Chinese culture views the heart, liver, lungs, spleen, and kidney all as instruments of knowledge.

Western civilization's split between mind and body and between reason and emotion—expressed in paradigmatic form in Descartes's *cogito*—has left a difficult legacy for philosophers, cultural critics, and psychological theorists to struggle with. As Paul Ricoeur has argued, Freud's drive metapsychology, which constitutes the bedrock of classical psychoanalytic theory, can be understood as an attempt to dethrone Descartes's *cogito*—to reintegrate the mind and body. Freud, however, could not escape the rationalist *Weltanschaung* in which he was writing, and his solution ultimately perpetuated the split he was trying to heal. Although he saw the tyranny of sexual repression as a major source of pathology, he believed that ultimately feelings and instincts must be controlled through reason. Since Freud, different psychological traditions have struggled with the mind–body, reason–emotion split in different ways.

Ego-analytic thinkers such as Hartmann, while arguing that the reality-oriented ego itself has an instinctual base, have retained Freud's conceptualization of the nonsocial nature of id impulses. Object relations theorists have emphasized the inherently interpersonal nature of human instincts, but have varied in terms of how trustful or mistrustful they ultimately are toward bodily felt experience. Melanie Klein, for example, emphasized the ongoing struggle between destructive and loving impulses, both of which are, in her view, instinctually derived. For her the tension becomes less one of instinct versus reason, than it is a struggle between different instincts.

Winnicott viewed the failure to become attuned to one's own bodily felt needs as the essence of psychological dysfunction. He believed that the individual who becomes overcompliant with perceived demands from the environment develops a split between the real self and a false self. Winnicott thus contrasts authentic and spontaneous living to living that is overly adaptational and reasonable in nature. His perspective is consistent in this respect with Kohut's self psychology and in many respects with experiential theorists (e.g., Rogers, Perls) who emphasize the importance of the "wisdom of the organism" and of maintaining contact with one's bodily felt experience.

The behavioral tradition that dominated academic psychology from the 1930s to the mid-1960s attempted to avoid the trap of dualism by considering mental processes to be inadmissible as scientific data. The rising popularity of cognitive psychology in the mid-1960s, however, returned the mind to center stage in psychological theory. Information-processing theory, however, has failed to address the question of how mind and body are related, and until recently has remained silent on the topic of emotions. In the therapeutic domain, cognitive therapy has viewed rationality and objectivity as the *sine qua non* of mental health. Although this perspective is beginning to change with the development of post-rationalist approaches, cognitive therapists have traditionally emphasized the importance of adopting a scientific stance toward one's experience as a way of controlling disruptive emotions.

In recent years an important shift has taken place in academic psychology. Theorists and researchers have begun to take up the challenge of reintegrating emotion and somatic experience back into the human organism. A parallel shift has begun to take place in the psychotherapy field as theorists and researchers from different traditions have begun to focus more systematically on the role of affective experience in the change process. Historically, those therapeutic approaches that have been most interested in the roles of emotion and bodily felt experience in the change process (e.g., neo-Reichian approaches, Gestalt therapy, bioenergetics, primal therapy) have not participated in academic discourse. Perhaps because of the anti-intellectual stance characteristic of these traditions, they have avoided participation in such dialogue.

Conversely, many academically oriented psychotherapy theorists have eschewed the topics of emotion and bodily felt experience, perhaps at least in part because of a suspiciousness of this realm of existence that resists elucidation through rational inquiry or mastery through intellectual control. With the current explosion of interest in emotion in academic psychology, however, the time is ripe for psychotherapy theorists and researchers to begin participating in dialogue with one another and with academic psychology in an attempt to heal the emotion–reason, body–mind split endemic to Western society.

In this book we have enlisted the aid of theorists from three different psychotherapy traditions (cognitive-behavioral, psychodynamic, and experiential) in the task of mapping out the various ways in which emotion plays a role in the process of change. In the past, psychotherapy theorists from different theoretical traditions have viewed the topic of emotion from different perspectives and have developed intervention strategies to facilitate a variety of different affective change processes. There has, however, been a failure to treat the topic of emotion in any kind of systematic fashion or to develop a theoretical framework to integrate insights deriving from different theoretical traditions.

The development of a transtheoretical approach to the topic of emotion in psychotherapy has been hindered by the absence of dialogue on the topic between psychotherapy theorists and researchers from different traditions. This dialogue in turn has been hindered by the fact that different theoretical traditions differ in terms of basic philosophical assumptions and styles of theoretical discourse that shape their evaluation of what constitutes good theory.

Behavioral thinking, which emphasizes the objective nature of psychological inquiry, has tended to be more linear and data-oriented in nature. Psychoanalytic theorizing often has a more literary tone to it. Theorists in the experiential tradition have intentionally adopted a more personal mode of expression, which is consistent with a more humanistic approach to human problems. These stylistic differences tend to block theoretical cross-fertilization. Behaviorists often dismiss experiential and psychoanalytic theory as unscientific. Psychoanalytic theorists often dismiss behavioral theory as mechanistic. Wholesale dismissals of this type impede the type of integration necessary for real theoretical progress.

Our objective in this book is to facilitate the type of dialogue between cognitive-behavioral, experiential, and psychodynamic theorists that will lead to a further articulation of the domain of emotional processing in psychotherapy. To this end, we have invited psychotherapy theorists from each of these traditions to present examples of affective change processes that they view as being important in their approaches to psychotherapy. They have been asked to provide clinical examples illustrating the relevant change processes and to speculate on the theoretical mechanisms under- lying these change processes.

The reader will find that the different contributions reflect the differ- ent philosophical, theoretical, and stylistic biases of the relevant theoreti- cal orientations. As editors of this volume, we have seen our job as one of providing a common theoretical task for the contributors, rather than one of homogenizing the style of theoretical discourse employed to accom- plish that task.

We have, however, attempted to synthesize the different theoretical contributions through the comments section of the book and our final chapter. By enlisting theorists from different traditions in the task of articulating the various ways in which emotion plays a role in the process of therapeutic change, our hope has been to contribute to a further articulation of the domain of emotion in the process of therapeutic change.

While some of the chapters may be more congenial to a particular reader's theoretical frame of reference than others, we believe that taken together the chapters allow for a broader perspective on the theme of emotion in psychotherapy than would otherwise be possible.

JEREMY D. SAFRAN
LESLIE S. GREENBERG

Contents

PART I

INTRODUCTION

1

Emotion in Human Functioning: Theory and Therapeutic Implications

JEREMY D. SAFRAN
Adelphi University

LESLIE S. GREENBERG
York University

This book is designed to extend and deepen an important knowledge domain—our understanding of the role of emotion in psychotherapeutic change. Psychotherapists and psychotherapy theorists have always recognized the centrality of emotion to the psychotherapeutic enterprise. Despite this recognition, however, there has been an absence of any systematic attempt to map the various ways that emotion influences the change process and to clarify the underlying theoretical mechanisms. There has been a tendency to apply a uniformity assumption to the domain of emotional processing in therapy and to lump diverse processes within general categories, such as emotional insight or catharsis.

This volume has been assembled as part of a systematic attempt to correct this situation; it is an attempt to map out the domain of affective processing and to clarify the theoretical mechanisms of processing (Greenberg & Safran, 1984, 1987, 1989; Safran & Greenberg, 1986, 1987, 1989). In some ways it can be thought of as a sequel to our earlier book on the topic, *Emotion in Psychotherapy* (Greenberg & Safran, 1987), but it stands on its own right.

It focuses on *affective change events* in psychotherapy. A change event is a pattern of therapeutic process leading to change, which occurs with sufficient regularity to make it worth investigation (Rice & Greenberg, 1984). It is a unit consisting of a particular client process, and the therapist intervention that activates it. An affective change event is one that involves the processing or expression of some form of emotional experience on the client's part. The emotional experience in this context is an active ingredient or an instrumental mechanism in the change process, rather than a by-product or an epiphenomenon.

This book has both practical and theoretical objectives. At a practical level it is designed to provide the clinician with detailed descriptions of a wide range of different intervention strategies for working with affective processes. At a theoretical level it is designed to clarify the underlying mechanisms through which these interventions work, and to encourage empirical research in this important domain.

In Part II, contributors from three different therapeutic traditions (cognitive-behavioral, psychodynamic, and experiential) have been asked to identify and describe affective change events that they believe are important in their approaches and to speculate about their underlying processes. We have asked for detailed descriptions of the relevant therapist-client interactions, as well as clinical transcripts illustrating the change processes. Part III contains comments on the preceding chapters and examines the theme of emotion in psychotherapy from the perspective of current developments in cognitive psychology and emotion theory. In Part IV, we provide a synthesis and critical analysis of previous chapters and speculate about a number of core affective processes leading to change.

An important development contributing to the feasability of the current enterprise has been the explosion of interest in the topic of emotion in academic psychology in recent years. In the same sense that the 1960s and 1970s have been deemed the era of the "cognitive revolution," the 1980s appear to have been the era of the "affective" revolution. Whether or not the current interest of academic psychology in emotions ultimately will have as much impact as the cognitive revolution remains to be seen, but the burgeoning interest in emotion and motivational processes in the past decade is undeniable. This interest is marked historically with Zajonc's (1980) classic article on "feeling and thinking," in which he drew attention to the fact that concentrated study of affective phenomena had by and large been ignored by academic psychologists. He urged theorists and researchers to recognize the centrality of emotion in human functioning and to begin to investigate emotion as an important phenomenon in its own right, rather than as a by-product of cognitive processes.

He also argued that affect and cognition operate within partly independent systems and that, contrary to the common view, affective reactions often occur prior to cognitive reactions. Zajonc's position sparked a lively debate regarding the relative primacy of affect and cognition (e.g., Lazarus, 1982, 1984; Zajonc, 1989). As Leventhal and Scherer (1987) conclude, this debate may ultimately be unproductive and will hopefully give way to more differentiated questions regarding the fundamental nature of cognitive and emotional processes. However, Zajonc's (1980) article and the responses to it have played important roles in beginning to shift the focus away from the prevailing view in which emotion was seen as an epiphenomenon of cognition.

Another influence on the growing interest in emotion has been the research of Gordon Bower and colleagues on mood and memory. A series of studies summarized in Bower (1981) demonstrated that people find it easier to learn about events that match their emotional state and find it easier to recall an event if their mood at the time of retrieval is the same as the mood at the time of encoding. In order to account for these phenomena, Bower et al. proposed a modified semantic network theory in which emotion is represented as a node in semantic memory. Although subsequent studies have failed to replicate the initial findings consistently (Blaney, 1986; Bower & Mayer, 1986; Ucros, 1989), this work stimulated an interest in emotion by cognitive psychologists and resulted in a clinically oriented extension of both the theory and the research paradigm by clinical psychologists.

The third important influence on the growing interest in emotion among academic psychologists has been the criticism from within the field of cognitive psychology itself that much of the theory and research of cognitive psychology lacks ecological validity. One of the more vocal and articulate critics in this respect has been Neisser (1976, 1982), who was himself a seminal influence on the development of cognitive psychology. Although Neisser has not focused on the topic of emotion, his cogent criticisms and assertions regarding the importance of understanding the human organism as it functions in the real world have drawn attention to the limitations of attempting to model cognitive processes without attempting to understand their relationship to emotional and behavioral processes. There is a growing recognition that any account of cognitive functioning that neglects emotions will necessarily be seriously incomplete (Oatley & Johnson-Laird, 1987). As Oatley (1987) argues: "The understanding of emotions, and the problems that surround them, will be one of the central issues for understanding intelligent systems" (p. 207).

THEORIES OF EMOTION

In the 1960s and early 1970s the theory of emotion that dominated psychological research was the cognition-arousal theory (Schacter & Singer, 1962). This model views emotion as the product of the interaction between nonspecific arousal and cognitive interpretation. Although empirical findings ultimately failed to support cognition-arousal theory, the view of emotions as the product of the cognitive interpretation of nonspecific arousal was very much consistent with the cognitive *Zeitgeist* of the times.

Although cognition-arousal theory dominated the field during this period two other lines of thought were developing at the same time. The first group of theories can be generally classified as evolutionary/expressive (Izard, 1977; Plutchik, 1980; Tomkins, 1980). These theories trace their roots back to Darwin's work (1872/1955) on emotion and expressive behavior in human beings and nonhuman species. The approach emphasizes the survival value of emotion in an evolutionary context, and in contrast to cognition-arousal theory, hypothesizes that different emotions are associated with different expressive-motor behavior. Another line of thought regarding emotion, represented by Arnold (1960) and Lazarus (1968), can be referred to as a cognitive appraisal theory. These theories emphasize the importance of emotional processes in providing the organism with feedback about the meaning of events for the individual, which can play an adaptive role in the functioning of the organism.

In recent years, a number of theorists have begun to articulate models of emotion that integrate different facets of the evolutionary/expressive and cognitive appraisal approaches with concepts and findings emerging from cognitive psychology and the field of nonverbal behavior (e.g., Buck, 1985; Ekman & Friesen, 1975; Frijda, 1986, 1988; Leventhal, 1982, 1984). Theory and research on emotion is beginning to converge to the extent that a common perspective on emotion is emerging in the field. In the following section a number of the features of this perspective are outlined. Subsequently we will outline some of the potential implications of this perspective for psychotherapy.

FEATURES OF EMOTION

1. *Emotions are adpative.* The emotional processing system has been wired into the human organism through an evolutionary process because of its adaptive significance in human functioning.

2. *Emotions motivate goal-directed behavior important to survival.* Emotions function to safeguard and satisfy the goals of the overall system (Frijda, 1988; Simon, 1967). These goals concern standards regarding what should and should not be. The fundamental ones are wired into the system (e.g., self-protection, hunger satisfaction, attachment needs, and procreation). Other goals or standards are derivatives of these more basic goals that develop as a result of learning. For example, specific beliefs about the way one needs to be, in order to maintain relatedness to other human beings, are standards that develop as a result of the interaction between the wired-in propensity for interpersonal relatedness (Fair-

bairn, 1962; Harlow, 1958) and the specific interactions the individual has with significant others (Safran, 1990a).

3. *Emotions provide action disposition information.* Emotions provide information regarding the readiness of the system to act in a certain way (Frijda, 1988). Emotions are thus a type of action disposition information (Arnold, 1960; Lang, 1983; Leventhal, 1982, 1984). There is an intrinsic connection between emotion and action. For example, anger provides information regarding the readiness of the system to protect itself in an aggressive fashion. Love provides information regarding the readiness for the system to act in an affiliative fashion.

4. *Emotion is motivational.* Emotion has a motivational aspect to it (Arnold, 1960; Izard, 1977; Plutchik, 1980). It not only provides information regarding the readiness of the system to act in a certain way, it also tends to push the system in a certain direction.

5. *Emotions organize systemic priorities through their salience.* Because of the role that emotions play in safeguarding important systemic goals, they have a compelling quality which overrides the entire system. Frijda (1988) refers to this as "control precedence." The idea here is that the action readiness associated with a particular emotion tends to override other considerations, such as long-term goals. For example, the experience of anger may override a rational decision to act in a more cautious fashion. A feeling of attraction for another person may override a more careful and rational evaluation of the potential hazards of becoming emotionally involved. This compelling quality of emotional experience is important to the optimal functioning of the human system. For example, in a life-threatening situation (e.g., being attacked by a predator) it is important for the mobilization of appropriate action (i.e., flight) to take precedence over any other goals the system might have (e.g., eating, socializing, etc.) Emotion thus provides a way of deciding between multiple and possibly incompatible goals by overriding the system in a fashion which is consistent with the system's priorities. Some of these priorities are wired in. Others are learned.

6. *Emotional responses are mediated by anticipated interpersonal consequences.* Although emotion has an involuntary, compelling quality to it, the emotional responses are always mediated by the individual's perception of the environmental response to that emotion. This is referred to by Frijda (1988) as the law of care for consequence. The particular fashion in which the individual perceives the environment responding will in turn be determined by the individual's life experiences.

7. *Emotions involve discrete expressive–motor patterns.* There is a fundamental expressive–motor component to emotional experience. This component is wired into the system and there are specific expressive–motor configurations (physiological, facial, postural, and vocal) corre-

sponding to specific primary emotions (Ekman & Friesen, 1975; Izard, 1977; Leventhal, 1984; Plutchik, 1980; Tomkins, 1980). It is this expressive-motor component that gives emotion its "feeling" quality and this is a primary feature distinguishing emotion from nonemotional information processing.

8. *Emotion is a primary communication system.* Emotion plays a primary role in human communication in a biological system that has evolved to meet the demands of an ecological niche that is characterized by interdependence with other human beings (Darwin, 1872/1955; Izard, 1977). The human system has evolved in a fashion that facilitates both the signaling to other human systems of its own action disposition or action readiness and the reading of the action dispositions of other human systems, as indicated by their emotional displays.

9. *Emotion is a form of meaning.* An important survival value of emotional processing is that it provides quick and economical information regarding the relevance of various contingencies to the system's overall standards and goals. The information provided is rapid, not requiring any time-consuming conceptual analysis. It is economical in the sense that a complex situational configuration and its relevance to the various goals and standards of the entire system can be summarized in an emotional experience. Thus emotional experience provides a condensed, unarticulated form of meaning (Frijda, 1986; Leventhal, 1979).

10. *Schematic emotional memory mediates emotional responding.* Primary processes involved in elaborating the goal and subgoal structure for the human system involve the cognitive processing of events that the individual participates in as well as the emotional responses that are evoked by the situation. From birth, the individual begins developing memory codings for specific events and the emotional responses that are evoked by them. Over time, he/she abstracts generic representations of specific types of events and specific expressive-motor behaviors, and patterns of autonomical arousal that have been evoked by these events (Lang, 1983; Leventhal, 1984). These generic representations provide affective records of the individual's experiences, which influence all future experiences. They thus play a central role in the individual's emotional life. Emotion is thus always a combination of more basic expressive-motor behaviors with cognitive appraisal at various levels of complexity and experience. As Leventhal and Scherer (1987) suggest, it is useful to distinguish between the cognitive processing involved in the activation side of the emotion response and the cognitive processing involved on the response side. On both sides, the cognitive processing involved can range along a continuum from very simple perceptual to more sophisticated conceptual analysis.

11. *Activation of emotion schemata produces emotional experience.* When the right match occurs between stimulus features in the

environment and a particular emotion schema, or an individual's internal processes and key features of a particular emotion schema, that schema will be activated (Leventhal, 1979; Lang, 1983). When this occurs, the information contained in the schema (including images, expressive-motor behaviors, and automatic arousal) will be run off. This information is in turn subjected to further information processing, as the individual attempts to make sense of his/her experience. This combination of processes results in the subjective experience of emotion.

12. *Emotion schemata are continually elaborated by new experience.* As new situations are encountered they activate existing emotion schemata; the entire configuration of the event and the information contained within the schema is processed in order to arrive at a holistic perception of the meaning of the event. This information is in turn encoded, thereby elaborating existing affective memories (Leventhal, 1984).

13. *Cognitive-affective processing provides a rapid but flexible response system.* Because emotion is intrinsically tied to action it provides a rapid way of mobilizing the system to respond in a potentially adaptive fashion in reaction to different contingencies. The expressive-motor component of emotional experience is similar in some ways to a reflex. As Leventhal and Scherer (1987) point out, however, emotion is more than a reflex. Unlike reflex actions, the expressive-motor component of emotion provides information that is subjected to further processing before a final decision regarding action is made. Thus as Sloman (1987) points out, although reflexes have survival value in that they are fast acting, they have the disadvantage of being "dumb." In contrast, emotional processing provides for quick but flexible responding.

THERAPEUTIC IMPLICATIONS

Having outlined some of the central features of the understanding of emotional experience developing in the field, we will now outline, in brief, some of the general implications of this perspective for psychopathology and for psychotherapy.

1. *Full awareness of emotions enhances adaptive functioning.* Since emotion provides information necessary to the optimal functioning of the system, incomplete or distorted emotional processing results in suboptimal functioning of that system (Greenberg & Safran, 1984, 1987; Safran & Greenberg, 1986, 1987). When, for example, an individual fails to learn to process accurately one class of emotional experiences because it conflicts with other goals, he/she will have poor access to information that may be relevant to optimal functioning. For example, when an indi-

vidual learns not to process action readiness information consistent with anger because it conflicts with the goal of attachment, this emotional processing bias may subsequently show up as a clinical problem.

2. *Emotion provides information regarding tacit values and standards.* Since emotion provides a wealth of information about the meaning of various events for the system, accessing and subjecting emotional information to further cognitive processing can provide important information about roles, standards, and values of the system that are not articulated in logical or conceptual form. Because of the compelling quality of emotion, it is difficult to challenge rationally (Safran & Greenberg, 1982a,b). For example, if an individual experiences overwhelming anger in a situation, it is difficult to "talk" the individual out of experiencing anger or for the individual to talk him/herself out of experiencing anger. In such a situation, the anger provides important information regarding the implicit meaning of that situation for the individual. Further assessment is required to clarify the particular idiosyncratic configuration of rules or standards that result in appraising the situation in a fashion that evokes anger.

3. *Awareness of the communicative impact of one's emotion enhances interaction.* Since emotion plays such a central role in interpersonal communication, people read and react to others' emotional displays without necessarily being aware of what they are responding to (Kiesler, 1986). In situations in which an individual is not fully processing affective information about his/her own action dispositions, others may nevertheless respond to an affective readout of the relevant action dispositions. An individual may thus elicit an unexpected and undesirable response in others without understanding what is being responded to. In such a situation, helping the individual to become aware of the action disposition information that he/she is transmitting can be an important part of the change process (Safran & McMain, in press; Safran & Segal, 1990).

4. *Maladaptive emotional responses can be learned.* Although the emotional hardwiring of the human system is designed for adaptive functioning, maladaptive learning experiences can result in dysfunctional programming of the system. Thus, for example, the fact that fear and the associated avoidance response plays a potentially adaptive role in the overall functioning of the system is not incompatible with the acquisition of a fear response to an innocuous situation.

Moreover, a particular standard or goal acquired by the system through learning may ultimately be dysfunctional. For example, one may learn to strive for perfection in everything in order to satisfy attachment needs. In such situations, emotions may function to safeguard dysfunctional goals. An emotional response that is adaptive when it is learned in the original context may be maladaptive in a new context.

5. *Emotional restructuring requires schema activation.* Because emotional experience is synthesized out of prototypical emotion memories that have developed, the modification of maladaptive emotional experience will not take place unless these emotion memories are accessed and in some way modified (Greenberg & Safran, 1987, 1989; Safran & Greenberg, 1986).

6. *Emotional experience presses for completion.* Because of the control precedence of emotional experience, the failure to express emotional experience fully may interfere with the ability to allocate processing capacity in an optimal fashion to other tasks. As Kuhl and Helle (1986) have demonstrated, the failure to implement an action disposition that has been activated results in a persevering emotional state; this intrudes into working memory, thereby claiming processing capacity that may be needed for the enactment of new goals and intentions.

7. *The therapeutic relationship is an important medium for changing emotion schemata.* Since the experience and expression of emotion is shaped by the anticipation of the interpersonal consequences of that emotion, a pivotal variable mediating the exploration and synthesis of new emotional experience in therapy will always be the quality of the therapeutic relationship. The therapeutic relationship thus provides an important medium for modifying emotion schemata (Safran, 1990a,b; Safran & Greenberg, 1989; Safran & Segal, 1990).

CONCLUSION

The preceding summary of theoretical axioms and their therapeutic implications can be thought of as a knowledge base, which, in theory, should be useful in understanding the mechanisms underlying the affective processes examined by the contributors to this volume. The reader may wish to keep them in mind while reading the next section, and to engage in an ongoing evaluation of the extent to which they are useful in refining one's understanding of the theoretical mechanisms underlying the various change processes that are examined. In the final chapter, we will make explicit reference to these axioms in an attempt to isolate underlying mechanisms of change.

In the past, theory development in the major psychotherapy traditions has by and large been divorced from theory development and research on general human functioning in mainstream psychology. Thus, for example, the psychoanalytic perspective has traditionally had its own models of human development and psychological functioning, which in many ways have been developed in isolation from general psychology. Similarily, the experiential tradition (client-centered psychotherapy and Gestalt therapy) has articulated its own theories of human functioning (including such concepts as self-actualization, wisdom of the organism, etc.) without contact with theoretical and empirical development in mainstream psychology.

Although the behavioral tradition attempted to maintain a link with mainstream experimental psychology, the applicability to clinical situations of simple learning models based upon animal experimentation has limitations. To deal with these limitations, behavior therapists at first developed their own more cognitively oriented models, without attending to developments in cognitive psychology (Mahoney, 1974). In the last decade, this situation has changed, as cognitive therapists have begun to borrow concepts from cognitive psychology. As indicated earlier, however, many developments in cognitive psychology have limited applicability to real-life situations (Neisser, 1976, 1982). In recognition of this problem, cognitive psychologists are beginning to attempt to deal with more ecologically valid concerns and to conceptualize the human organism in a holistic fashion, which considers cognition, emotion, and action as integrated aspects of the biological organism. This is resulting in the seeds of an integration between cognitive psychology and emotion theory—two subdisciplines that have traditionally been distinct. This in turn increases the potential applicability of mainstream academic psychology to the field of psychotherapy.

An important question to ask, however, is whether current theory and research in cognitive psychology and emotion theory will ultimately contribute to our understanding of the emotional change processes in psychotherapy, or simply provide another language for reformulating ideas with which clinicians are already familiar. There is no simple answer to this question. On the one hand it can be argued that reframing old psychotherapeutic concepts in the language of contemporary academic psychology provides the advantage of creating a bridge between the two domains. This has the virtue of increasing the possibility that the field of psychotherapy will be open to new, empirically based developments emerging from academic psychology. Moreover, by increasing the dialogue between academic psychology and psychotherapy theory, it increases the possibility that new developments in academic psychology will be ecologically valid. Another possible advantage is that by simply focusing our attention in a systematic fashion on the domain of affective processing in psychotherapy, the possibility of developing a more systematic and differentiated perspective, which will ultimately lead to a more refined understanding of the relevant phenomenon, emerges.

Ultimately, however, the onus will be upon those who wish to establish a link between emotion theory and psychotherapy theory and research, to demonstrate that this enterprise leads to genuinely novel therapeutic implications. Our assessment is that at this stage it is too early to render a final verdict. Hopefully, however, the contributions to this volume will demonstrate that there is promise.

REFERENCES

Arnold, M. B. (1960). *Emotion and personality.* New York: Columbia University Press.

Blaney, P. (1986). Affect and memory. *Psychological Bulletin, 99,* 229-246.

Bower, G. H. (1981). Mood and memory. *American Psychologist, 36,* 129-148.

Bower, G. H., & Mayer, J. D. (1986). *In search of mood dependent retrieval.* Unpublished manuscript.

Buck, R. (1985). Prime theory: An integrated view of motivation and emotion. *Psychological Review, 97,* 398-412.

Darwin, C. (1955). *The expression of emotions in man and animal.* New York: Philosophical Library. (Original work published 1872)

Ekman, P., & Friesen, W. V. (1975). *Unmasking the face.* Englewood Cliffs, NJ: Prentice-Hall.

Fairbairn, W. R. D. (1962). *An object relations theory of personality.* New York: Basic Books.

Frijda, N. H. (1986). *The emotions.* New York: Cambridge University Press.

Frijda, N. H. (1988). The laws of emotion. *American Psychologist, 43,* 349-358.

Greenberg, L. S., & Safran, J. D. (1984). Integrating affect and cognition: A perspective on the process of therapeutic change. *Cognitive Therapy and Research, 8,* 559-578.

Greenberg, L. S., & Safran, J. D. (1987). *Emotion in psychotherapy.* New York: Guilford.

Greenberg, L. S., & Safran, J. D. (1989). Emotion in psychotherapy. *American Psychologist, 44,* 19-29.

Harlow, H. F. (1958). The nature of love. *American Psychologist, 13,* 673-685.

Izard, C. E. (1977). *Human emotions.* New York: Plenum.

Kiesler, D. J. (1986). Interpersonal methods of diagnosis and treatment. In J. D. Cavenar (Ed.), *Psychiatry.* Philadelphia: Lippincott.

Kuhl, J., & Helle, P. (1986). Motivational and determinants of depression: The degenerated intentions hypothesis. *Journal of Abnormal Psychology, 95,* 247-251.

Lang, P. J. (1983). Cognition in emotion: Concept and action. In C. Izard, J. Kagan, & R. Zajonc (Eds.), *Emotions, cognition and behavior.* New York: Cambridge University Press.

Lazarus, R. S. (1968). Emotions and adaptation: Conceptual and empirical relations. In W. J. Arnold (Ed.), *Nebraska Symposium on Motivation* (pp. 175-266). Lincoln, NE: University of Nebraska Press.

Lazarus, R. S. (1982). Thoughts on the relations between emotion and cognition. *American Psychologist, 37,* 1010-1019.

Lazarus, R. S. (1984). On the primacy of cognition. *American Psychologist, 39,* 124-129.

Leventhal, H. (1979). A perceptual–motor theory of emotion. In P. Pliner, K. Blankenstein, & I. Spigel (Eds.), *Advances in the study of communication and affect.* New York: Plenum.

Leventhal, H. (1982). The integration of emotion and cognition: A view from the perceptual–motor theory of emotion. In M. S. Clarke & S. T. Fiske (Eds.), *Affect and cognition.* Hillsdale, NJ: Erlbaum.

Leventhal, H. (1984). A perceptual–motor theory of emotion. In L. Berkowitz (Ed.), *Advances in experimental social psychology* (Vol. 17, pp. 117–182). New York: Academic Press.

Leventhal, H., & Scherer, K. (1987). The relationship of emotion to cognition: A functional approach to a semantic controversy. *Cognition and Emotion, 1,* 3–28.

Mahoney, M. J. (1974). *Cognition and behavior modification.* Cambridge, MA: Ballinger.

Neisser, U. (1976). *Cognition and reality.* San Francisco: W. H. Freeman.

Neisser, U. (1982). *Memory observed.* San Francisco: W. H. Freeman.

Oatley, K. (1987). Editorial: Cognitive science and the understanding of emotions. *Cognition and Emotion, 1,* 209–216.

Oatley, K., & Johnson-Laird, P. N. (1987). Towards a cognitive theory of emotions. *Cognition and Emotion, 1,* 29–50.

Plutchik, R. (1980). *Emotion: a psychoevolutionary synthesis.* New York: Harper.

Rice, L. N., & Greenberg, L. S. (Eds.). (1984). *Patterns of change: Intensive analysis of psychotherapy process.* New York: Guilford.

Safran, J. D. (1990a). Towards a refinement of cognitive therapy in light of interpersonal theory: I. Theory. *Clinical Psychology Review, 10,* 87–105.

Safran, J. D. (1990b). Towards a refinement of cognitive therapy in light of interpersonal theory: II. Practice. *Clinical Psychology Review, 10,* 107–121.

Safran, J. D., & Greenberg, L. S. (1982a). Cognitive appraisal and reappraisal: Implications for clinical practice. *Cognitive Therapy and Research, 6,* 251–258.

Safran, J. D., & Greenberg, L. S. (1982b). Eliciting "hot cognitions" in cognitive behavior therapy: Rationale and procedural guidelines. *Canadian Psychology, 23,* 83–87.

Safran, J. D., & Greenberg, L. S. (1986). Hot cognition and psychotherapy process: An information processing/ecological perspective. In P. C. Kendall (Ed.), *Advances in cognitive-behavioral research and therapy* (Vol. 5, pp. 143–177). New York: Academic Press.

Safran, J. D., & Greenberg, L. S. (1987). Affect and the unconscious: A cognitive perspective. In R. Stern (Ed.), *Theories of the unconscious* (pp. 191–212). Hillsdale, NJ: Analytic Press.

Safran, J. D., & Greenberg, L. S. (1989). The treatment of anxiety and depression: The process of affective change. In P. C. Kendall & D. Watson (Eds.), *Anxiety and depression: Distinctive and overlapping features* (pp. 455–489). San Diego: Academic Press.

Safran, J. D., & McMain, S. (in press). Therapy from a cognitive–interpersonal perspective for personality disorders. *Cognitive Psychotherapy: An International Quarterly.*

Safran, J. D., & Segal, Z. V. (1990). *Interpersonal process in cognitive therapy*. New York: Basic Books.

Schacter, S., & Singer, J. E. (1962). Cognition, social and physiological determinants of emotional state. *Psychological Review, 69,* 379-399.

Simon, H. A. (1967). Motivational and emotional controls of cognition. *Psychological Review, 74,* 29-39.

Sloman, A. (1987). Motives, mechanisms and emotions. *Cognition and Emotion, 1,* 217-223.

Tomkins, S. S. (1980). Affect as amplification: Some modifications in theory. In R. Plutchik & H. Kellerman (Eds.), *Emotion: Theory, research and experience* (Vol. 1). New York: Academic Press.

Ucros, C. G. (1989). Mood state-dependent memory: A meta-analysis. *Cognition and Emotion, 3,* 139-167.

Zajonc, R. B. (1980). Feeling and thinking: Preferences need no inferences. *American Psychologist, 35,* 171-175.

Zajonc, R. B. (1989). On the primacy of the affect. *American Psychologist, 39,* 117-123.

PART II

AFFECTIVE CHANGE EVENTS

Section A

Cognitive–Behavioral Approaches

Traditionally behavior therapists and cognitive–behavior therapists have focused on the reduction of undesirable affective states, such as anxiety and depression. Theorists in the behavioral tradition tended to view anxiety as a conditioned response that could be unlearned through various procedures such as systematic desensitization, flooding, and exposure. Depression has been conceptualized as resulting from an absence of interpersonal skills instrumental in obtaining environmental reinforcement. Techniques such as pleasant events scheduling, skills training, and assertion training have thus been employed to help clients develop impoverished skills and obtain missing reinforcement. With the development of more cognitively oriented approaches, the role of dysfunctional cognitive processes in producing anxiety and depression has been emphasized, and various cognitive procedures for modifying dysfunctional thinking have been developed.

The chapters in this section represent two relatively recent developments in cognitive–behavioral approaches to emotion. Foa and Kozak articulate a cognitive information-processing approach to the conceptualization of the development and treatment of anxiety disorders. Following developments articulated by theorists such as Jack Rachman and Peter Lang, they conceptualize anxiety disorders as resulting from fear structures (i.e., emotional memories that are encoded at levels of both imagery and expressive–motor behavior). This type of formulation is consistent with the type of emotion schema conceptualization articulated in Chapter 1 of this volume. In their chapter they examine the way in which the activation and reprogramming of emotion structures of this type can play a role in the treatment of anxiety disorders.

Guidano, writing from a cognitive-constructivist perspective, provides a good example of some of the newer developments in the cognitive conceptualization of the role of emotion in psychotherapy. In contrast to more traditional behavioral and cognitive-behavioral conceptualizations of emotion, Guidano emphasizes the adaptive role that emotional processing plays in the human biological system. In his chapter, he explores the informational function of emotional processing in the human organism as well as the role that such processing can play in systemic change.

2

Emotional Processing: Theory, Research, and Clinical Implications for Anxiety Disorders

EDNA B. FOA
MICHAEL J. KOZAK
Medical College of Pennsylvania

THEORY AND EMPIRICAL EVIDENCE

Emotional experiences can often be relived well after the original emotional events have occurred. Vivid recall seems to involve the re-experiencing of emotion itself, including details of the original situation. This phenomenon is clearly exemplified by the common experience of recurring grief following the loss of a loved one. Memories of the lost person coinciding with the sadness as felt at the time of loss are labeled emotional re-experiencing. It seems that people more often report reliving of unpleasant memories than of pleasant ones. A crime victim, when remembering the crime, is more likely to get in touch with the horror and the helpless sensation that he/she had felt than is a prize-winner to re-experience the euphoria that accompanied the winning of a large sum. Likewise, one is more likely to be sad when thinking about the death of a friend than elated when remembering a friend's wedding. Therefore, in clinical practice, incomplete emotional processing of negative emotional events predominates.

Mostly, the frequency and intensity of emotional re-experiencing decrease over time. A mother who has lost her child may, at first, sob uncontrollably when reminded of it. With the passage of time, the pain lessens, although perhaps never entirely disappears. Rachman (1980), in his classic paper on emotional processing, has alerted us to the significance of processes underlying the decline of emotional revivification; when these are impaired, psychopathology emerges. Accordingly, the index of unsuccessful emotional processing is "the persistence or return of intrusive signs of emotional activities such as obsessions, nightmares, pressure of talk, phobias, inappropriate expressions of emotions" (Rachman, 1980, p. 51).

As noted by Rachman, classical accounts of neurosis (Freud, 1910) construe symptoms as remnants of traumatic experiences. Presumably, such memories are too painful to be entertained, and thus, remain for the most part out of consciousness. Psychoanalytic therapy focuses on bringing early painful experiences into awareness, thereby reducing their current emotional impact. In behavior therapy, too, experiences of negative affect are often seen as necessary for the reduction of neurotic symptoms. Thus, Wolpe (1978) explained certain unsuccessful cases of fear reduction by systematic desensitization as stemming from patient's inability to experience fear while they imagined their feared situations. Convergently, Lang (1977) argued that phobics who profited most from desensitization were those best able to experience anxiety during their imagery, suggesting that the affective component of imagined scenes "may be a key to the emotional processing which the therapy is designed to accomplish" (p. 863).

If some kind of emotional processing is hypothesized to occur during psychotherapy to mediate the reduction of neurotic symptoms, this construct requires elaboration. Toward this end, Foa and Kozak (1985, 1986) integrated available concepts of fear, relevant experimental data, and clinical investigations. In this chapter, we will first discuss this theory and consider recent data pertinent to it. Next, we will examine implications of the theory for treatment of anxiety, particularly obsessive–compulsive disorder.

Emotion and Cognition

Colloquially, people seem to label states of heightened physiological activity as emotional when the context is perceived as especially good or bad. Psychological theorists have for the most part adopted the notion that emotion is physiology plus interpretation. They differ, however, in their focus. Cognitive theorists (Lazarus, 1966; Mandler, 1975; Schachter & Singer, 1962) emphasize the importance of interpretive aspects. Somatic theorists (Ekman & Friesen, 1974; James, 1890; Leventhal, 1980) focus on the physiological aspects of emotions. Regardless of emphasis, both schools view cognitive and somatic events as necessary components of affects. Coexistent with these ideas in psychology is the view that affect is distinct from cognition. Zajonc (1980) and Zajonc and Markus (1984) have advocated this distinction, proposing that affect and cognition are served by parallel, separate, and at least partly, independent systems. Furthermore, at least some affect is seen as independent of cognitive events and as strictly physiological:

> In the pure case, the analysis of feelings attends primarily to energy transformations, for example, the transformation of chemical or physical energy at the sensory level into autonomic or motor output. In contrast, the analysis of thoughts focuses principally on information transformations . . . affects is always present as a companion of thought, whereas the converse is not true for cognition. (p. 154)

A dichotomy of affect and cognition may be forced by two related assumptions: (1) an often implicit equation of cognition and awareness, and (2) an assumption that cognition must be semantically coded. If one equates awareness and cognition, and also accepts that emotions can be expressed unconsciously (e.g., see Zajonc & Markus, 1984), one must conclude that emotion can occur without cognition. Similarly, if cognitions are always semantically coded, but emotion is not always expressed semantically, one must conclude that emotion need not be cognitive. There are, however, difficulties with both assumptions. There is evidence from experimental literature (Horton & Kjeldergaard, 1961; Nisbett & Wilson, 1977) that cognitive changes occur in the absence of awareness about the underlying processes. Second, ample evidence of nonsemantic cognitive representations also refutes the second assumption. For example, the far greater recognition capacity for pictures compared with that for words (Shepard, 1967; Standing, Conezio, & Haber, 1970) indicates that "subjects must have remembered something about pictures other than simple verbal descriptions of them" (Klatzky, 1975, p. 200). Similarly, memory for musical pattern can occur in the absence of knowledge of musical symbols or semantic labels for the composition.

If one abandons the requirement that cognitions be available to introspection, the need to dichotomize cognition and emotion disappears. Thus, we view emotional expression as controlled by special types of cognitive structures that are characterized by response elements and intense positive or negative valence. Our focus here will be on fear and its reduction via exposure therapy, but our conceptualization is potentially applicable to other emotions as well.

The Cognitive Structure of Fear

Adopting Pylyshyn's (1973) construal of a propositional network as an organization of concepts related to one another by other concepts, Lang (1977, 1979) suggested an analysis of the fear structure into propositions.

Accordingly, fear is represented as a network in memory that includes three kinds of information: (1) information about the feared stimulus situation, (2) information about verbal, physiological, and overt behavioral responses, and (3) interpretive information about the meaning of the stimulus and response elements of the structure. This information structure is conceived of as a program for escape or avoidance behavior.

We have proposed that if the fear structure is indeed a program to escape danger, then it must involve information that stimuli and/or responses are dangerous, as well as information about physiological activity preparatory for escape. Thus, a fear structure is distinguished from other information structures, not only by response elements, but also by certain "meaning" information it contains. For example, the programs for running ahead of a baton-carrying competitor in a race and for running ahead of a club-carrying assailant on a racetrack are likely to involve similar stimulus and response information. What distinguishes the fear structure is the meaning of the stimuli and responses: Only the fear structure involves escape from threat.

The Structure of Pathological Fear

Most people experience fear in some circumstances, thus implying the *running* of a program for fear. Normal fear occurs with the perception of real threat and disappears when the danger is removed. Sometimes, fear occurs in the absence of danger, but decreases when the person discovers that the situation is safe. We consider fear to be pathological when it is disruptively intense and persists despite information that is unrealistic. In other words, pathological structures involve excessive response elements (e.g., avoidance, physiological activity) and are resistant to modification. A fear is considered to be unrealistic when its underlying memory structure contains stimulus–stimulus (S-S) associations which do not accurately represent relationships in the world. For example, for many obsessive–compulsive washers, floors are strongly associated with feces (and therefore are highly contaminated), whereas in reality, feces are rarely encountered on floors. Another disordered stimulus-stimulus link is that of germs on doorknobs and skin cancer. Any associations between harmless stimuli and responses (S-R) preparatory to escape or avoidance are also disordered: Escape from doorknobs does not enhance an organism's survival. Embedded in these disordered S-S and S-R associations is some of the erroneous meaning of the pathological fear structure. Additional erroneous meaning can be coded semantically as interpretive elements in the structure.

Several types of evaluations can characterize the fear structures of those anxiety-disordered individuals. First, there is a reluctance to engage in fear-provoking experiences because of one's evaluation that anxiety will persist until escape is realized. Second, the fear stimuli and/or responses are estimated to have an unrealistically high potential for causing psychological (e.g., going crazy, losing control) or physical (e.g., dying, being ill) harm. Third, the anticipated consequences have a relatively high negative valence; that is, they are extremely aversive for the individual.

The anxiety disorders can be viewed as representing different fear structures. For example, the presence of a relationship between certain situations and fear responses in panicky agoraphobics or simple phobics indicates a disordered link among stimulus and response elements of their underlying fear structures. However, what distinguishes the agoraphobic structure from that of simple phobia and other anxiety disorders is erroneous evaluation of the fear responses. Agoraphobics commonly perceive anxiety itself to be dangerous, the risks being of either physical harm (e.g., heart attacks) or psychological harm (e.g., going crazy, being embarrassed). Stimulus elements (e.g., supermarkets) are not evaluated as intrinsically dangerous: The danger is perceived to lie in the anxiety that they evoke. In contrast, for simple phobics, the potental harm does stem from the stimulus situation itself (e.g., snakes, wasps, dogs). An agoraphobic fear structure is schematically illustrated in Figure 2.1.

Unlike agoraphobics who fear their own responses, obsessive–compulsive washers, like simple phobics, mistakenly interpret certain harmless stimuli as harmful. For the person who fears infection from even indirect contact with feces and urine, the fear structure represents three types of conceptual errors: S-S associations, S-R associations, and associations between semantic elements and stimulus elements. Figure 2.2 illustrates such a structure.

Not all elements of an emotional structure are accessible by introspection. Although individuals may be aware of some aspects of their fear, their knowledge is surely imperfect. Just as a person may be unaware of some response information in a fear structure (e.g., information that underlies increased blood pressure), so also may one be unaware of the meaning of those responses. Theories of emotions must take into account what people tell us about their emotions, but these reports must be treated with caution. Two types of errors in conceptualizing introspective data can arise: One extreme is to ignore the inherent meaning of people's interpretation of their experiences, or to reject a priori their validity. Researchers who hold this position might allow that self-reports could evidence some hypothetical construct but that the reports themselves have no content validity. At the other extreme, the content validity of subjective reports is taken for granted and becomes the basis for theories of emotion.

A satisfactory theory would encompass the content of self-reports without theoretical dependency on introspective explanations, since such explanation may or may not be valid. Indeed, people report beliefs and evaluations that necessarily reflect elements of their cognitive structures,

SCHEMATIC AGORAPHOBIC FEAR NETWORK

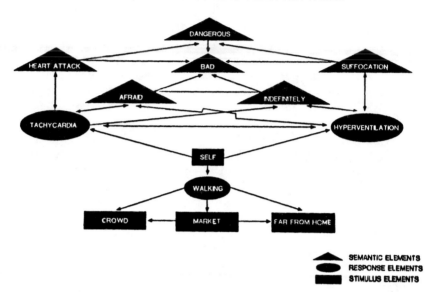

FIGURE 2.1.   Connecting vectors suggest directions for the various conceptual relations among the elements; for example, tachycardia causes heart attack, heart attack brings tachycardia, self is walking in the market. From "Emotional Processing of Fear: Exposure to Corrective Information" by E. B. Foa and M. J. Kozak, 1986, *Psychological Bulletin, 99,* 20–35. Copyright 1986 by the American Psychological Association. Reprinted by permission.

and therefore, must be taken into account by a satisfactory theory of emotion. On the other hand, because of people's imperfect knowledge about their emotions, nonintrospective assessment of emotional structures is also required. Traditionally, psychophysiological measurement constituted one such assessment. However, in addition to recorded physiology, nonverbal behavior such as facial expressions, postural adjustments, overt actions, and so on, would also be expected to reflect some elements. Any of these data can complement subjective reports as bases for hypotheses about emotional structures.

Empirical Evidence

The fear structure of agoraphobics has gained considerable attention with the emergence of the *fear of fear* hypothesis (Goldstein & Chambless, 1978; Weekes, 1973). This hypothesis holds that agoraphobics, but not simple phobics, fear interoceptive cues that they interpret as signaling

A SCHEMATIC FEAR NETWORK
OF AN OBSESSIVE-COMPULSIVE WASHER

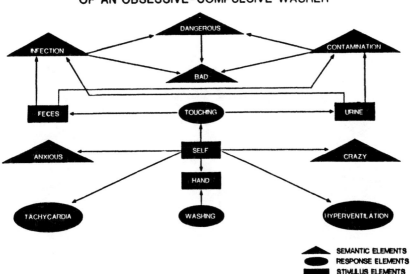

FIGURE 2.2.   Connecting vectors suggest directions for the various conceptual relations among the elements; for example, touching feces causes infection, touching urine causes contamination, contamination is dangerous.

pending disasters, for example, death. Support for this hypothesis was found in retrospective data reported by Goldstein and Chambless (1978).

In a prospective study by Dattilio and Foa (1987), the association of interoceptive responses with danger was compared in different anxiety disorders. One hundred subjects were studied, with 20 in each of the following conditions: specific phobias, generalized anxiety disorder, panic disorder with and without agoraphobia, nonanxious. All received questionnaires assessing fear of fear. On the Anxiety Sensitivity Index (Reiss, Peterson, Gursky, & McNally, 1986) and the Body Sensations Questionnaire (Chambless, Caputo, Bright, & Gallagher, 1984) in which individuals were asked to rate their concern with certain anxiety-related physical sensations and their anticipated consequences, panic-disordered groups scored higher than the other three groups. A consistent picture emerged for all these measures: panic-disordered groups showed greater response-harm associations than the other groups. Some questionnaires assessed both fear of interoceptive cues and of situations that would be fearful to non-anxiety-disordered individuals, for example, "getting mugged but not seriously hurt." Both of the panic-disordered groups overestimated the probabilities that feared interoceptive responses would occur, but they did not differ from the other groups in anticipating general fear events. The same pattern emerged for ratings of valence: Panic-disordered groups rated feared interoceptive responses as more aversive than did the other groups, but general fear items were rated similarly by all groups.

Associations among events and threat were also examined by having subjects rate imagined vignettes, each of which could be interpreted as either dangerous or nondangerous. Some scenarios focused on interoceptive cues, others on external events. Panic-disordered groups interpreted more situations as dangerous regardless of the type of events involved. The ratings of ambiguous situations converged with those of the other questionnaires to support the hypothesis that panic-disordered patients exhibit especially strong associations among physiological responses and harm. Notably, however, the different questionnaires yielded divergent findings about general fear situations. On brief-item questionnaires, panic-disordered groups, as expected, did not differ from the other groups. When presented with more elaborate scenarios, however, the panic-disordered groups scored higher on general fear items than the other groups. Perhaps imagined vignettes are more successful in evoking fear than brief questions, regardless of fear content. If so, once the physiology of fear is evoked in panic-disordered patients, response–harm associations are accessed, priming an association of harm with contextual stimulus events.

Further evidence that agoraphobics, but not simple phobics, show especially strong associations between interoceptive responses and threat comes from a psychophysiological study of imagery with eight agoraphobics and eight simple phobics (Mansueto, Grayson, & Foa, 1987). Subjects were presented with four types of scenes: (1) external fear stimuli such as supermarkets or snakes, constituting each person's most feared object or situation, (2) interoceptive fear responses such as heart rate or breathing changes, constituting the responses most associated with fear for each individual, (3) stimulus plus response scenes, combining the external and interoceptive propositions for each person, and (4) neutral (nonfear) stimuli. Self-report, skin conductance, spontaneous fluctuations, and heart rate were used to assess fear. Agoraphobics were fearful while imagining external, interoceptive, and combined scenes, but not neutral material; simple phobics, however, were fearful only while imagining external and combined material, but not interoceptive material. These psychophysiological results converge with the questionnaire data of Dattilio and Foa (1987) to suggest that agoraphobic fear structures, unlike those for simple phobias, are characterized by the particular interpretive meaning that interoceptive responses are dangerous. This convergence of introspective and physiological data indicates that people's beliefs about the nature of their fears can reflect elements of their fear structures.

Further support for the hypothesis of particular response–threat associations in the fear structures of agoraphobics emerges in a study comparing nine normal controls and nine untreated agoraphobics with nine agoraphobics who had been successfully treated via exposure and anxiety management techniques (McNally & Foa, 1987). All three groups received questionnaires with items pertaining to fear of interoceptive cues and the harm anticipated from them, as well as items about general fear situations that might also disturb non-anxiety-disordered individuals. The questionnaires were the same as those used by Dattilio and Foa (1987) above, and the results of the two studies were consistent. Untreated agoraphobics scored higher than normals when asked to estimate the probability and cost of interoceptive cues, but not of external fear situations. Also, as in the other study, when asked to consider scenarios describing either interoceptive responses or external stimuli, this group interpreted *both* types as more threatening than did normals. Interestingly, the treated agoraphobics did not differ from normals on any of the measures. These results not only evidenced a connection between the hypothesized agoraphobic fear structure and symptoms, but also suggested that change in the fear structure may explain therapy outcome.

Modifying the Fear Structure

Assuming that therapy for anxiety disorders is modifying fear structures, we have proposed that regardless of the type of therapy selected, two conditions are required for the reduction of fear (see Foa & Kozak, 1986). First, fear-relevant information must be made available in a manner that will activate the fear memory. Accordingly, as also suggested earlier by Lang (1977), if the fear structure remains in storage but unaccessed, it will not be available for modification. Next, information made available must include elements that are incompatible with some of those that exist in the fear structure, so that a new memory can be formed. This new information, which is at once cognitive and affective, has to be integrated into the evoked information structure for an emotional change to occur. This change in the fear structure constitutes emotional processing. Behavioral treatments for anxiety are designed to provide information that is sufficiently incompatible with the fear structure to reduce fear.

We have identified three indicators of emotional processing that are associated with successful outcome of exposure treatment for anxiety. First, patients who improve with therapy show physiological responses and self-reports of fear that evidence activation of anxiety. Second, their reactions decrease *gradually* within exposure, that is, during confrontation with feared objects or situations. Third, initial reactions to the fear at each exposure session decrease across sessions. Support for the validity of these indicators comes from clinical outcome studies and experiments that have been reviewed by Foa and Kozak (1986). Recent data further buttress the argument for their validity.

Kozak, Foa, and Steketee (1988) explored the relationship between the three indicators and therapy outcome with obsessive–compulsives who were treated by exposure and response prevention. Treatment outcome was evaluated via ratings of target symptoms by the therapist, patient, and independent assessor. Processes during therapy were assessed through self-report of anxiety as well as by cardiac and electrodermal responses. The first indicator, activation of anxiety, was evident in both self-report and physiological measures during exposure sessions, and predicted posttreatment improvement. As expected, treatment was successful overall, and the second indicator, habituation within sessions, was also evident in both self-report and physiology for the group as a whole. This indicator did not, however, predict individual differences in outcome, perhaps because most patients habituated within sessions. The third indicator, habituation across sessions, was found for the group only in self-report, but individual differences on this indicator (both heart rate and self-report) predicted outcome. In summary, the three hypothesized indicators of emotional processing were evidenced either by the group means or the correlations. The association among successful outcome and the three indicators supports our claim that these indicators reflect mechanisms of emotional processing.

The above results converge with those of another investigation of the process and outcome of therapy (Schwartz & Kaloupek, 1987) in which speech-anxious volunteers were treated with imaginal exposure. Outcome was evaluated by self-report, observations of speech performance, and cardiac and electrodermal activity. Process of therapy was assessed by self-report and physiological measures during imaginal exposure sessions. Greater responding and greater habituation within and/or between sessions predicted better outcome of therapy.

Variables That Influence Affective Change

Content of the Evocative Information

A fear memory is thought to be accessed when a fearful individual is presented with fear information that matches some of the information structure in memory (Lang, 1977). This information may be about the feared situation, the person's responses in the situation, or their meaning. Lang (1977) suggested that some critical number of information units must be matched for the entire fear memory to be activated, and that some information elements may be especially important in evoking the fear structure. Intense phobias, he proposed, may be characterized by strongly coherent structures that can be evoked with minimally matching information. For example, the sight of a coiled garden hose may elicit intense fear in a snake phobic. Likewise, a warm sensation may evoke a panic attack in the agoraphobic who fears certain physiological sensations.

In studying variables that influence the accessing of fear structures, Lang and his associates found that descriptions of both stimulus and response propositions (e.g., "your heart pounds as you see a green snake on a rock") evoked greater fear than did descriptions of stimulus material only (Lang, Kozak, Miller, Levin, & McLean, 1980). The effects of combining stimulus and response material were amplified when fear-relevant scenes were presented to phobics (Lang, Levin, Miller, & Kozak, 1983) and to nonphobic good imagers (Miller et al., 1988). These results suggest that response elements are important aspects of fear memory, and evocative material including them constitutes a better match and thereby promotes fear accessing.

How does the stimulus content of exposure influence fear accessing, and hence, its modification? The above experiments focused on how the response structure of evocative material increases accessing. The match between stimulus material and the stimulus structure of a fear memory would also seem important. Experimental results bearing on this hypothesis were reported by Foa, Steketee, Turner, and Fischer (1980) with obsessive-compulsives who had checking rituals. Disaster scenarios constitute a central component of checkers' fears, but of course are not realized during *in vivo* exposure. The information delivered in *in vivo* exposure does not constitute such a good match for their fear structure and, thus, would alone be expected to produce less improvement than when combined with imagery of disasters. Indeed, the group that received both imaginal and *in vivo* exposure maintained its gains, whereas some relapse was evident for those who received *in vivo* exposure only. Notably, at follow-up, the variance in the relapsing group was larger: Some patients did not relapse at all, whereas others showed complete relapse. Perhaps those who did not need imaginal exposure to maintain their gains were able to use the limited information presented *in vivo* to call up other relevant elements in the structure, that is, disaster scenarios. Conversely, when *in vivo* presentation failed to access these elements, emotional processing was impeded and fear returned.

Evocative Medium

An obvious way to access a fear memory is confrontation with an actual feared situation. However, *in vivo* exposure is not the sole mode of information input that activates fear. Evocative information can be delivered via a variety of audio or visual media.

The relative efficacy of a particular medium for activating fear may depend on how well it can depict the elements of the fear structure, as well as on a person's willingness or ability to engage in the recall process. For example, actual (*in vivo*) presentation of a feared situation is more likely to evoke a fear response than imaginal exposure for simple phobics. Indeed, Watson, Gaind, and Marks (1972) found that for simple phobics, the average initial heart rate response during fear-relevant images was 8 beats/minute, whereas the average response during *in vivo* exposure to these same stimuli was 28 beats/minute. With obsessive–compulsives, however, *in vivo* exposure does not seem to be superior in evoking fear. Equivalent increases in self-report and autonomic measures of fear have been found for both imaginal and *in vivo* exposure with ritualizers. Boulougouris (1977) reported heart rate increases of just under 3 beats/minute during both imaginal and *in vivo* exposure; Kozak et al. (1988) found increases of 4 beats/minute for imaginal exposure and 2 beats/minute for subsequent *in vivo* exposure. Thus, simple phobics may differ from obsessive–compulsives in the magnitude of their heart rate responses during exposure, and in the evocative potency of imaginal versus *in vivo* procedures.

At least two alternative hypotheses can be advanced to explain the different responses during imaginal and *in vivo* exposure for the two disorders. First, the physiological responding represented in obsessive–compulsive fear structures may simply be of smaller magnitude than in simple phobics, such that less responding is observed even when fear is fully evoked. In this case, the lower ceiling for obsessive–compulsives might mitigate differences among evocative media. Secondly, excessive response elements are equivalent but compulsives may have less coherent fear structures than simple phobics so that they are more difficult to evoke under the constraints of the laboratory environment. This would also yield truncated fear responses and the ceiling effect described above.

Clinical observations favor the first hypothesis: Simple phobics seem more likely to describe intense physical fear reactions than do obsessive–compulsives. Given this, one would expect a stronger relationship of physiological activation and habituation to outcome for simple phobics than for obsessive–compulsives. Notably, the correlations found for simple phobics by Lang, Melamed, and Hart (1970) among heart rate activation, habituation, and outcome were higher (.75 to .91) than those found among these variables by Kozak et al. (1988) for obsessive–compulsives (.36 to .54).

This hypothesized difference in fear structure implies that for simple phobics, it is practically sufficient to focus on treatment variables that promote activation and habituation of fear such as content and duration of exposure. In contrast, for obsessive–compulsives, treatment should probably encompass variables that engage other mechanisms besides physiological activation and habituation, such as certain aspects of the meaning represented in the fear structure, for example, probability of harm, subjective valence.

Duration of Exposure

The finding that longer duration exposure produces better outcome of therapy is robust across both diagnostic groups and types of exposure (Chaplin & Levine, 1980; Rabavilas, Boulougouris, & Stefanis, 1976; Stern & Marks, 1973). During exposure treatment, gradual decreases in autonomic responding and reported fear have been repeatedly observed to occur over time, and such decreases have been related to success of treatment. Of course, since habituation requires time, longer duration exposure would be expected to yield more habituation, and thus, superior therapy outcome.

Notably, the length of exposure required for habituation differs across disorders. Chaplin and Levine's speech phobics started to habituate to fear imagery after 25 minutes, whereas the agoraphobics in the Foa and Chambless (1978) study began to habituate after 50 minutes. During *in vivo* exposure with agoraphobics, heart rate decreases after 60 minutes were observed (Stern & Marks, 1973), whereas with specific phobics, decreases after about 20 minutes were found (Watson et al., 1972). It is plausable to view the fears of agoraphobics as generally more pervasive, intense, and complex than those of simple phobics. Thus, it appears that the more intense or pervasive the fear, the longer the exposure time required to achieve habituation within sessions and the consequent change in the fear structure.

If emotional processing is construed as the modification of an emotional memory through the incorporation of corrective information, an obvious prerequisite is sensory encoding of the information presented. Two studies of exposure treatment of fear suggest that attention promotes fear-relevant images with or without instructions to relax. Relaxed subjects benefited more from treatment by exposure than did nonrelaxed ones, reported greater imagery vividness, showed larger initial heart rate responses during imagery, and more habituation (Borkovec & Sides, 1979). The authors suggested that these seemingly diverse effects become coherent if relaxation is seen to enhance attention to fear-relevant information. Indeed, if a relaxed subject is better able to encode the available information, he/she would be expected to access his fear structure more fully; habituation to the fear content can then take place and emotional processing should occur. With obsessive–compulsives, Grayson, Foa, and Steketee (1986) found that during exposure with distraction instructions, no habituation of heart rate occurred, whereas with attention instructions, the customary heart rate decreases appeared.

Mechanisms for Emotional Processing

We have embraced the view that fear is represented as a propositional network in memory, which serves as a program for fear behavior. Pathological fear, we suggested, includes erroneous elements and/or associations among elements. It follows, then, that change in the pathological network is the target of psychotherapy for anxiety disorders. Such change, which we have called emotional processing, requires the integration of information that is incompatible with the pathological elements of the structure. We have described indicators of emotional processing and discussed variables that influence treatment outcome. If we hypothesize that psychotherapy of fear promotes structural changes, it is incumbent upon us to specify what cognitive representations must be changed, that is, what needs to be learned.

Dissociation of Response Elements

Earlier, we proposed that pathological fear structures are characterized by S-R associations in which the responses preparatory to escape or avoidance are unwarranted by the context. Exposure leads to physiological habituation within sessions, which involves decreases in such preparatory responding. The absence of this responding in the fear context constitutes information that is incompatible with the existing structure, thereby weakening the pre-existing links between stimulus and response elements. Disordered response–response associations, as found in panic disorders, are also hypothesized to succumb to habituation. Accordingly, the association between dizziness and tachycardia can be weakened in the same way as that between feces and tachycardia.

Meaning

In addition to promoting changes in the S-S and S-R links of a fear memory via short-term physiological habituation, harmless confrontation with a feared situation also changes both semantic and nonsemantic aspects of meaning. Such changes involve a reduction in the exaggerated probability associated with the feared harm and/or a change in the representation of its valence.

Reduction in probability of harm might occur in two ways: One obvious process is incorporation of new contingencies, for example, a barking puppy dog on one's lap is not followed by painful bites, and thus, the association between bites and dogs is weakened. This type of change can be construed as weakening of S-S associations. Another way of modifying semantic representations of probability is via their replacement with incompatible content. For example, the instruction that AIDS cannot be communicated through handshakes changes the perceived probability of AIDS, given handshaking. Perhaps weakening the S-S associations requires neither conscious awareness nor language, whereas modification of semantic representation of probability may require both.

Just as with probabilities, modification of negative valence can occur in two ways: weakening of S-S or S-R associations and changing semantic representations. In the case of harmless exposure to a dog, the weakened association between dog and biting results not only in representation of decreased probability of a bite from the dog, but also of decreased negative valence: Dogs are unlikely to bite, dogs are not bad. Likewise, habituation of fear responses results in weakening associations between fear stimuli and responses. The power of the stimulus to evoke the responses decreases. If the fear responses themselves are aversive, then their dissociation from the stimulus renders it less negatively valent. From these two examples, it is apparent that although probability of harm and valence are conceptually distinct, in practice they seem to covary with changes in strength of S-S and S-R associations. Such covariance may not occur when valence of probability is modified semantically, either by direct instruction or through observation. For example, the negative valence of contracting syphilis remains high even with the instruction that it is not contracted from toilet seats: The likelihood of syphilis changes but not the valence. Conversely, when one is instructed that syphilis is readily cured, the disease becomes less negative, regardless of its probability of occurrence.

Indirect support for the notion that meaning also changes through unconscious S-S weakening comes from experiments on extinction of generalization gradients in aversive conditioning (Hoffman & Fleshler, 1961). Pigeons received shocks signaled by 1,000-Hz tones and the generalization of extinction to different tones was then tested. Extinction was minimal to the original tone but increased gradually as the test tones grew less similar to the 1,000-Hz conditioned stimulus. This sharpening gradient of extinction developed without either previous or concurrent differential reinforcement. This paradigm can be interpreted as analogous to exposure therapy procedures in which a feared stimulus is presented repeatedly. Accordingly, associated fear stimuli would be expected to lose potency more readily than the target stimulus itself. For example, imaginal exposure to a house fire for an obsessive–compulsive would lead to more reduced fear of electrical appliances than of a destructive house fire itself. This illustrates how imaginal exposure to disaster scenarios may change the valence of associated events more than it changes the valence of the disaster itself.

TREATMENT OF PATHOLOGICAL FEAR: THE EXAMPLE OF OBSESSIVE–COMPULSIVE SYMPTOMS

Symptoms and Fear Structure

In DSM-III-R (American Psychiatric Association, 1987), the official diagnostic manual of the American Psychiatric Association, obsessive–compulsive disorder is listed among the anxiety disorders. Requisite for this diagnosis is the presence of obsessions and/or compulsions. Obsessions are recurrent and persistent thoughts or images experienced as intrusive, unwanted, and senseless. They are recognized by the person as a product of the mind, and not imposed externally on him/her. Typically, the individual attempts to ignore or suppress them. The most common obsessions include repetitive thoughts of violence, contamination, and doubt.

Compulsions are repetitive and purposeful behaviors performed according to certain rules or in a rigid stereotyped fashion. The compulsive act is not an end in itself; rather, it is an attempt to neutralize or prevent discomfort arising from an event or situation that is feared unrealistically. Usually, the individual is able to recognize and acknowledge the excessive and irrational nature of the compulsion. Obsessions and compulsions produce marked distress, are time consuming, and can interfere markedly with social and occupational functioning. Among the most common compulsions seen clinically are repetitive handwashing, counting, checking, and touching.

Obsessive–compulsive disorder includes both cognitive and behavioral aspects. Conventional formulations of this disorder typically refer to thoughts, images, and impulses as obsessions, whereas repetitious overt actions are defined as compulsions or ritualistic behavior. This distinction poses conceptual problems that become apparent when the functional relationship of symptoms to anxiety is considered. For example, one patient reported as much discomfort from physical contact with chicken soup as from the mere thought of it. Both prompt anxiety, yet one is a cognitive event and the other, overt. The patient relieved the former discomfort by washing, an overt ritual, and the latter by the thought "palmolive," a cognitive ritual. In a second case, the number "3" provoked anxiety, while the number "7" reduced it. Although the numbers are similar in form, they had quite different results. These observations point out the inadequacies of the traditional definitions and suggest that alternative conceptualizations are needed.

The above considerations have led Foa and Tillmanns (1980) to propose a definition of obsessions and compulsions based on the functional relationship between obsessive–compulsive symptoms and anxiety. According to their model, *obsessions* or *ruminations* are defined as thoughts, images, or actions that generate anxiety. *Compulsions*, on the other hand, are conceived of as attempts to alleviate the anxiety aroused by the obsessions. They take the form of either overt actions or covert, *neutralizing*, events; they are functionally equivalent (Rachman, 1976).

DSM-III-R endeavors to specify symptoms descriptive of obsessive-compulsive disorder while refraining from theoretical concepts. However, these symptoms might be understood as reflecting certain fear structures. Elsewhere, we have hypothesized several forms of fear structures to occur in obsessive–compulsives (Foa & Kozak, 1985). The patient who fears contracting venereal disease from public bathrooms and exhibits washing rituals has a fear structure that includes disordered associations among stimulus and response elements as well as mistaken evaluations about the harm from the stimulus situation. This fear structure resembles that of simple phobia. The woman who feels contaminated by her mother and avoids even the most indirect contact with her for fear that the ensuing anxiety would make her crazy, is similar in her fear structure to an agoraphobic. For other obsessive–compulsives, fear responses are associated with evaluative elements rather than with a particular stimulus set. For example, patients who are disturbed by perceived asymmetry and reduce anxiety by rearranging objects, do not fear the objects themselves, nor do they usually anticipate disaster from the asymmetry. This latter form does not resemble the fears of agoraphobics or simple phobics.

It appears from the examples cited that no one form of fear structure is common to obsessive–compulsives. One unifying variable, however, may be an impairment in the interpretive rules for making inferences about harm. Typically, obsessive–compulsives base their beliefs about danger on the absence of disconfirming evidence and often fail to make inductive leaps about general safety from specific disconfirmations regarding danger. Consequently, although rituals are performed to reduce the likelihood of harm, they do not provide lasting safety and, therefore, must be repeated. In observing obsessive–compulsive checkers, one is impressed by a seeming memory deficit for their own actions *vis-à-vis* danger situations. Rather than reflecting a memory deficit, however, a patient's doubt about the status of the just-checked gas burners may reflect an impairment in evidential rules for inferring danger. The epistemological idiosyncrasies of obsessive–compulsives seem to foster the resistance of their fear structures to modification.

Exposure and Response Prevention

Employing prolonged exposure to obsessional cues with strict prevention of ritualistic behavior, Meyer (1966) reported successful outcome in two cases and later in 10 of 15 cases; only two relapses occurred after a 5- to 6-year period (Meyer & Levy, 1973; Meyer, Levy, & Schnurer, 1974). Not surprisingly, such remarkable results with a severely dysfunctional group of patients provoked considerable interest in this treatment. Variants of this method have now been examined in many controlled and uncontrolled studies. Findings have been remarkably consistent: Approximately 65% to 76% of more than 200 patients who have undergone this procedure were improved and stayed so at follow-up (for reviews, see Foa, Steketee, & Ozarow, 1985; Rachman & Hodgson, 1980).

The treatment consists of patients exposing themselves for long periods (45 minutes to several hours) to circumstances that provoke discomfort. Typically, exposure is graded so that moderately disturbing situations precede more upsetting ones. Ten to 20 daily sessions are held. Patients with washing rituals touch their particular "contaminated" objects; those with checking compulsions confront situations that evoke urges to check (e.g., exiting through the door, using the stove). They must refrain from ritualizing regardless of the strength of their urges to do so.

The effects of treating obsessions and compulsions with exposure only, response prevention only, or their combination were examined by Foa and colleagues (Foa, Steketee, Grayson, Turner, & Latimer, 1984; Foa, Steketee, & Milby, 1980; Steketee, Foa, & Grayson, 1982). At both posttreatment and follow-up, combined treatment was clearly superior to the two individual components employed separately. The component treatments produced different benefits: Exposure affected primarily the anxiety about contaminants while response prevention mostly influenced ritualistic behavior. The superiority of employing both procedures simultaneously was thus established.

The advantage of exposure *in vivo* rather than in imagination has been demonstrated for simple phobics. For obsessive–compulsives and for agoraphobics, the picture is less clear: The available evidence does not strongly support the superiority of *in vivo* versus imaginal procedures (for a review, see Foa & Kozak, 1985). Moreover, if it is important to include exposure to all types of fear cues, then patients who fear disastrous consequences from contact with external situations (e.g., contracting a disease from bathroom germs or being responsible for the outbreak of a fire) should improve more when imaginal exposure is included in the behavioral treatment. Therefore, Foa, Steketee, Turner, and Fisher (1980) tested the effects of combined *in vivo* and imaginal exposure versus *in vivo* exposure only. Although at the end of treatment, no differences between groups were observed, the *in vivo* plus imaginal exposure group better maintained its gains. This finding suggests that for those patients who focus largely on anticipated harm, the addition of imaginal exposure is indicated.

Assessment of the Fear Structure

The first step is to identify the distinguishing elements of the patient's fear structure. Accordingly, interviewing is directed at the discovery of: (1) ideas and situations that provoke fear, (2) fear responses including avoidance and rituals, (3) concepts of the relationship between feared situations, their responses, and harm.

The following narrative[1] exemplifies information gathering about situations that provoke fear:

THERAPIST: Can you tell me why you wash so much?

PATIENT: My car is dirty. Every time I use the car, I have to wash a lot so that I don't spread it all around.

T: What is it about the car that is dirty?

P: I'm not sure, I just know it feels dirty to me and everything in it is dirty. I have to be very careful about cleaning it.

T: What else besides the car and the things that touch the car are dirty?

P: Some of my furniture.

T: What furniture?

P: There's a cupboard and a table.

T: If you clean them well, will they be clean?

P: I can clean the dishes that are in them and that's okay, but I can't seem to get the furniture itself clean enough.

T: What about the car? Can you clean it?

P: No, I can never get it clean enough but I keep from spreading it by cleaning the things in it. I wash the clothes I wear and shower after I was in the car.

T: And you don't know why the car feels dirty?

P: No, I'm sorry.

T: When did it start?

P: About 7 years ago when I lived in a basement apartment in New York. It was flooded with a sewage backup.

T: What happened?

P: I cleaned it but it never felt really clean like it used to. I moved after 4 months because I never got used to the dirty feeling.

T: Did the furniture that bothers you come from that apartment?

P: Yes, I think so.

T: Did you have any other things from that apartment?

P: No, I got rid of them. But I couldn't afford to get rid of everything.

T: Would you feel contaminated by sewers in general?

P: No, that never occurred to me.

T: What would happen if I asked you to go back to your apartment?

P: I could never do that.

T: So the thing you are most afraid of is to return to your apartment. Is it that the furniture and your car are dirty because of that apartment?

P: Maybe, I didn't think about it.

Below is an example of an inquiry about fear-evoking ideas.

T: You've told me that there are certain thoughts that make you feel you have to wash. Can you tell me about them?

P: I wash if I pass Fifth Avenue.

T: What is it that makes you wash? What are your thoughts?

P: I can't talk about it.

T: I really need to know about them. It's important for your treatment.

P: I've never told them to anyone. I can't make myself say them. They are really awful. You wouldn't want to talk to me if you knew.

T: We all have thoughts we're ashamed of, mostly sexual or religious ones. Or sometimes we get urges to hurt someone and this can be pretty upsetting. Are your thoughts similar to any of the ones I just mentioned?

P: I really don't want to say.

T: I understand your reluctance to share thoughts you yourself don't approve of, but I'm afraid the treatment will not be good enough if we do not take into consideration what upsets you most. Remember, everyone of us gets shameful thoughts. I promise that I will continue to talk to you even after you tell me about them.

P: I'm afraid that if I talk about them, they might come true.

T: As you yourself know, it's unlikely that saying them will make them come true. But in any case, even if it were remotely possible, you will have to take this risk in order to get better.

The patient's responses, both physiological and overt, constitute another important area for assessing the fear structure. Below is a dialogue to illustrate the fear responses of a patient who fears contamination by AIDS as well as nonspecific diseases transmitted by animals and by "street" people.

T: When you think you have been contaminated by a dead rat, what sensations do you have?

P: I get very upset and I want to wash.

T: I understand. What bodily sensations do you notice when this happens?

P: You mean like knots in my stomach?

T: Exactly. What other sensations do you notice?

P: If I'm really upset, I can sometimes feel my heart racing but usually I calm down after I wash.

T: I see. So you do a lot of washing. Tell me about it.

P: You see, when it started, I used to feel clean with just soap and water. But then it wasn't doing me any good. I washed and washed and I still felt dirty. So I started to use rubbing alcohol. I figured it cleans better than water because they use it in hospitals.

T: How many times per day do you wash?

P: Depends on the day. Sometimes I wash a lot. Other days I don't wash more than five, or maybe, ten times. But mostly I use the alcohol.

T: How does it work?

P: I get up in the morning and I sterilize the spigots before I take my shower.

T: What special things do you do in the shower?

P: I always wash my feet last. They are more dirty, you know. Then I brush my teeth. So I need more alcohol to make sure my hands are clean. I don't want this dirt inside me.

Guiding the patient through a description of daily activities helps to reveal the rituals that are performed to reduce the anxiety. Next, avoidance patterns are identified.

T: Is there anything that you avoid so that you won't get dirty?

P: Because of AIDS, I don't go to 13th Street anymore. You know the kind of people that you see there. Also, I don't go to restaurants where the waiters seem to be gay.

T: What about your contamination by animals? How do you avoid them?

P: This is a real problem. They are everywhere. Well, of course I stay away from parks; but also they are all over the streets. So I watch where I walk. And car tires, they are very dirty. I make sure I don't touch them.

Another aspect of the fear structure is the meaning ascribed to the feared situation. Of particular interest is the perception of harm that may ensue if avoidance and rituals are not performed. Many obsessive–compulsives believe that unless they take proper precautions, some harm will befall them or their loved ones. They vary, however, in how clearly they construe this harm.

T: What do you think will happen if you don't get clean after visiting 13th Street.

P: Well, of course, I'll get sick. Germs cause disease, don't they? They don't even know how you get AIDS, so you have to be careful.

T: And what about the dead animals?

P: I'm not sure. I don't really know what will happen. I just know that they carry diseases.

Not all patients fear an environmental disaster. About half of the washers deny any concern about physical harm stemming from contamination. Rather, it is the intense unpleasant emotional state that they find intolerable. Without their rituals, they fear that the experience of high anxiety will be unending and will ultimately destroy them emotionally. This sort of fear may be viewed as a special type of anticipated harm. While most patients are aware of the senselessness of their fears, when questioned carefully, a rare few will assert that the disastrous consequences they anticipate (e.g., dying from contact with a leukemic patient's water glass) will in fact occur.

T: Rationally, how likely is it that you will get cancer if you touch a person with cancer and you don't wash? What is the percent likelihood that this will actually happen? Give me a number from 0 to 100.
P: Oh, it feels really dangerous.
T: I'm not asking you about your feelings. I know that you *feel* that it's dangerous or you wouldn't go to the lengths you do to avoid these situations. Ignore your feelings for a moment and just use logic. How likely is it that you'll get cancer from touching your neighbor who has leukemia?
P: Not that high, maybe 40%.
T: You mean that of 10 people who touch her, 4 will get cancer?
P: No, that's not right. If you put it like that, it's probably less than 1%.

Most obsessive–compulsives will respond in the above manner. Some, however, are convinced that their fears are realistic. The following dialogue is typical of these individuals who have been called overvalued ideators (Foa, 1979).

P: If I go to a cancer hospital and I touch my children without washing real well, they will get cancer.
T: How certain are you that they'll get it?
P: One hundred percent.
T: How likely is it that I'd get cancer if I went there?
P: I'm not sure, probably less than my kids. I'm not sure I'd get it either. We're probably stronger than they are. But I'm sure they would get it.

In addition to finding out the patient's subjective estimate of the probability of harm, one needs to assess its valence. The aversiveness of contracting AIDS is widely accepted. However, the perceived harm in other events can vary greatly across individuals. As we proposed earlier, one characteristic of anxiety disorders is excessively negative valence associated with anticipated harm.

T: How terrible will it be if you make a mistake in signing a check?
P: It would be very embarrassing for the check to be returned. I know people who work at the bank and I'm sure they'll think I'm an idiot. I don't like to make mistakes—that's my problem.

Assessment of Pathological Inferences about Harm

The development of pathological fear structures may stem from some disorder in the process of making inferences about harm. That is to say that these rules are not part of the structures themselves, but rather, operate to produce them.

A widespread error among obsessive-compulsives is the assumption that in the absence of evidence for safety, events are dangerous.

T: I noticed that you were careful not to touch me when we met. What would bother you about that?

P: I think it is toilet germs, really.

T: What gives you the idea that I carry toilet germs?

P: I figure that people aren't careful enough after using the bathroom. You know, they don't wash their hands properly.

In this case, in the absence of evidence of cleanliness, the patient assumes that the therapist's hands are contaminated.

In some instances, obsessive-compulsives construe the threat in a way that it *cannot* ever be disconfirmed. For example, the disaster is anticipated in the far distant future, or perhaps, after death.

T: Both you and your children have touched flea collars but you have not gotten cancer from this.

P: That's right, but it takes time for cancer to develop, maybe years. You now how people work with chemicals and it's 30 or 40 years before they get sick. Maybe it's like that with flea collars.

A common fear is punishment from God, especially after death. This is a particularly difficult hypothesis to disconfirm.

Mistaken estimates of the probability of harm may stem from a general deficit in estimating probabilities. Lack of knowledge about rules for calculating probabilities may underlie this deficit.

T: What are the chances of drawing a king from an ordinary deck of 52 playing cards? What are the chances of rolling a "6" using only one of a pair of dice? What are the chances of getting *heads* in a single coin toss?

Patients' answers to these and similar questions will reveal whether they have the rudimentary knowledge of how to calculate possibilities. Clearly, without such knowledge, one's estimates of the probability of harm are unlikely to be accurate.

Even though general knowledge about probability estimates is available, other errors in estimating danger can be made. One such error stems from overemphasizing readily available information (cf. Tversky & Kahneman, 1974) in estimating threat. For example, the patient who reads in a newspaper that more cases of venereal disease have appeared in local hospitals, takes more care to avoid touching doorknobs. The focus on the salient newspaper story leads to an overestimate of the likelihood of harm. Whereas for most people, such an *availability* error would be transient, disappearing when the bad news becomes *passé*, for obsessive-compulsives and for other anxiety-disordered patients, it would usually be more stable. Phobics tend to be *hypervigilant* for fear-relevant stimuli, which therefore, stand out more for them. This could lead to chronic overestimates of the probability of harm from these feared stimuli (e.g., Burgess, Jones, Robertson, Radcliffe, & Emerson, 1981; Foa & McNally, 1986; Mathews & MacLeod, 1985).

Another class of errors often encountered in obsessive-compulsives is that of interpretation and classification. One such type includes errors of degrees and exaggeration. These occur when people do not consider the amount of the feared stimulus when estimating its danger. The washer who refrains from using insecticides for fear of getting poisoned exemplifies this error. This error reflects a failure to discriminate between lethal and harmless quantities of the chemical.

Extreme fear leads to yet another mistake in information interpretation: that the feared stimulus is harmful as authoritative irrespective of its source. Basically, obsessive-compulsives tend to believe information that their feared stimulus is dangerous and dismiss information suggesting it is harmless. This error is exemplified by the credence given to manufacturers' warning labels that are found on containers of household chemicals, notwithstanding that they were designed to protect the manufacturer.

Threat is commonly construed as a product of the estimated probability and the valence of the harm (e.g., Carr, 1974; Mathews & MacLeod, 1985). Thus, the perceived threat of AIDS stems from its high cost despite the low probability of contracting it; threat of a common cold is much lower, despite its high probability because of its low cost.

In their eagerness to protect themselves from their feared harm, obsessive-compulsives often fail to include fear irrelevant gains and losses in calculating the expected value of a "risky" action. The person who protects him/herself from AIDS by avoiding all contact with homosexuals will be constrained in many areas of interaction and movement, such as having any job requiring public contact.

Directions for Further Research

We have argued earlier that exposure and response prevention change fear structures including meaning aspects. Does this treatment also address the pathological cognitive processes that may underlie the erroneous elements of the structure? As formally described in the literature (Marks, 1987; Rachman & Hodgson, 1980), this treatment is not designed for this purpose. Recently, since we have focused on information-processing impairments in obsessive-compulsives, we have introduced informal training to correct thinking habits during exposure procedures. For example, we discuss the distinction between large and small amounts of contaminants and their relationship to actual danger. We often read the warning labels on cans and analyze the incentives for manufacturers to exaggerate danger. We repeatedly point out the necessity for evidence of danger for conclusions that a given situation involves threat. In effect, we practice informal *cognitive therapy* during exposure, in that we help patients to examine ways in which they evaluate threat and to develop inferential processes that lead to more realistic conclusions.

We have not studied the efficacy of training in inferential reasoning with the obsessive–compulsive disorder. However, results from two controlled trials of cognitive therapy with obsessive–compulsive disorder are available. Self-instructional training has been found ineffective (Emmelkamp, Van der Helm, Van Zanten, & Plochg, 1980). More recently, however, rational–emotive therapy was found helpful and equivalent to self-controlled exposure *in vivo* (Emmelkamp, Visser, & Hoekstra, 1988). Our cognitive therapy procedures resemble rational–emotive therapy in that they challenge mistaken fearful beliefs and analyze the process by which the beliefs are formed.

When obsessive–compulsive disorder is treated with rational–emotive therapy fear structures are not deliberately evoked. When we challenge the mistaken beliefs of obsessive–compulsives during exposure, fear usually has been evoked. The extent to which fear evocation is needed for the therapeutic efficacy of arguments about mistaken beliefs is unknown and is thus a fertile area for research.

We do not expect that our hypotheses about cognitive impairments in obsessive–compulsive disorder constitute an exhaustive list. Rather, they represent preliminary attempts to identify distinctive features of obsessive-compulsive thinking. Historically, clinicians have observed the often bizarre ideas and behavior of obsessive–compulsives, leading to assertions that they were latent schizophrenics (Rosen, 1957). Also, it was hypothesized that obsessive–compulsive symptoms were mechanisms of defense against schizophrenic decompensation. Clinical observations, however, contraindicate this conceptualization. The great majority of obsessive–compulsives do not become schizophrenic (Lewis, 1966). Moreover, treatment by exposure and response prevention usually reduces obsessive–compulsive symptoms but without accompanying schizophrenic decompensation.

Although there is general agreement that obsessive–compulsives are not schizophrenic (Rachman & Hodgson, 1980), they seem to show thinking deficits not seen in other anxiety-disordered individuals. In this chapter, we have hypothesized some information-processing deficits that may underlie the development and maintenance of the pathological fear networks by which we understand obsessive–compulsive symptoms. Understanding the nature of impaired thinking should allow the development of more effective psychological treatments for the obsessive–compulsive disorder. The first step, however, is the empirical testing of these hypotheses, which we are currently pursuing in our laboratory.

NOTE

1. Patient–therapist narratives are not verbatim transcripts of actual therapy sessions from any one patient but rather are representative of this type of dialogue, abstracted from many patients treated by the authors.

REFERENCES

American Psychiatric Association. (1987). *Diagnostic and statistical manual of mental disorders* (3rd ed.—rev.). Washington, DC: Author.

Borkovec, T. D., & Sides, J. (1979). The contribution of relaxation and expectancy for fear reduction via graded imaginal exposure to feared stimuli. *Behaviour Research and Therapy, 17,* 529-540.

Boulougouris, J. C. (1977). Variables affecting the behavior modification of obsessive–compulsive patients treated by flooding. In J. C. Boulougouris & A. D. Rabavilas (Eds.), *The treatment of phobic and obsessive-compulsive disorders.* New York: Pergamon.

Burgess, I. S., Jones, L. M., Robertson, S. H., Radcliffe, W. N., & Emerson, E. (1981). The degree of control exerted by phobic and nonphobic verbal stimuli over the recognition behavior of phobic and nonphobic subjects. *Behaviour Research and Therapy, 19,* 233-243.

Carr, A. T. (1974). Compulsive neurosis: A review of the literature. *Psychological Bulletin, 81,* 311-318.

Chambless, D. L., Caputo, G. C., Bright, P., & Gallagher, R. (1984). Assessment of fear of fear in agoraphobics: The Body Sensations Questionnaire and the Agoraphobic Cognitions Questionnaire. *Journal of Consulting and Clinical Psychology, 52,* 1090-1097.

Chaplin, E. W., & Levine, B. A. (1980). The effects of total exposure duration and interrupted versus continuous exposure in flooding. *Behavior Therapy, 12,* 360-368.

Dattilio, F. M., & Foa, E. B. (1987). *Fear of fear: A comparison of generalized anxiety disorder, panic disorder with and without agoraphobia, and simple phobia.* Unpublished manuscript.

Ekman, P., & Friesen, W. V. (1974). Nonverbal behavior in psychopathology. In R. J. Friedman & M. M. Katz (Eds.), *The psychology of depression: Contemporary theory and research.* New York: Wiley.

Emmelkamp, P. M. G., Van der Helm, M., Van Zanten, P., & Plochg, I. (1980). Contributions of self-instructional training to the effectiveness of exposure *in vivo. Behaviour Research and Therapy, 18,* 61-66.

Emmelkamp, P. M. G., Visser, S., & Hoekstra, R. J. (1988). Cognitive therapy vs. exposure *in vivo* in the treatment of obsessive–compulsives. *Cognitive Therapy and Research, 12,* 103-114.

Foa, E. B. (1979). Failures in treating obsessive–compulsives. *Behaviour Research and Therapy, 17,* 169-176.

Foa, E. B., & Chambless, D. L. (1978). Habituation of subjective anxiety during flooding in imagery. *Behaviour Research and Therapy, 16,* 391-399.

Foa, E. B., & Kozak, M. J. (1985). Treatment of anxiety disorders: Implications for psychopathology. In A. H. Tuma & J. D. Maser (Eds.), *Anxiety and the anxiety disorders.* Hillsdale, NJ: Erlbaum.

Foa, E. B., & Kozak, M. J. (1986). Emotional processing of fear: Exposure to corrective information. *Psychological Bulletin, 99,* 20-35.

Foa, E. B., & McNally, R. J. (1986). Sensitivity to feared stimuli in obsessive–compulsives: A dichotic listening analysis. *Cognitive Therapy and Research, 10,* 477-485.

Foa, E. B., Steketee, G. S., Grayson, J. B., Turner, R. M., & Latimer, P. R. (1984). Deliberate exposure and blocking of obsessive–compulsive rituals: Immediate and long-term effects. *Behavior Therapy, 15,* 450-472.

Foa, E. B., Steketee, G. S., & Milby, J. B. (1980). Differential effects of exposure and response prevention in obsessive–compulsive washers. *Journal of Consulting and Clinical Psychology, 48,* 71-79.

Foa, E. B., Steketee, G. S., & Ozarow, B. (1985). Behavior therapy with obsessive–compulsives: From theory to treatment. In M. Mavissakalian (Ed.), *Obsessive-compulsive disorder.* New York: Plenum.

Foa, E. B., Steketee, G. S., Turner, R. M., & Fischer, S. C. (1980). Effects of imaginal exposure to feared disasters in obsessive–compulsives checkers. *Behaviour Research and Therapy, 18,* 449-455.

Foa, E. B., & Tillmanns, A. (1980). The treatment of obsessive–compulsive neurosis. In A. Goldstein & E. B. Foa (Eds.), *Handbook of behavioral interventions: A clinical guide.* New York: Wiley.

Freud, S. (1910). The origin of psychoanalysis. In J. Rickman (Ed.), *A general selection from the works of Freud.* London: Hogarth Press.

Goldstein, A. J., & Chambless, D. L. (1978). A reanalysis of agoraphobia. *Behavior Therapy, 9,* 49-57.

Grayson, J. B., Foa, E. B., & Steketee, G. S. (1986). Exposure *in vivo* under distracting and attention focusing conditions: Replication and extinction. *Behaviour Research and Therapy, 24,* 475-479.

Hoffman, H. S., & Fleshler, M. (1961). Stimulus factors in aversive control: The generalization of conditioned suppression. *Journal of the Experimental Analysis of Behavior, 4,* 374.

Horton, D. L., & Kjeldergaard, P. K. (1961). An experimental analysis of associative factors in mediated generalizations. *Psychological Monographs, 75,* 515.

James, W. (1890). *The principles of psychology* (Vol. 1). New York: Henry Holt.

Klatzky, R. (1975). *Human memory: Structures and processes.* San Francisco: W. H. Freeman.

Kozak, M. J., Foa, E. B., & Steketee, G. (1988). Process and outcome of exposure treatment with obsessive-compulsives: Psychophysiological indicators of emotional processing. *Behavior Therapy, 19,* 157-169.

Lang, P. J. (1977). Imagery in therapy: An information processing analysis of fear. *Behavior Therapy, 8,* 862-886.

Lang, P. J. (1979). A bio-informational theory of emotional imagery. *Psychophysiology, 16,* 495-512.

Lang, P. J., Kozak, M. J., Miller, G. A., Levin, D. N., & McLean, A. (1980). Emotional imagery: Conceptual structure and pattern of somatic-visceral response. *Psychophysiology, 17,* 179-192.

Lang, P. J., Levin, D. N., Miller, G. A., & Kozak, M. J. (1983). Fear behavior, fear imagery, and the psychophysiology of emotion. The problem of affective response integration. *Journal of Abnormal Psychology, 92,* 276-306.

Lang, P. J., Melamed, B. G., & Hart, J. (1970). A psychophysiological analysis of fear modification using an automated desensitization procedure. *Journal of Abnormal Psychology, 76,* 220-234.

Lazarus, R. S. (1966). *Psychological stress and the coping process.* New York: McGraw-Hill.

Leventhal, H. (1980). Toward a comprehensive theory of emotion. In L. Berkowitz (Ed.), *Advances in experimental social psychology* (Vol. 13). New York: Academic Press.

Lewis, A. J. (1966). Obsessional disorder. In R. Scott (Ed.), *Price's textbook of the practice of medicine* (10th ed.). London: Oxford University Press.

Mandler, G. (1975). *Mind and emotion.* New York: Wiley.

Mansueto, C. S., Grayson, J. B., & Foa, E. B. (1987). *Assessment of the "fear of fear" component in agoraphobic versus specific phobic patients.* Unpublished manuscript.

Marks, I. M. (1987). *Fears, phobias, and rituals.* New York: Oxford University Press.

Mathews, A., & MacLeod, C. (1985). Selective processing of threat cues in anxiety states. *Behaviour Research and Therapy, 23,* 563-569.

McNally, R., & Foa, E. (1987). Cognition and agoraphobia: Bias in the interpretation of threat. *Cognitive Therapy and Research, 5,* 567-581.

Meyer, V. (1966). Modification of expectations in cases with obsessional rituals. *Behaviour Research and Therapy, 4,* 273-280.

Meyer, V., & Levy, R. (1973). Modification of behavior in obsessive-compulsive disorders. In H. E. Adams & P. Unikel (Eds.), *Issues and trends in behavior therapy.* Springfield, IL: Charles C. Thomas.

Meyer, V., Levy, R., & Schnurer, A. (1974). A behavioral treatment of obsessive-compulsive disorders. In H. R. Beech (Ed.), *Obsessional states.* London: Methuen.

Miller, G. A., Levin, D. N., Kozak, M. J., Cook, W., McLean, J., & Lang, P. (1988). Individual differences in imagery and the psychophysiology of emotion. *Cognition and Emotion, 4,* 367-390.

Nisbett, R. E., & Wilson, T. P. (1977). Telling more than we know: Verbal reports on mental processes. *Psychological Review, 84,* 231-279.

Pylyshyn, Z. W. (1973). What the mind's eye tells the mind's brain: A critique of mental imagery. *Psychological Bulletin, 80,* 1-22.

Rabavilas, A. D., Boulougouris, J. C., & Stefanis, C. (1976). Duration of flooding sessions in the treatment of obsessive–compulsive patients. *Behaviour Research and Therapy, 14,* 349–355.

Rachman, S. (1976). The modification of obsessions: A new formulation. *Behaviour Research and Therapy, 14,* 437–443.

Rachman, S. (1980). Emotional processing. *Behaviour Research and Therapy, 18,* 51–60.

Rachman, S., & Hodgson, R. (1980). *Obsessions and compulsions.* Englewood Cliffs, NJ: Prentice-Hall.

Reiss, S., Peterson, R., Gursky, D., & McNally, R. (1986). Anxiety sensitivity, anxiety frequency, and the prediction of fearfulness. *Behaviour Research and Therapy, 24,* 1–8.

Rosen, I. (1957). The clinical significance of obsessions in schizophrenia. *Journal of Mental Science, 103,* 773–786.

Schachter, S., & Singer, J. (1962). Cognitive, social, and physiological determinants of emotional state. *Psychological Review, 69,* 379–399.

Schwartz, S. C., & Kaloupek, D. G. (1987). Acute exercise combined with imaginal exposure as a technique for anxiety reduction. *Canadian Journal of Behavioural Science, 19,* 151–166.

Shepard, R. N. (1967). Recognition memory for words, sentences, and pictures. *Journal of Verbal Learning and Verbal Behavior, 6,* 156–163.

Standing, L., Conezio, J., & Haber, R. N. (1970). Perception and memory for pictures: Single-trial learning of 2560 visual stimuli. *Psychonomic Science, 19,* 73–74.

Steketee, G. S., Foa, E. B., & Grayson, J. B. (1982). Recent advances in the treatment of obsessive–compulsives. *Archives of General Psychiatry, 39,* 1365–1371.

Stern, R. S., & Marks, I. M. (1973). Brief and prolonged flooding: A comparison in agoraphobic patients. *Archives of General Psychiatry, 28,* 270–276.

Tversky, A., & Kahnemen, D. (1974). Judgment under uncertainty: Heuristics and biases. *Science, 185,* 1124–1131.

Watson, J. P., Gaind, R., & Marks, I. M. (1972). Physiological habituation to continuous phobic stimulation. *Behaviour Research and Therapy, 10,* 269–271.

Weekes, C. (1973). A practical treatment of agoraphobia. *British Medical Journal, 2,* 469–471.

Wolpe, J. (1978). Cognition and causation in human behavior and its therapy. *American Psychologist, 33,* 437–446.

Zajonc, R. B. (1980). Feeling and thinking: Preferences need no inferences. *American Psychologist, 35,* 151–175.

Zajonc, R. B., & Markus, H. (1984). Affect and cognition. The hard interface. In C. Izard, J. Kagan, & R. Zajonc (Eds.), *Emotions, cognition and behavior.* New York: Cambridge University Press.

3

Affective Change Events in a Cognitive Therapy System Approach

VITTORIO F. GUIDANO
Center for Cognitive Therapy, Rome

INTRODUCTORY NOTES

The evolution of Western scientific thought coincides in many aspects with the history of empiricism, that is, the epistemological perspective, whose rise, about four centuries ago, enhanced the formation of a scientific methodology. The basic concept of empiricism is the existence of a unique, objectively given external reality that can be known as such through the senses. As Bacon claimed, sensations never lie; like "snapshots" of reality, they give an unbiased reproduction of the objective order in which we live.

Applied to psychology, this principle originated a basic perspective shared by both behaviorism and pragmatic relational approaches, by which organisms, basically passive, were only considered as "responding" to an external given order in which a "sense of things" was already objectively contained. On the grounds of this primacy of environment the study of organisms could be reduced to a description of the organism–environment interaction (the so-called black box hypothesis), and any psychological activity could be thought of as a sequence of behavioral and/or relational responses to specific environmental stimuli.

This basic perspective, which is still deeply rooted in contemporary psychology, has met a period of progressive crisis in the last two decades, especially when the concomitant interdisciplinary boom (systems approach, evolutionary epistemology, irreversible thermodynamics, cognitive science, etc.) questioned the fundamental assumptions of the empiricistic method. It is worth remarking that the decline of the traditional psychological perspective is not simply the result of what could be considered an ordinary alternation of hypotheses and theories within a single scientific discipline, but rather an expression of the profound change that has been intervening in every field of science in the last ten years, altering the very nature of scientific knowledge. In other words, the breakdown of empiricism—linked until recently to the notion of science itself—is what triggered the epistemological transformation that contemporary science as a whole is undergoing.

Thanks to the interdisciplinary convergence that has occurred in recent years, the outlines of what has come to be known as the "epistemology of complexity," in contrast to empiricism, have progressively appeared (cf. Atlan, 1979; Hayek, 1952, 1964: Jantsch, 1980; Nicolis & Prigogine, 1977; Prigogine & Stengers, 1984; Varela, 1979; Weimer, 1982, 1983; Winograd & Flores, 1986). Rather than being a new theory or a new discipline, this is a way of viewing things, a different perspective from which existent hypotheses and data can be reconsidered. Its basic element is a change in the notion of reality and of the observer, and therefore, ultimately, a radical change in the observer-observed relationship.

Reality is no longer conceived of as univocal and ultimately objective, but it is seen as a network of intertwined processes, articulated along multiple levels of interaction, which are simultaneously present, yet irreducible to one another. The observer, in turn, is no longer in the privileged Baconian position of one who is watching from the outside and would therefore be capable of perceiving the object's objective features and characteristics. On the contrary, his/her observation introduces into the network of intertwined processes an order by which all of the possible ambiguities caused by the multiple, simultaneous interactions acquire, to his/her eyes, an univocal and necessary character. In other words, any observation—far from being external and therefore "neutral"—is *self-referential*; it always reflects itself, that is, the perceiving order on which it is based rather than the intrinsic qualities of the perceived object. Consequently, the order and regularity with which we habitually deal with things, as well as with ourselves, are not external and objectively given, but rather a product of our active interactions with ourselves and the world.

This overturn in the observer-observed relationship brings about some rather relevant epistemological, psychological, and therapeutic consequences that will be briefly examined in the paragraphs that follow.

THE NOTION OF SELF-ORGANIZED COMPLEXITY

As we have seen in recent years, a broad interdisciplinary convergence as well as a range of thematic changes—in the way of conceptualizing behavior and experience—have led to a perspective in which a human knowing system should be considered essentially as a self-organizing complexity. In a nutshell, the crucial aspect of such a framework consists of considering the self-organizing ability of a human knowing system as a self-referent evolutionary constraint that, through maturational ascendance to higher cognitive levels of information processing, makes possible the progressive structuring of a full sense of personal identity with the inherent feelings of uniqueness and historical continuity. The availability of a stable and structured personal identity allows a continuous and coherent self-perception and self-evaluation in the face of temporal becoming and mutable reality; this, in turn, makes possible the scaffolding of experience along a unitary and consistent dimension of personal meaning. In other terms, in a perspective where human systems are seen as self-referential and self-organizing units, the role exerted by knowing processes in the construction of that ordering of reality, which we commonly call "personal experience," is one of absolute centrality; the personal identity perceived by the subject is not simply received from an objectively ordered external reality, but it is actively built by the knowing subject him/herself. Thus, far from merely reflecting an outside order, the ordering of reality in a set of predictable, and therefore intelligible regularities, is the autonomous construction of a system that, by scaffolding its own order within an ongoing flow of every changing stimuli, defines at the same time its individuality and identity as a system.

The self-referential logic underlying systems' self-organization also enables us to reformulate the notion of autonomy. A self-referential knowing system is autonomous, for in the course of its temporal becoming, it subordinates any possible change and/or transformation to the maintenance of the identity it has been able to elaborate. The maintenance of a sense of individuality and personal uniqueness throughout the life span results from the individual autopoietic activity (Maturana & Varela, 1980; Varela, 1979; Zeleny, 1981): an ongoing, generative process of self-renewal by which perturbations arising from exchanges with the world are transformed into more complex and integrated levels of self-identity and self-consciousness.

A complex knowing system is therefore *organizationally closed*, as it will not admit alternatives to the "experiential order" (personal meaning) on which are based the continuity and coherence of its sense of self, and it is *autonomous*, as in order to maintain and renew that order, it needs nothing else but to constantly refer to itself.

To view a system's autonomy from this perspective necessarily implies an equally radical reformulation of another basic notion, that is, adaptation. To the common empiricist outlook, which traditionally attributes a primacy to environment, adaptation is a progressive modeling of an organism's responses to environmental pressures; whereas, if primacy is given to self-organizing capabilities the resulting concept of adaptation is, in a way, overturned. A self-referential system is adapted to the extent that it is able to transform perturbations arising from interaction with the environment into information that is meaningful to its internal order (personal meaning). In other words, the only way a system can maintain adaptation is by preserving its own inner coherence at the expense of the environment, even if it means producing irreversible changes in the latter. Therefore, the adaptive adequacy of a self-organizing system does not reflect in any way the intrinsic qualities and features of its environment, which explains why the concept of *viability* in representations of self and world has become much more important, in recent evolutionary epistemology, than the one of *validity* (Maturana & Varela, 1980; Varela, 1979).

Quite evidently, in the light of this perspective, basic regulative mechanisms of personality are no longer connected to motivational aspects (whether meant as drives or hedonistic determination) but rather to the self-referentiality of individual knowledge processes, that is, the tendency to maintain the systemic coherence of one's personal meaning processes. The resulting image of the human being is no longer that of a hedonistic animal whose behavior is regulated step by step by rewards and punishments, but rather that of an epistemological animal whose adaptive adequacy coincides with the viability and effectiveness of his/her understanding of self and reality (Guidano, 1987).

Finally, in an evolutionary epistemology perspective, knowledge and mind-like behaviors appear to be an emergent property of the information-processing ability exhibited by every living system, able to assume different levels of organized complexity according to their respective evolutionary levels. Thus, knowledge is no longer seen solely as cognitive activity aimed at objectifying experience through analytical logic and rationality, but mostly as emotional and motor activity able to provide an immediate, overall (analogical) apprehension of relevant features in the surrounding reality. This is why the terms *tacit* and *explicit knowledge* are currently and increasingly being used to indicate two different modes of information processing within an individual knowing system (Airenti, Bara, & Colombetti, 1982a,b; Franks, 1974; Hayek, 1978; Polanyi, 1966; Shevrin & Dickman, 1980; Van Den Berg & Eelen, 1984; Weimer, 1973, 1977).

The emotional–affective system (tacit knowledge) is undoubtedly the most archaic and phylogenetically structured information-processing system, and for this reason the most deeply rooted in all animal species. Emotional reactivity is universally present in all living beings and represents the immediate "knowing response" to an environmental perturbation, enabling any organism to enact the strategies most effective for survival (*primacy of affect*; Eibl-Eibesfeldt, 1972; Ekman, 1984; Plutchik, 1980, 1983; Zajonc, 1980, 1984). This immediate knowing response has maintained its primary role in information processing, even in humans, and in spite of the emergence of language and of the new cognitive abilities connected to it (conceptual thought, etc.). In particular, the emotional modulation accompanying any cognitive and motor activity provides in a totally tacit and immediate way the apperceptive scaffolding (i.e., the invariant key perceptual features of constraining personal meaning processes) within which a specific individual comes to comprehend an endless range of environmental situations.

The logical–conceptual system (explicit knowledge) is the most sophisticated and specialized form of knowledge to ever appear, but on the other hand—and for this very reason—it is inevitably partial and needs the constant support of an immediate, overall knowledge as the tacit one. In other words, tacit processes provide the apperceptive scaffolding in which conscious selective attention is constrained, allowing the insertion and manipulation of deep-ordering rules into explicit procedures of thought representation (e.g., theories, beliefs, problem-solving strategies, etc.). Cognition, therefore, is the emergent result of the ongoing match between incoming data and contextual schemata resulting from the tacit and explicit levels of interaction. The matching procedure is biased by a tendency to first recognize and then scaffold incoming data into available, pre-existing knowledge structures, while the possibility of modifying the available decoding structure is mainly triggered by emotional perturbations arising from the discrepancies connected to the performance of recognition trials.

It should be emphasized that tacit and explicit levels of knowing should not be regarded as two polarities occupying the extremes of a single continuum or dimension, but rather as two independent and irreducible dimensions occurring in constant reciprocal interaction. Because of the irreducibility and oscillative tension between these two dimensions, each individual life-span is an open-ended, generative process, in which no special state of maturity or ultimate stable equilibrium is ever reached.

SELF-ORGANIZING SYSTEMS AND LIFE-SPAN DEVELOPMENT

As we have gathered, the key feature underlying a self-organizing system's autonomy consists in the latter's ability to transform into self-referential order the randomness of perturbations coming from both the environment and its own inner oscillations (the so-called "order-from-noise" principle; Atlan, 1981). The life-span of such a system will therefore acquire several relevant characteristics.

In the first place, the temporal evolution of an individual knowing system appears to be an ongoing process whose dynamic equilibrium delineates a progressive, generative directionality, in which more structured and integrated levels of self-referential order discontinuously emerge along the entire life-span; the principle underlying this dynamic equilibrium is known as "order through fluctuations," as the emergence of more structure is always the result of the assimilation of disequilibriums and discrepancies previously produced (Brent, 1978; Dell & Goolishian, 1981; Prigogine, 1976).

Finally, the construction of a sense of personal identity and uniqueness seems to be the distinctive characteristic of the way an individual system builds its self-referential order, so much so that the progressive differentiation of a sense of self appears from the start to be connected to the equally progressive cognitive/emotional development. In other words, mechanisms underlying identity are closely related to those underlying knowledge (Varela, 1979) and, consequently, the discontinuous emerging in an individual lifetime of more structured levels of self-referential order ultimately results in a progressive surfacing of more integrated levels of personal identity and self-consciousness.

We can now proceed to a closer analysis of: (1) the mechanisms with which a system constructs a specific sense of self (self-identity) throughout maturational stages; and (2) once development is completed, the mechanisms that underlie the maintenance of a coherent sense of self—allowing at the same time a continuous assimilation of experience.

Looking-Glass Effect

According to a line of thought commonly ascribed to sociologists of the early 20th century (Cooley, 1902; Mead, 1934) human beings are believed to acquire self-knowledge only by interacting with others. Moreover, supported by increasing evidence from neurophysiological and neuropsychological data, we may legitimately assume that children growing up in complete isolation never come to full self-consciousness. This phenomenon, known as *looking-glass effect* (or looking-glass self), is concisely explained by Popper and Eccles (1977) as follows: "Just as we learn to see ourselves in a mirror, so the child becomes conscious of himself by seeing his reflection in the mirror of other people's consciousness of himself" (p. 110).

In other words, if—as in a mirror—the child elaborates through others a specific self-image, it does not remain as a mere sensorial datum to be stored as such, but it orients and coordinates ongoing cognitive and emotional processes until the child can perceive him/herself consistently with the self-image that he/she has been able to abstract from family environment. If others play such a primary role, it is easy to see how important attachment processes (Bowlby, 1969, 1973, 1980) and their development can be for the construction of personal identity.

In human species, attachment and contact with parents are marked by some distinctive features, unprecedented in the rest of evolutionary scale. On the one hand, the entire process extends throughout a long period, usually far beyond adolescence and youth; on the other, attachment itself becomes more and more articulated in the course of development. From physical attachment of infancy, through childhood and adolescence, an increasingly complex emotional bond is established, able to foster more specific and structured processes of self-referential ordering, such as modeling and identification. Thus, throughout maturational stages and matching the development of cognitive abilities, the self-referent logic of attachment processes becomes more complex and integrated, until at adolescence it progressively changes into a highly structured vehicle through which unlimited and increasingly abstract information about self and world becomes available.

The most outstanding aspect of the development of self during maturational stages is by far the graduality of cognitive growth, that is, the relatively slow unfolding of explicit knowledge (Flavell, 1977; Piaget, 1951). Similar to what we have noticed to occur in the course of evolution, tacit knowledge is undoubtedly the first information-processing level to appear in the course of individual development. Because of the slow unfolding of cognitive abilities, childhood and preschool years are essentially marked by a global and immediate understanding of self and world, in which verbal and abstracting abilities, as well as self-consciousness, are absolutely irrelevant. Still similar to what occurred during evolution with the onset of higher cortical activities, the gradual emerging of logical–formal cognitive abilities progressively distances and decenters the subject's thinking from the concrete immediacy of experience.

Individual development is therefore characterized by a temporal gap between the subject's functioning levels of tacit and explicit knowledge. The organization of experience that takes place during infancy and childhood entails the elaboration of increasingly complex sets of self-referential ordering tacit rules (personal meaning); on the other hand, the slow unfolding of cognitive abilities enables the subject to become at least partly aware of such rules only at a more advanced stage, generally in late adolescence and youth. Only in this phase can the tacit/explicit knowledge relationship undergo a reorganization by which prelogical, immediate aspects of the sense of self that have been elaborated can be restructured in a conscious self-image able to direct one's life planning actively.

However, as the "cognitive revolution" takes place in adolescence and youth, attachment (though shifting toward a more abstract level) maintains its fundamental interdependence with selfhood processes and personal meaning. Because attachment to significant others is central to the structuring of self-knowledge throughout development, during adulthood new kinds of attachment emerge (e.g., intimate, love relationships) that acquire the function of confirming, supporting, and further expanding personal reality. In a word, assuming a systems perspective and trying to explain how a human being comes to elaborate an exclusive and specific sense of his/her individuality, attachment can no longer be considered as a mere structural device for the maintenance of proximity and contact with a significant figure, as is usually the case in descriptive methodologies based on empiricist principles (Trevarthen, 1980, 1984). Within an explicative, process-oriented methodology, attachment becomes the self-referential system that pre-eminently underlies the development and maintenance of personal identity, and consequently, an adult attachment style can be seen as a self-referent pattern aimed at preserving the systemic coherence of an individual's personal meaning through the production of emotional experiences consistent with his/her perceived sense of self (Guidano, 1987; Marris, 1982). If the continuity and systemic coherence of personal meaning processes rests on a balanced interplay between individuals and their interpersonal network, we can legitimately anticipate that the most disrupting emotions able to trigger the deepest changes in one's personal experience, are those activated in the course of establishing, maintaining, and breaking affectional bonds (Bowlby, 1977; Brown, 1982; Brown & Harris, 1978; Henderson, 1982; Henderson, Byrne, & Duncan-Jones, 1981).

Orthogenetic Perspective

How can an individual knowing system's evolution in time be viewed, when—having reached a complete cognitive maturation—it has elaborated a fully articulated, sufficiently abstract, and above all, stable sense of self?

The traditional empiricist outlook regards the trend of an individual life-span after developmental stages as a sort of "plateau," as if adulthood consisted virtually in nothing more than maintaining indefinitely the optimal equilibrium that is thought to be attained by the end of the maturational period. This point of view, known as the homeostasis perspective, identifies the fundamental aim of adaptation in the maintenance at any cost of the feedback equilibrium established with the environment. Quite obviously, such a perspective excludes any generative progression in development, reducing adulthood to a passive and cumulative process of data remodeling regulated at any moment by contingency relationships established with the environment.

Oppositely, in a systems perspective the life-span of a self-organizing system is characterized by the so-called *orthogenetic progression* (Werner, 1948, 1957); that is, the system's inner complexity increases in time as a consequence of the ongoing assimilation of experience, giving rise to a discontinuous emerging of more articulated and integrated levels of knowledge of self and world. The self-regulating ability exhibited by a system in proceeding along orthogenetic directionality is expressed by that particular dynamic equilibrium known as order through flucuations (Brent, 1978; Prigogine, 1976); a series of continuous, progressive shifts of the point of equilibrium are the only way to maintain the systemic coherence underlying the continuity of one's sense of self, and, at the same time, to assimilate perturbations that inevitably arise as a result of the personal experience thus produced.

Moreover, the increase in a system's complexity throughout its life-span does not have a linear course; on the contrary, it is a rather unpredictable process that unfolds through critical, discontinuous emergences. Because of such critical increases in complexity, the system can maintain its internal order only by carrying out a more or less thorough reorganization of its experiential order. Unlike maturational stages, whose course appears more linear and uniform, development in adulthood proceeds by crises that are reminiscent in many aspects of the pattern of "punctuated equilibria" proposed by the post-Darwinian pluralistic evolutionary approaches (cf. Gould, 1980). Periods of apparent stability in which the system seems only concerned with the maintenance of its status quo, becoming thus extremely predictable, are followed by very intense periods in which the slightest environmental changes unexpectedly trigger major existential crises and deep reorganizations of personal experience.

It must be remarked, on the other hand, that the notion of order through fluctuations clearly implies the continuous presence in the system of an essential tension generated by the interdependence and reciprocal regulation between opponent processes—such as the ones that, during a crisis, urge for the maintenance at all cost of the status quo, versus the ones making pressures for a revision of one's conception of the world. Contradictions and discrepancies occurring in a system's internal coherence seem, therefore, to be the essential push and pull underlying the orthogenetic directionality of any individual life-span. As Brent (1984) clearly states:

> The most important feature of this mode . . . is its postulation that each new level of structural organization is a synthesis of previously antithetical forces. Thus, the occurrence of internal conflicts between different aspects of an organized system is a fundamental impetus for the process or organic development itself. Thus within this model tension, conflict, and stress among the constituents of a structure is not in itself indicative of a problem within that structure, but merely the sign of the ongoing process of organic development. (p. 163)

Adulthood should therefore be regarded as an open process of experience assimilation bringing about "punctuated" reorganizations of personal meaning; consequently, no specific moment of a life-span can be identified as the one in which an ultimate, exhaustive understanding of oneself is achieved, nor is there any indication, within the system's orthogenetic directionality, of the existence of a "right" or "optimal" equilibrium, or of anything suggesting that an ultimate stage of maturity has been reached. On the other hand, it is quite evident that no reorganization—not even if it brings about a truly deep personal growth—is completely painless, as, in any case, it always requires a change in the habitual way of seeing reality; this implies a massive activation of intense emotions that result, at least at first, neither readily intelligible nor easily controllable.

A system's level of self-awareness exerts, therefore, a crucial role in orienting an ongoing reorganization process toward a direction of personal growth or toward one of existential breakdown more or less intermingled with emotional disturbances. For this reason the "symptoms" a system may display in any stage of its life-span must be considered as full-fledged knowing processes highlighting unsuccessful attempts to change, whose origin traces back to a poor and/or distorted level of awareness preventing a complete and coherent assimilation of the personal experience produced thus far. Both clinical and basic research should therefore be more and more preferentially oriented toward (1) the study of the variables underlying the development of awareness in self-organizing systems, and (2) the study of the relationship existing between a system's level of awareness and its possibilities of assimilating and reorganizing its personal experience.

EMOTIONAL AND THERAPEUTIC CHANGE

If the role of emotionality in personal knowing is viewed within the conceptual framework described, the key function of affect in change processes should become more easily understandable. Besides evolutionary considerations set forth in preceding paragraphs, the primacy of affect is equally evident throughout the entire course of an individual's life-span development.

The very organization of human knowledge processes shows unmistakably that emotions are an essential requirement for the structuring of any kind of experience. In other words, tacit knowledge and emotion are closely intertwined, and, as the tacit level steadily provides the first apprehensional frame without which no conscious conceptual understanding would be possible, we can confidently conclude that emotionality is involved in every aspect of mental processing. In perception, attention, remembering, understanding, and so on, the ongoing emotional modulation provides the apperceptive scaffolding that constrains the kinds of experiences one has to expect and seek at the conscious level of interaction with the world (Leventhal, 1980, 1984, 1986; Van Den Berg & Eelen, 1984; Zajonc, 1980, 1984).

Moreover, even at the conscious level, analytical thought processes (deductive reasoning, decision making, etc.) succeed in transforming incoming information into personal experience, thanks to the emotional background with which they are interdependent. The very capability of abstract objectification and logical consequentiality make thought procedures rather impersonal; their main function is to isolate and analyze accurately all the possible aspects of incoming data. Such aspects would, however, remain fragmentary if the ongoing emotional modulation did not provide a feeling of self-reference from which they immediately acquire a specific configuration in the subject's pre-existing personal experience. The meaningfulness of potentially available incoming data seems therefore to be closely correlated to the degree of self-referentiality, that is, to the extent and quality of personal meaning experienced by the subject.

On the other hand, proceeding from the general aspects of human knowledge processes on to the trend of an individual life-span, the key role of affect is made evident by several considerations.

The organizational unity of one's emotional domain—underlying the coherence of personal meaning processes—grows during maturational stages out of an array of living attachments; throughout adulthood it undergoes a process of maintenance and constant articulation based on a progressive self-referent ordering of one's interpersonal domain. The notion that knowledge relies on others goes far beyond the concrete and immediate aspects of affective relationships. Since any category discovered in other people can also apply to oneself, and vice versa, even in adult life the perceived, imagined, or remembered experience of significant others is a necessary condition for supporting and further expanding one's personal reality; that is, self-referent emotional modulation matched with the continuous interplay with others' experience represents the basic process underlying the continuity and coherence of personal identity and self-awareness.

The orthogenetic directionality of a life-span development unfolds into an order through fluctuations based on a dynamic process that progressively integrates critical perturbations triggered by inevitable discrepancies resulting from the continuous assimilation of experience. As a consequence, emotional perturbations discontinuously emerging within the steady, coherent unfolding of any life-span's orthogenetic progression are undoubtedly the most remarkable set of challenging pressures for a reorganization of personal meaning processes. The quality and generativity of such reorganizations, and whether they represent progressive or regressive shifts, compared with the subject's specific orthogenetic directionality, depend to a large extent on the structure and quality of self-awareness that he/she has been able to elaborate until that moment (Guidano, 1987).

No change seems possible without emotions (this might explain why no spontaneous change can occur in a computer's inner organization). Throughout life-span development the continuity and coherence of per-

sonal meaning processes rely on the organizational unity of the individual's emotional domain; the self-regulation between core affective themes
provides a focus and direction in organizing the individual's thoughts,
feelings, and actions along dimensions of abstract and integrated knowledge compatible with his/her self-awareness. In addition, while ideational
themes (i.e., dimensions of abstract knowledge) usually undergo a more or
less continuous process of differentiation, recombination, and integration,
basic affective themes seem much more constant in time and exhibit a
different rate and different mechanisms of change, compared with cognitive structures (cf. Haviland, 1984). The well-known hypothesis according
to which a change in cognitions entails a correspondent change in emotions is, therefore, groundless, insofar as self-regulation and self-develop-
ment of core affective themes seem not to be as affected by logical rules of
differentiation and integration as ideational themes are. In other words, it
appears even more evident that *while thinking usually changes thoughts,
only feeling can change emotions*; that is, only the emergence of new
emotional experiences, by adding new tonalities of feelings to the unitary
configuration of core emotional themes, can affect their self-regulation
facilitating a reordering in personal meaning processes. As a consequence, the causes of a "crisis" are always within the system itself, and
therefore they should not be sought in a supposed specificity of certain
stressful life-events, but rather in the specific nature of personal meaning
that determines the range of events that are discrepant for one particular
individual. On the other hand, the critical role that a life-event can play
does not necessarily imply that such meaning needs to be consciously
elaborated, because often what appears as nonsense at the conscious level
is in fact critical, challenging information from the unconscious level
(Atlan, 1981; Serres, 1976); the relatively autonomous emergence of
critical emotions signaling an ongoing change in the individual's apperceptive scaffolding is made possible exactly by the irreducibility and oscillative tension between tacit and explicit dimensions. In other words, the
transformation of tacit ordering rules as well as the elaboration of new
abstract rules are not initiated and controlled by the the conscious mind;
the latter can only aim at discovering (i.e., explicitation and procedures of
thought representations) the ordering rules that are already biasing its
functioning (Hayek, 1978; Miró & Belloch, 1986; Weimer, 1982). However, although the surfacing of challenging perturbations is a necessary
condition for triggering a reorganization process, it cannot go as far as
determining the kind of change that can be achieved once reorganization
is completed.

   *The structure and quality of change depend to a large extent on the
level and quality of self-awareness with which the subject carries out
the reorganization process.* To make the tacit become explicit should not
be viewed simply as a verbal and imaginal translation of deep ordering

rules onto a monitor (Marcel, 1983; Reber & Lewis, 1977). Conscious explicit knowing, therefore, is not to be conceived of as a mere cognitive epiphenomenon, for example, like a beam of light displaying an already well-arranged and complete configuration of elements, with the only purpose of acknowledging their existence. As an example, a "personal revolution" (i.e., a successful deep reorganization; Mahoney, 1980) and a clear-cut "clinical syndrome" (i.e., an unsuccessful deep change), although both triggered by a deep challenging perturbation, are the outcome of different explicit reordering processes, which in turn result from different qualitative levels of self-awareness and conscious thought.

How are the above considerations reflected by the therapeutic strategy of a systems, process-oriented cognitive therapist?

In the first place, for such strategy to prove effective, the client must experience during the therapeutic process some affect-laden event able to exert pressures toward a reorganization. Throughout this process, the therapist must be able to provide tools of analysis and self-observation which, by increasing the flexibility and plasticity of the client's levels of awareness, will enable him/her to accomplish gradually a progressive reorganization, one where the problematic perturbation is assimilated and understood in a more abstract and integrated conception of self and world, not involving any particular intense emotional distress.

Finally, the therapeutic relationship is the absolutely specific context where it becomes possible for the therapist both to set off affective events and to aim at orientating the reorganization process that they activate. As the therapeutic relationship is in all respects a *real, living interaction*, that is, one in which cognitive and emotional aspects are continuously intertwined, its emotional aspects produce a facilitating effect for the assimilation of new data or the reframing of existing ones.

To give a more specifically articulated form to these observations, we will begin by reporting two therapeutic settings that exemplify the role of affective-laden situations, and proceed to outline a possible explanation of the close correlation between affective events and change processes; lastly, it may be useful to conclude by illustrating briefly the essential aspects of the therapeutic methodology on which the data and comments of the two preceding paragraphs are based.

CASE REPORTS

Once the therapeutic relationship that has been structured is perceived as valid and reliable by the client, the therapist's approach in facilitating the production of emotionally involving situations to trigger a reorganizing effect should of course be directed at what the client perceives as his/her major existential concern. It hardly needs pointing out that an arousal of emotional perturbations in less-relevant domains of personal meaning elicited by paradoxical or openly provoking attitudes exhibited by the therapist is not only ineffective in activating a reorganization, but it can also seriously compromise the client's reliance on the therapeutic relationship. Through appropriate techniques of assessment and developmental analysis—an opportunity to provide the client with principles and techniques of self-observation—the therapist should therefore accurately reconstruct the client's present disequilibrium, with special reference to the set of affective-laden discrepancies existing between his/her conscious self-image and the challenging perceived sense of self of which the client is not fully aware (Guidano, 1987, 1988). In many cases it is possible to act on those very discrepancies that emerge in the course of assessment by reconstructing them with the client, and gradually (adjusting the timing to his/her rhythms of understanding) bringing them within one's range of self-awareness. If this procedure generates in the client a point of view about his/her essential concern that is both discrepant and alternative to the one he/she is used to, a fast change in the perception of self and world (as the one obtained with Necker's cubes; Mahoney, 1980, 1985) is very likely to occur and to activate a reorganizing effect.

Gordon

Gordon, a 35-year-old industry manager, in the past 3 years has been suffering from phobic symptoms centered on a haunting fear of an imminent heart attack; this reduced his freedom of movement enough to hinder his work seriously. Though inwardly convinced of having an organic disease (he saw his cardiologist almost every day, whenever he was free from work), he accepted the doctor's insistent advice to undergo psychotherapeutic treatment. As had been thoroughly discussed elsewhere (Guidano, 1987; Guidano & Liotti, 1983, 1985), agoraphobics' blindness to emotions makes them sensitive only to their physical, sensorial (i.e., "quantitative") aspects, while the subjective, "qualitative," content of emotional states (i.e., images accompanying them, feeling tones, mood oscillations, etc.) is largely neglected up to the point of not being noticed and focused at all. Therefore, training clients to focus the content of the "negative" emotions experienced becomes the basic procedure to provide the client with meaningful cues (e.g., affective polarity perceived, domain of personal experience involved, etc.) that, though overlooked, are essential in facilitating a more exhaustive comprehension of the critical emotions experienced and, in the last analysis, their reordering.

Gordon was a very bright and open-minded man and, despite his prejudicial stance toward psychotherapy, he was decidedly cooperative from the beginning; within a few months it was possible, on the one hand, to reconstruct his personal history and, on the other, to train him in self-observation so that he could focus both the structure of his disturbing feelings and the variations, however slight, of the environmental context that accompanied their onset.

It then became more and more evident, even to Gordon's astonished eyes, that—although the accompanying images ranged greatly—his distressing feeling presented the one common theme of loneliness and that all anxiety-causing environmental variations were invariably connected to a perceived physical and/or affectional detachment on the side of his wife. Discussing it with Gordon, whose initial surprise was slowly giving way to a sort of disquieting curiosity, we felt it was legitimate to investigate the possible connection between disturbing emotions and the attachment style he had developed toward significant figures.

The series of ten or so sessions that followed were for Gordon strongly charged with emotions; little by little he began to see as clearly as in a film how the fear of physical abandonment and love withdrawal had been a constant feature of his infancy and childhood until the threshold of adolescence; he was thus able to evoke and focus memories that had long been obsolete—the times when, as a child, he used to lie awake in terror, waiting for his parents to come home from their evenings out, and each time he had a foreboding they would never come back; or his panic when, a few years older, his parents' resentful and detached attitude in consequence of a mediocre school performance convinced him that he had forever lost their affection and protection. When we came to the point of reconstructing the attachment patterns toward his wife, the level of emotional involvement that had characterized this series of crucial sessions quite suddenly reached a peak. Gordon realized at once that his symptoms had begun almost at the exact time when he had learned by chance and from indirect sources that his wife had had a short but extremely intense affair with an office colleague. It was as if the representation of his life acquired, as it approximated the present time, a consequentiality and logic typical of detective stories, and enabled him to understand in its entirety the relationship that he had with his wife and the disturbing sense of uncertainty that it gave him, and that he had only occasionally perceived in the course of therapy. The new ordering of personal experience that Gordon elaborated going back and forth through his developmental history was matched by a parallel restructuring of his conscious range of perceived emotions; the internal states triggered by the attitudes of his wife were no longer perceived as "strange" and "extraneous" feelings merely signaling an impending physical disaster, but as personal meaningful experiences modulating the oscillations in the level of emotional involvement that he experienced in the relationship with his wife.

From that moment onward, his attitude toward what he perceived in his wife as physical and affectional detachment radically changed; not that he had become indifferent to these matters, but in place of the usual panic and anxiety, they now elicited a wholly different set of emotions, such as sadness and dejection for what has happened, regret for their earlier times together, resentment for the wife's different view of life and love relationships, and so on. All this was, of course, accompanied by a dissolution of symptoms, and, by making possible a shift toward a reformulation of the problem in terms of reorganizing his married life and affectional style, it essentially opened a new phase in Gordon's psychotherapy.

Needless to say, we are not always confronted with situations as simple and relatively uncomplicated from the point of view of therapeutic strategy as the one reported above. In certain circumstances, the severity of symptoms, clients' high degree of unawareness, and most of all their extreme reluctance to accept that the therapeutic situation may become a means of cooperation and exploration, force the therapist to assume a much more active role, and often severely test his/her capacities and experience. The therapist's task consists basically in acting upon the emotional aspects of the therapeutic relationship in an attempt to trigger a discrepant effect "à la Necker's cube," able to set off a reorganization process. In this regard, it is worth reporting a highly emotional therapeutic situation experienced by the author many years ago during the treatment of a seriously anorexic female client.

Jessica

At 21, Jessica suffered from severe anorexia: about 5 feet 8 inches tall, she weighed barely 90 pounds; she had been amenorrheic for 4 years and took about 150 to 200 laxative pills a day. She was sent to me by a colleague of a nearby university after a series of therapeutic failures that had made her even more skeptical and diffident than she had been in the past toward therapists and psychotherapy.

The first 6 weeks or so (five or six sessions) were spent entirely in an effort to establish a cooperative relationship. Her doubts, uncertainties, and constant oscillations between the convenience of facing the problem versus trying to live with it, however, made it difficult to come to define in any way what would be her commitment to the therapy, so that the real therapeutic work could begin. We then agreed to go on, with no commitment on her side, to a phase of general investigation and exploration of possible psychological factors at the origin of her problem. Hence, I began to inquire in a very soft, reassuring way about the kind of family environment, relationships with peers, and school (intentionally overlooking the "hot topics," such as eating style, use of laxatives and so on, that she could very easily have felt as exceedingly intrusive). However, Jessica seemed absent; she was very vague and undetermined in her answers, and above all, never talked about herself and the emotions that she felt in connection to what she was reporting. We carried on like this for another 6 weeks or so in a situation of constant uncertainty and ambiguity; Jessica seemed, on the one hand, totally uninterested in what was said in our conversations and considered it a waste of time, but, on the other hand, she attended the sessions regularly and punctually (she even lived in another city and came to Rome specifically for the therapy) and never even hinted at the possibility of interrupting them.

After a short time Jessica's attitude gradually changed. She was more and more openly seductive toward me, at first by making broad remarks such as "my only problem is to find the right man." But soon she began to convey (as a joke in the beginning, then less so) that the "right man" could be me. Though I recognized and appreciated that somehow her emotions were beginning to show, the situation remained critical since she still rejected any attempt on my side to switch to a more abstract level of explanation that could allow us to define her seductive attitude within a wider perspective.

Jessica then went into a true "seductive escalation": she wrote to me every day (some days more than once) and arrived with a present for me at every session. Letters and presents were unquestionably intimate, the kind a girl gives to her boyfriend. On the other hand, Jessica was obviously handling the situation in such a way as to bring upon herself a probable bitter disappointment, which would surely worsen her anorexic attitude; one day, for instance, after the usual letter written on pink paper, I received a telegram: "999 men out of 1,000 are disappointing. You will never disappoint me."

My position was becoming more and more difficult. Because of the impossibility of shifting the level of analysis and interpretation, I was forced to take a stand within her own way of setting the problem, that is, to have or not to have an affair with her, and in both cases the situation would clearly become unbearable and would inevitably have consequences on her emotional disorders. At this point, events came to a head in a dramatic session; Jessica had come absolutely determined to get an answer out of me, and after a few minutes of small talk she came straight to the point. The climax of this session is worth reporting verbatim:

JESSICA (*ironical and defiant*): It seems to me you're making yourself ridiculous by still pretending to ignore how I feel about you. What is this, the proverbial male indifference and superiority toward a woman's supposed fragility? (*after a short pause*) Or are you just one of those kindhearted gentlemen who pretend not to see, to spare a woman the humiliation of a refusal?

THERAPIST (*staying as self-possessed as possible*): Not in the least. I am simply trying to understand the meaning of what you say you feel and its relation to the problem we have met about and on which we are trying to work.

J (*repressing a sarcastic smirk*): Ha! Sure enough, there you go again with your pompous air. Do you expect me to be fascinated or something, to admire your commitment to professional duty and all that kind of trash! (*getting harsher and more aggressive*) It's nothing but a lot of trash, you hide yourself like a coward behind this nonsense to avoid telling me the truth. And the truth is that you reject me, you don't give a damn about me. I feel insulted because you must think I'm a fool not to realize it. (*jumping to her feet and threateningly leaning across my desk*) But let me inform you that you won't find a way out this time. You have used all possible nonsense and I won't get out of this room until you tell me right to my face whether you like me as a woman or no.

T (*jumps to his feet; banging his fist on the desk and dropping his self-control, calls her by her first name*): Now I'm sick and tired of being annoyed by a boring, impudent brat. I'm sick and tired of your making a fool of me with love proposals that are just ridiculous, since you're skin and bones, you haven't had your period for 4 years and a gust of wind is enough to make you take off. What if I did say yes, how could I ever go to bed with you without being afraid of breaking your bones? (*Jessica is visibly upset; the therapist, staring into her eyes, in a mocking, challenging tone*) Look, sweetheart, I'm a grown-up man, not some character in a fairy tale. If ever you should put yourself in a condition where I can see you as a woman I assure you we could discuss matters again in a different way. (*He drops down on his armchair as if exhausted.*)

J (*first weeps silently while the therapist is still speaking, then her crying becomes louder, her sobs are mixed with curses and threats*): I knew I shouldn't trust you either . . . You're as cowardly and selfish as everybody else . . . You're mean and cruel . . . No human being can be told the things you just told me . . . The conscientious doctor, indeed! You're a monster with a computer instead of a heart . . . (*Sobbing, she leaps to her feet and goes to the door.*) I don't want to see you again; never, never again . . . I wish you all the harm you have done me . . . (*She goes out banging the door loudly and leaves.*)

Less than 10 minutes later, as I was still confused and concerned about the recent scene, the telephone rang: It was Jessica. In a matter-of-fact tone, as if nothing had happened, she wanted to know if our next appointment was confirmed, since in the haste she had forgotten to ask.

From that moment, the change in Jessica's attitude was really impressive; of her own accord (we had never explicitly talked about these subjects) she went back to eating more regularly and gradually reduced the laxatives; she resumed her university studies and started to make plans to leave her family and go live on her own. As to the therapy, Jessica became extremely cooperative and after a short period of training in self-observation she selected as a therapeutic target her excessive sensitivity to other people's judgment, something she was now becoming more and more aware of.

Twelve years have passed, and after completing her therapy (it went on for about a year after the session reported above) I have kept in touch with her. Although she lived in another city, she called regularly, and every time she was in Rome she never failed to come to see me. In these 12 years, Jessica has gone through difficult, stressful situations (death of both her parents, a painful divorce as an end to a marriage that meant much to her, failure in her career, etc.) but she has never again manifested the slightest anorexic reaction. Of course she had not "toughened" in the face of misfortune but—as for Gordon—misfortune now triggered a different range of emotions; for example, during the divorce proceedings she suffered from intense anxiety reactions intermingled with psychosomatic disorders and after the end of her marriage she experienced a phase of depression that required a mild drug treatment. In the light of more than a decade of follow-up, it is therefore reasonable to assume that the discrepant effect she felt during our turbulent session has somehow triggered in the perception of herself and the world a reorganization process that has remained relatively stable.

AFFECTIVE EVENTS AND CHANGE PROCESSES

How can we explain the close correlation between affective events and change processes on the basis of the proposed psychological model and case reports? In the first place, the essential requisite facilitating a therapeutic change appears to be the simultaneous occurring of two processes, the intensity and structure of which range widely: (1) a *discrepancy effect* (deriving from explanations offered by the therapist) able to trigger an appreciable modification of the client's point of view toward him/herself, and (2) a consistent level of *emotional involvement* in the therapeutic relationship. A deeper analysis of these processes may help to clarify their reciprocal correlation.

Discrepancy Effect

The efficacy of therapeutic explanations and interpretations depends more on their degree of discrepancy, compared with clients' usual perception of themselves, than on the specific contents of knowledge they provide (Claiborn, 1982; Claiborn & Dowd, 1985). Thus, in contrast to the traditional assumption, the crucial effect rather than being identified with the transmission of more rational knowledge contents, should be traced back to a forced reappraisal of one's self-image triggered by a critical perturbation experienced in one's ongoing apperceptive scaffolding of self and reality. Such reappraisal, in turn, involves a modification of the current level of self-awareness, whose constructive and generative effect unfolds through a reorganization of the relationships established between items contained in individual consciousness.

Of course, the patterns that a discrepant effect may assume within a therapeutic setting range widely, and the clinical cases reported in the previous section represent, in a way, the two extremes. In Gordon's case the discrepant effect coincided with his assimilation of self-observation techniques that led him—without his fully realizing it—to give the flow of daily events an entirely different construction from the usual one; on the contrary, in Jessica's case, the therapist was unable to act upon self-observation procedures and had to exploit the inconsistencies and ambiguities of her attitude to build up a "paradoxical response," in which the perturbing effect consisted in disclosing brusquely the insubstantiality of her requests. However, even if the availability of explanations conveying discrepant effects is a necessary condition to activate a challenging perturbation, it is not sufficient in itself to trigger a reorganizing effect.

Emotional Involvement

An appreciable level of emotional involvement in the therapeutic relationship puts the client in a condition where he/she cannot in any way avoid facing a challenging point of view constraining him/her to an immediate, overall self-referent attribution that generates the very perception of discrepancy. In other words, regardless of its specific content, a challenging perspective can produce a discrepant effect only through the level of self-referentiality that it acquires within an adequate emotional context. As common experience shows, a message penetrates more or less according to the quality of ongoing interaction; criticism from someone to whom we are indifferent generally leaves us disturbed (and often even has a "paradoxically" confirming effect), whereas the same remark from a very significant person is most likely to upset us deeply. The emotional involvement that Jessica was experiencing toward the therapist worked as the self-referential attributive framework that constrained her to perceive the therapist's response as an intense, unbearable challenge capable of reordering her current sense of self.

However, the necessity for an emotional involvement should not be thought of as a concern only to the client; the therapist's involvement in the setting exerts a crucial role in activating in the client that condition of unavoidability and self-referentiality previously described. Indeed, the centrality of commitment in the structure of language acts seems to be one of the most innovative aspects promoted by linguistics in the last decade:

The essential presupposition for the success of an illocutionary act consists in the speaker's entering into a specific *engagement*, so that the
hearer can rely on him. An utterance can count as a promise, assertion,
request, question, or avowal, if and only if the speaker makes an offer that
he is ready to make good insofar as it is accepted by the hearer. The
speaker must engage himself, that is, indicate that in certain situations he
will draw certain consequences for action. (Habermas, 1979, quoted by
Winograd & Flores, 1986, p. 59)

Going back to Jessica's dramatic session, it should be quite evident that
what made the therapist's paradoxical intervention discrepant was his
losing his temper. The emotional involvement of the therapist made it
evident that he considered himself as engaged in a "real" relationship and
this, in turn, made his attitude reliable to Jessica's eyes; that is, that there
was an effective possibility for an alternative explanation and experiencing
of her present problems, and that the therapist was "ready to make good
his offer if only it was accepted by her." Most likely if the same paradoxical
response had been formulated with professional composure it would have
produced very little effect, except perhaps an irreparable deterioration of
the ongoing relationship.

It should be kept in mind that we can only aim at conditions capable
of triggering a reorganization process, but we cannot determine the ways
and times of its occurring, nor its outcome. As Dell and Goolishian (1981)
put it: "One can intervene in such systems and push them to the point of
instability, but one cannot control precisely when they reorganize, nor
can one control in what fashion they reorganize" (p. 179). As Jessica's
case shows, everything that took place in her after that session was completely out of my planning and control; I was, so to speak, assisting in an
incessant springing of new decisions and changes of attitude, and did
nothing but corroborate her capabilities of self-observation so that she
could feel increasingly certain of what she felt and thought. On the other
hand, in these 12 years Jessica herself—although we have discussed it at
length on many occasions—has never been able to find an exhaustive,
ultimate explanation for a change that still astounds her.

As a conclusion of our analysis, consideration will now be given to the
methodological changes entailed by a cognitive therapy systems approach.

METHODOLOGICAL REMARKS FOR COGNITIVE THERAPY

The adoption of a systems, process-oriented perspective has considerable
repercussions on the conceptualization of change and, consequently, on
therapeutic methodology.

In traditional cognitive approaches, still solidly bound to the notion of
adulthood as a plateau, therapeutic change is mainly regarded as recovery

of the adaptive equilibrium that existed prior to the onset of symptoms (Beck, 1976, 1985; Ellis, 1962, 1985; Goldfried, 1982; Meichenbaum, 1977). Such recovery essentially coincides with an increase of self-control skills with respect to discrepant emotions, and with an enactment of more rational problem-solving procedures toward critical situations and attitudes.

Cognitive approaches whose orientation is more systemic and structural, on the contrary, prevalently regard adulthood as an orthogenetic progression of individual knowledge, and thus the fundamental question about change comes to be reformulated on another basis: How can clients' awareness of their own functioning be modified so that, moving along their orthogenetic directionality, they can assimilate the present disequilibrium and shift toward a more progressive dynamic equilibrium? (Guidano, 1987, 1988; Guidano & Liotti, 1983; Mahoney, 1980, 1985, 1991; Mahoney & Gabriel, 1987; Reda, 1986; Rice & Greenberg, 1984; Safran, 1990).

I will now briefly try to highlight the methodological relevance of such a perspective, making reference to basic themes currently debated by different cognitive trends.

The Problem of "Objectivity"

In the traditional cognitive approach, rationality is conceived of as a set of universally valid standard axioms that make up the external, univocal, and objective order against which we can assess if and to which extent any behavior is problematic or inconsistent. So the therapist, as a trustee and warrantor of such axioms, is able to impersonate, in the therapeutic relationship, the role of an outside impartial observer who can "objectively" criticize the irrationality of clients' conduct, while inducing in different ways more rational beliefs and behaviors.

As a result of this therapeutic approach, ordinary cognitive therapies end up turning the relationship with the client into a sort of didactic course, with a scientific, philosophic, or pedagogic orientation according to the therapist's personal background. Apart from the obvious impoverishment of the therapeutic relationship, the actual limit of this position is that more emphasis is given to formal characteristics of problematic behaviors (i.e., comparison with standard rational axioms) than to their knowledge contents. For instance, as far as so-called negative emotions are concerned (anxiety, sadness, helplessness, etc.), relevance is usually attributed to their fitness with a standardized style of life, and subsequently to the most convenient rational procedures to control them; the fact that the content of these emotions (images, bodily perceptions, feeling tones, etc.), once properly focused, can provide to the client essential cues on the dynamics of his/her personal meaning, is generally overlooked. In other words, if the perspective endorsed is centered on an objective, immutable outside order that univocally rules the trend and sense of human events, the therapeutic relationship cannot but become an order-establishing instrument, rather than a means for clients' personal explorations and a path for their gradual grasping—through the apparent senselessness of their disturbing emotions—of the rules that constrain the rigid coherence of their personal meaning.

On the other hand, if the ordering of reality into personal experience is a system's autonomous construction, we cannot expect to identify any objective outside point of view by which to evaluate the degree of rationality and validity of observed problematic behaviors. Rather than being an absolute criterion to judge an attitude in itself, rationality is instead intrinsically relativistic and, as such, simply enables definition of the degree of adequacy of a given attitude *if the latter is referred to the system that generated it and to which it belongs.* From an evolutionary point of view, rationality appears to be an emerging property of self-organizing systems and since the very beginning it is connected with the elaboration of specific rules for the development of increasingly effective, purpose-directed behaviors. Therefore, if rationality is essentially "action," it cannot refer to logical categories as true or false (Weimer, 1987). Thus, rationality merely evidentiates the self-referentiality of adaptive processes in a given system, specifying that adaptation itself consists not so much in attaining a "right" or "true" purpose, but rather in pursuing an aim whose possible usefulness is such only from the standpoint of the system involved.

In other terms, through the tacit oscillation between boundaries of meaning underlying his/her perceived identity, every subject is able to structure a simultaneously stable and dynamic demarcation between what is real and what it is not. A systems, process-oriented therapist, therefore, will consider "rational" for a given individual, the set of tacit rules, emotional schemata, thought processes, and so on, that provide internal coherence to his/her personal meaning, regardless of their adherence to the laws of classical logic. It is clear that in a perspective of this kind the therapist's attitude toward the client is considerably modified. Within a therapeutic relationship intended to be essentially a tool of exploration, the therapist will accurately avoid confronting the problematic emotions with a critical and/or worried attitude, that would inevitably confirm to the client the sense of extraneousness with which he/she usually perceives such emotions, and would thus further decrease the possibilities of their assimiliation. On the contrary, by gradually reconstructing the internal coherence ("rationality" existing beyond the apparent illogic of disturbing emotions) the therapist will aim at showing the client with growing clarity how such emotions, far from being alien to his/her nature, contain fundamental information, the understanding and assimilation of which may very likely facilitate the overcoming of the current existential stalemate.

Self-Control versus Reorganization of Personal Reality

Self-control (regaining of the existing but temporarily lost equilibrium) and reorganization of personal experience (construction of a new equilibrium, not yet existent), being based on different conceptions of individual life-span development, correspond to basically different methods of therapeutic intervention.

The approach aimed at self-control adopts a strategy oriented toward the client's *persuasion*, whereas the therapist, playing the role of "enlightened sage" or "devil's advocate," according to case, tries with every available means to convince the client of the irrationality of his/her problematic attitudes while constantly giving instructions how to strengthen more adaptive behaviors. The most suitable operational setting for such a procedure is a more or less pressing dialectical confrontation, and persuasion technically consists of an intervention of the client's representational surface structures (imagery, beliefs, internal dialogue, etc., directed at modifying the semantic aspects of cognitive processes), while leaving syntactic rules at the basis of these same processes totally unchanged.

In agoraphobic subjects, while basic syntactic rules keep the clients perceiving themselves as defenseless in a menacing, hostile world, the intervention is focused, for instance, on the way they represent to themselves a panic attack in traffic, and is accompanied by a series of instructions that they must introduce in their inner dialogue whenever they face the feared situation again. No doubt clients will obtain a better control on anxiety in feared situations if they will keep telling themselves: "I must remember the doctor told me nothing can happen to me. . . ," "I must keep calm, it's all my imagination. . . ," "Nobody ever died from waiting at a traffic light. . . ." Undeniably, though, the meaning of anxiety attacks remains unchanged for clients, and, furthermore, they still find no explanation for their being so "strangely" oversensitive and vulnerable to unimportant situations of constriction and/or loneliness. If the intervention is limited to a modification of the cognitive appraisal, the disturbing emotional reaction is in no way changed in tone, even if its intensity can be better controlled (cf. Zajonc, 1984). Critical emotions remain alien to the subject who, instead, has acquired skills in controlling them "from the outside." In other words, rather than a reorganization of personal meaning, what occurs is only a semantic change inside the same meaning tonality.

Quite clearly, to obtain a significant therapeutic change a therapist cannot limit him/herself to being a "hidden persuader," inducing more adaptive attitudes through relational or behavioral maneuvers (paradoxical prescriptions, challenging dialectic disconfirmations, etc.). On the contrary, since clients' attainment of a more accurate and exhaustive *understanding* of their functioning represents the central variable for a more adequate assimilation of the problematical experience, the therapist will no longer have any interest in inducing behavioral modifications *beyond the client's awareness.* Therefore, since the aim consists not so much in changing, at any cost, clients' beliefs, but rather in their becoming aware of their way of elaborating beliefs, the therapist orients from the very beginning toward a gradual reconstruction and comprehension of basic syntactic rules underlying the invariant aspects of critical emotions and representations. If at the beginning of therapy such a strategy is carried on through self-observation techniques prevalently focused on the *hic et nunc*, as comprehension gradually increases, it will progressively include a reconstruction of personal developmental history.

The process of making clients repeatedly go over their developmental history undoubtedly produces the highest possible levels of distancing and decentering from certain emotional schemata and cognitive patterns closely connected to the perceived sense of self. The new patterns of self-awareness thus emerging activate further reorganizations of past data, which in turn trigger further comprehending processes, and so on. In other words, by so proceeding, the therapist works on clients' memories (that is to say, on their way of selecting and ordering their life events so as to obtain a meaning specifically consistent with their ongoing internal coherence) with the result of activating a reordering and reframing of their constructions (Bara, 1984). An analysis of significant changes occurring during psychotherapy (so-called deep or central changes) shows that such changes are invariably matched by substantial changes in clients' memory.

As a conclusion to these notes, a few comments should be dedicated to the role played by emotional aspects of the therapeutic relationship in triggering change.

At the present state of knowledge, it seems more and more evident that emotional perturbations arising from the therapeutic relationship—especially in case of clients' "positive" involvement—have an absolutely primary role in activating modifications in ongoing levels of self-awareness enabling clients to elaborate alternative representations of themselves. On the other hand, we are far from having attained an exhaustive theory of the mind that is able to explain the close interdependence between emotions and cognitions and, in particular, in what way affect facilitates the assimilation of experience; therefore a therapist's ability in using relational dynamics to promote change cannot but remain, presently at least, more an art than a science.

Anyhow, from this perspective, the emerging image of the therapist is one of a person who, in pursuing the task of "technically" aiming at modifying clients' awareness patterns, is extremely alert in using ongoing emotional oscillations observed in clients to facilitate a comprehension of what is being reconstructed. But clearly a more exhaustive definition of the therapist's role as a *strategically oriented perturber* will require that psychotherapeutic research be more and more focused upon the elaboration of patterns exemplifying how the emotional oscillations that take place during the comprehension of critical data can enhance the acquisition of new data and/or the reframing of existing ones.

Finally, it should be noted that this problem appears to be even more complex today than in the past because the radical change in the observer–observed relationship results in a direct involvement of the therapist in contrasting and, until now, unpredictable ways. The fact that the therapist can no longer be considered as an outside, impartial observer is not only indicative of the influence of his/her conceptual aspects on the collection and elaboration of observed data, but also of the influence that his/her emotional aspects exert on the course of the relationship, and, therefore, on the definition of therapeutic reality itself. On the one hand, the therapist is forced to take into account his/her own emotional oscillations, which accompany and modulate the ongoing perception and understanding of the client's problems. But, on the other hand, such oscillations, though triggered by the interaction with the client, inform not so much on the latter's functioning, as on the therapist him/herself.

In other words, if therapists renounce the role of "trustees of an objectivity principle" and accept to enter in the game of self-referentiality, then inside any order they are able to perceive they cannot but grasp the contour of their own image. Far from evoking the usual solipsistic ghosts, this means that any knowledge is intrinsically interactional and "participatory," that is, is based on the reciprocal negotiation of a mutual agreement rather than on mere transmission of data from one system to the other. Along these same lines, Robert Musil, with his usual epistemological keenness, wrote in his diaries many years ago: "Is there such a thing as the knowledge of men? We shall remember, from time to time, that understanding a man is nothing but reacting psychically to him in a well determined manner" (1980, p. 128).

REFERENCES

Airenti, G., Bara, B. G., & Colombetti, M. (1982a). Semantic network representation of conceptual and episodic knowledge. In R. Trappl (Ed.), *Advances in cybernetics and system research* (Vol. 11). Washington: Hemisphere.
Airenti, G., Bara, B. G., & Colombetti, M. (1982b). A two level model of knowledge and belief. In R. Trappl (Ed.), *Proceedings of 6th E.M.C.S.R.* Amsterdam: North-Holland.
Atlan, H. (1979). *Entre le cristal et la fumée.* Paris: Seuil.
Atlan, H. (1981). Hierarchical self-organization in living systems. In M. Zeleny (Ed.), *Autopoiesis: A theory of living organization.* New York: North-Holland.

Bara, B. G. (1984). Modifications of knowledge by memory processes. In M. A. Reda & M. J. Mahoney (Eds.), *Cognitive psychotherapies.* Cambridge, MA: Ballinger.

Beck, A. T. (1976). *Cognitive therapy and the emotional disorders.* New York: International Universities Press.

Beck, A. T. (1985). Cognitive therapy, behavior therapy, psychoanalysis, and pharmacotherapy: A cognitive continuum. In M. J. Mahoney & A. Freeman (Eds.), *Cognition and psychotherapy.* New York: Plenum.

Bowlby, J. (1969). *Attachment and loss: Vol. 1. Attachment.* New York: Basic Books.

Bowlby, J. (1973). *Attachment and loss: Vol. 2. Separation: anxiety and anger.* New York: Basic Books.

Bowlby, J. (1977). The making and breaking of affectional bonds: (1) Etiology and psychopathology in the light of attachment theory. *British Journal of Psychiatry, 130,* 201-210.

Bowlby, J. (1980). *Attachment and loss: Vol. 3. Loss, sadness and depression.* London: Hogarth Press.

Brent, S. B. (1978). Prigogine's model for self-organization in nonequilibrium systems: Its relevance for developmental psychology. *Human Development, 21,* 374-387.

Brent, S. B. (1984). *Psychological and social structures.* Hillsdale, NJ: Erlbaum.

Brown, G. W. (1982). Early loss and depression. In C. M. Parkes & J. Stevenson-Hinde (Eds.), *The place of attachment in human behavior.* London: Tavistock.

Brown, G. W., & Harris, T. (1978). *Social origins of depression.* London: Tavistock.

Claiborn, C. D. (1982). Interpretation and change in counseling. *Journal of Counseling Psychology, 29,* 439-453.

Claiborn, C. D., & Dowd, T. E. (1985). Attributional interpretations in counseling: content versus discrepancy. *Journal of Counseling Psychology, 32,* 188-196.

Cooley, C. H. (1902). *Human nature and the social order.* New York: Scribner.

Dell, P. F., & Goolishian, H. A. (1981). "Order through fluctuations": An evolutionary epistemology for human systems. *Australian Journal of Family Therapy, 2,* 175-184.

Eibl-Eibesfeldt, I. (1972). *Love and hate: The natural history of behavior patterns.* New York: Holt, Rinehart & Winston.

Ekman, P. (1984). Expression and the nature of emotion. In K. R. Scherer & P. Ekman, (Eds.), *Approaches to emotion.* Hillsdale, NJ: Erlbaum.

Ellis, A. (1962). *Reason and emotion in psychotherapy.* New York: Lyle Stuart.

Ellis, A. (1985). Expanding the ABC's of rational-emotive therapy. In M. J. Mahoney & A. Freeman (Eds.), *Cognition and psychotherapy.* New York: Plenum.

Flavell, J. H. (1977). *Cognitive development.* Englewood Cliffs, NJ: Prentice-Hall.

Franks, J. J. (1974). Toward understanding understanding. In W. B. Weimer & D. S. Palermo (Eds.), *Cognition and the symbolic processes.* Hillsdale, NJ: Erlbaum.

Goldfried, M. R. (Ed.). (1982). *Converging themes in psychotherapy.* New York: Springer.

Gould, S. J. (1980). *The panda's thumb: More reflections in natural history*. New York: Norton.

Guidano, V. F. (1987). *Complexity of the self*. New York: Guilford.

Guidano, V. F. (1988). A systems, process-oriented approach to cognitive therapy. In K. S. Dobson (Ed.), *Handbook of cognitive–behavioral therapies*. New York: Guilford.

Guidano, V. F., & Liotti, G. (1983). *Cognitive processes and emotional disorders*. New York: Guilford.

Guidano, V. F., & Liotti, G. (1985). A constructivistic foundation for cognitive therapy. In M. J. Mahoney & A. Freeman (Eds.), *Cognition and psychotherapy*. New York: Plenum.

Habermas, J. (1979). What is universal pragmatics? In J. Habermas, *Communication and the evolution of society*. Boston: Beacon Press.

Haviland, J. (1984). Thinking and feeling in Woolf's writing: from childhood to adulthood. In C. E. Izard, J. Kagan, & R. B. Zajonc (Eds.), *Emotions, cognition, and behavior*. Cambridge, England: Cambridge University Press.

Hayek, F. A. (1952). *The sensory order*. Chicago: University of Chicago Press.

Hayek, F. A. (1964). The theory of complex phenomena. In M. Bunge (Ed.), *The critical approach to science and philosophy: Essays in honor of K. R. Popper*. New York: Free Press.

Hayek, F. A. (1978). *New studies in philosophy, politics, economics, and the history of ideas*. Chicago: University of Chicago Press.

Henderson, S. (1982). The significance of social relationships in the etiology of neurosis. In C. M. Parkes & J. Stevenson-Hinde (Eds.), *The place of attachment in human behavior*. London: Tavistock.

Henderson, S., Byrne, D. G., & Duncan-Jones, P. (1981). *Neurosis and the social environment*. New York: Academic Press.

Jantsch, E. (1980). *The self-organizing universe*. New York: Pergamon.

Leventhal, H. (1980). Toward a comprehensive theory of emotion. In L. Berkowitz (Ed.), *Advances in experimental social psychology* (Vol. 13). New York: Academic Press.

Leventhal, H. (1984). A perceptual motor theory of emotion. In K. R. Scherer & P. Ekman (Eds.), *Approaches to emotion*. Hillsdale, NJ: Erlbaum.

Leventhal, H. (1986). Emotion: Today's problems. *Annual Review of Psychology, 37*, 565–610.

Mahoney, M. J. (1980). Psychotherapy and the structure of personal revolutions. In M. J. Mahoney (Ed.), *Psychotherapy process*. New York: Plenum.

Mahoney, M. J. (1985). Psychotherapy and human change processes. In M. J. Mahoney & A. Freeman (Eds.), *Cognition and psychotherapy*. New York: Plenum.

Mahoney, M. J. (1991). *Personal change processes: The scientific foundations of psychotherapy*. New York: Basic Books.

Mahoney, M. J., & Gabriel, T. (1987). Psychotherapy and cognitive sciences: An evolving alliance. *Journal of Cognitive Psychotherapy, 1*, 39–59.

Marcel, A. J. (1983). Conscious and unconscious perception: an approach to the relations between phenomenal experience and perceptual processes. *Cognitive Psychology, 15*, 238–300.

Marris, P. (1982). Attachment and society. In C. M. Parkes & J. Stevenson-Hinde (Eds.), *The place of attachment in human behavior*. London: Tavistock.

Maturana, H. R., & Varela, F. (1980). *Autopoiesis and cognition: The realization of the living*. Dordrecht, Netherlands: Reidel.

Mead, G. H. (1934). *Mind, self, and society*. Chicago: University of Chicago Press.

Meichenbaum, D. (1977). *Cognitive-behavior modification*. New York: Plenum.

Miró, M., & Belloch, A. (1986). *Selfhood processes as an approach to personality: Preliminary remarks*. Paper presented at the third European Conference on Personality Psychology, Gdansk, Poland.

Musil, R. (1980). *Diari* (Vol. 1). Turin, Italy: Einaudi.

Nicolis, G., & Prigogine, I. (1977). *Self-organization in nonequilibrium systems: From dissipative structures to order through fluctuations*. New York: Wiley.

Piaget, J. (1951). *Psychology of intelligence*. London: Routledge & Kegan Paul.

Plutchik, R. (1980). A general psychoevolutionary theory of emotion. In R. Plutchik & H. Kellerman (Eds.), *Emotion: Theory, research, and experience* (Vol. 1). New York: Academic Press.

Plutchik, R. (1983). Emotions in early development: A psychoevolutionary approach. In R. Plutchik & H. Kellerman (Eds.), *Emotion: Theory, research, and experience*. New York: Academic Press.

Polanyi, M. (1966). *The tacit dimension*. Garden City, NY: Doubleday.

Popper, K. R., & Eccles, J. C. (1977). *The self and its brain*. New York: Springer.

Prigogine, I. (1976). Order through fluctuations: Self-organization and social systems. In E. Jantsch & C. H. Waddington (Eds.), *Evolution and consciousness: Human systems in transition*. Reading, MA: Addison-Wesley.

Prigogine, I., & Stengers, I. (1984). *Order out of chaos: Man's new dialogue with nature*. New York: Bantam.

Reber, A. S., & Lewis, S. (1977). Implicit learning: An analysis of the form and structure of a body of tacit knowledge. *Cognition, 5*, 333–361.

Reda, M. (1986). *Sistemi cognitivi complessi e psicoterapia*. Roma: NIS.

Rice, L. N., & Greenberg, L. S., (Eds.). (1984). *Patterns of change: Intensive analysis of psychotherapy process*. New York: Guilford.

Safran, J. D. (1990). Towards a refinement of cognitive therapy in light of interpersonal theory: I. Theory. *Clinical Psychology Review, 10*, 87–105.

Serres, M. (1976). Le point de vue de la biophysique. In Critique, Paris, *La psychoanalyse vue de dehors* (special issue, March), 265–277.

Shevrin, H., & Dickman, S. (1980). The psychological unconscious: A necessary assumption for all psychological theory? *American Psychologist, 35*, 421–434.

Trevarthen, C. (1980). [Review of *The making and breaking of affectional bonds*, by John Bowlby]. *British Journal of Psychiatry, 137*, 390.

Trevarthen, C. (1984). Emotions in infancy: Regulators of contact and relationships with persons. In K. R. Scherer & P. Ekman (Eds.), *Approaches to emotion*. Hillsdale, NJ: Erlbaum.

Van Den Berg, D., & Eelen, P. (1984). Unconscious processing and emotions. In M. A. Reda & M. J. Mahoney (Eds.), *Cognitive psychotherapies*. Cambridge, MA: Ballinger.

Varela, F. (1979). *Principles of biological autonomy.* New York: North-Holland.
Weimer, W. B. (1973). Psycholinguistics and Plato's paradoxes of the Meno. *American Psychologist, 28,* 15–33.
Weimer, W. B. (1977). A conceptual framework for cognitive psychology: Motor theories of the mind. In R. Shaw & J. D. Bransford (Eds.), *Perceiving, acting, and knowing.* Hillsdale, NJ: Erlbaum.
Weimer, W. B. (1982). Hayek's approach to the problems of complex phenomena: An introduction to the theoretical psychology of the sensory order. In W. B. Weimer & D. S. Palermo (Eds.), *Cognition and the symbolic processes* (Vol. 2). Hillsdale, NJ: Erlbaum.
Weimer, W. B. (1983). *Spontaneously ordered complex phenomena.* Paper prepared for Committee 1 of the 12th International Conference on the Unity of the Sciences, Chicago.
Weimer, W. B. (1987). *Rationality in complex orders is never fully explicit nor instantly specifiable.* Unpublished manuscript.
Werner, H. (1948). *Comparative psychology of mental development.* New York: International Universities Press.
Werner, H. (1957). The concept of development from a comparative and organismic point of view. In D. E. Harris (Ed.), *The concept of development.* Minneapolis: University of Minnesota Press.
Winograd, T., & Flores, F. (1986). *Understanding computers and cognition.* Norwood, NJ: Ablex.
Zajonc, R. B. (1980). Feeling and thinking: Preferences need no inferences. *American Psychologist, 35,* 151–175.
Zajonc, R. B. (1984). On primacy of affect. In K. R. Scherer & P. Ekman (Eds.), *Approaches to emotion.* Hillsdale, NJ: Erlbaum.
Zeleny, M. (Ed.). (1981). *Autopoiesis: A theory of living organization.* New York: North-Holland.

Section B

Psychodynamic Approaches

The chapters in this section represent some of the more current developments in the psychodynamic conceptualization of the role of emotion in psychotherapy. Freud initially saw affect as the expression of psychic energy—a quasiphysiological instinctive source of energy that must be maintained at a constant level in order to maintain psychological health. As Butler and Strupp point out in their chapter, this led to therapeutic models emphasizing the discharge, conversion, repression, and sublimation of psychic energy. More recent psychodynamic formulations have attempted to retain Freud's more important insights about both the nature of human psychological functioning and the therapeutic process, while reformulating psychoanalytic metatheory in a fashion more consistent with contemporary developments in biological and psychosocial sciences. Strupp and Binder's chapter represents some important trends in contemporary psychodynamic theory. First, the chapter is consistent with the general movement away from classical drive metapsychology toward more relational or interpersonal formulations in psychodynamic theory. Second, they emphasize the role of "corrective emotional experience" as a mechanism of change rather than insight. Third, following Roy Schafer's attempt to reformulate psychoanalytic metatheory in terms of an "action language" approach, they conceptualize emotion as a type of action. This emphasis is consistent with contemporary developments in emotion theory as discussed in Chapter 1 of this volume, as well as some of the more recent developments in the cognitive–behavioral conceptualization of emotion (as represented in the chapters of Foa and Kozak, and Guidano in this volume).

Silberschatz and Weiss emphasize the informational function that emotional appraisal plays in the human organism and the role that pathogenic beliefs about interpersonal relationships play in preventing access to potentially adaptive emotional experience. Their systematic research program has played an important role in clarifying the fashion in which the therapeutic relationship can play a role in disconfirming such pathogenic beliefs. Their chapter illustrates the fashion in which the emergence of painful, disavowed emotion in a client can be facilitated through the therapist's disconfirmation of pathogenic beliefs, and lead to a reorganization in the client's view of both him/herself and others.

Dahl in his chapter provides an update of his psychoanalytic model of motivation (originally articulated in 1978) and applies this model to the examination of the process of change in a long-term psychoanalytic case. In his model, Dahl has attempted systematically to remedy a number of shortcomings in the classical psychoanalytic theory of motivation. He attempts to integrate certain ego-analytic developments in the conceptualization of motivation with various developments in both contemporary emotion theory and cognitive psychology in order to develop a systematic psychoanalytic theory of emotion. Dahl emphasizes both the action evoking and the appraisal functions of emotional experience. His model is complex, but the chapter represents a serious attempt to apply empirically a systematic model of emotion to the analysis of a change process in psychotherapy.

4

The Role of Affect in Time-Limited Dynamic Psychotherapy

STEPHEN F. BUTLER
Brookside Hospital, Nashua, New Hampshire

HANS H. STRUPP
Vanderbilt University

INTRODUCTION

Affect or emotional response held a central role in psychoanalytic thinking in the earliest days of that tradition. Breuer and Freud's (1895) classic *Studies on Hysteria*, which presented the first full statement of a psychoanalytic theory of neurosis, proposed that the root of hysterical symptoms was strong emotion that had been "strangulated." *Abreaction* was the process by which the patient was able to achieve direct expression of these affects, resulting in the cure, or *catharsis*, conceptualized as a draining off of emotional energies (Strupp, 1967). As pivotal theoretical constructs, abreaction and catharisis soon became controversial, and, while interpretation became increasingly central in psychoanalytic thinking, the role of affect was accorded less attention. Often the role of affective experience seems to have been taken for granted by many psychoanalytic theorists, mentioned in passing as an inevitable, perhaps even undesirable, accompaniment of the therapeutic process (Strachey, 1934).

What was once a rather monolithic body of psychoanalytic theory and technique has, over the years, spawned a number of different approaches to psychotherapy, subsumed under the generic term, dynamic psychotherapy. Each of these approaches emphasizes different aspects of the complex phenomena of psychotherapy, including the role of affect in psychotherapy and how affect is to be conceptualized. Recently, Strupp and Binder (1984) introduced a new model of psychotherapy, called Time-Limited Dynamic Psychotherapy (TLDP), which is an integration of earlier dynamic approaches presented in the form of a therapy "manual." In this chapter we will: (1) present a brief introduction to the principles and strategies of TLDP, (2) examine the theoretical roots of our current thinking on the role of affective experience in psychotherapy, (3) explicitly integrate these theoretical positions into the principles and technical considerations of TLDP, (4) present vignettes illustrating how TLDP therapists address two different affective problems, and (5) discuss some theoretical and research implications inherent in our view of emotional experience in psychotherapy.

TIME-LIMITED DYNAMIC PSYCHOTHERAPY

TLDP represents an approach to individual psychotherapy that integrates clinical concepts from a variety of psychodynamic perspectives and attempts to provide a conceptually coherent framework for viewing psychotherapy. Accordingly, TLDP is rooted in psychoanalytic conceptions and reformulations by contemporary theorists. Augmenting the psychoanalytic foundation is the interpersonal perspective of Harry Stack Sullivan, members of the neo-Freudian school (Horney, Erikson), and contributions of modern interpersonal theorists (Anchin & Kiesler, 1982). The effort has been to synthesize this material into a coherent approach while staying as close as possible to clinical observations, unencumbered by metapsychological jargon.

The impetus for the creation of TLDP, as a particular psychotherapy model, came from two sources: First was the growing recognition in the field of the necessity for specific descriptions of treatment modalities, the so-called treatment manuals (e.g., Beck, Rush, Shaw, & Emery, 1979; Klerman, Rounsaville, Chevron, Neu, & Weissman, 1984; Luborsky, 1984). Such specification was deemed essential to advance significantly the scientific study of psychotherapy (Bergin & Strupp, 1972; Strupp & Bergin, 1969). Secondly, observations made at Vanderbilt's Center for Psychotherapy Research comparing patient–therapist interactions evidenced in good and poor outcome cases, found that treatment failures tended to be associated with negative therapeutic relationships (Strupp, 1980a,b,c,d). The major deterrents to the formation of a good working alliance seemed to be not only the patient's characterological distortions and maladaptive defenses but, equally important, the therapist's personal reactions to these difficulties as manifest in the therapeutic relationship. As Strupp (1980d) pointed out, "In our study we failed to encounter a single instance in which a difficult patient's hostility or negativism were sucessfully confronted or resolved" (p. 954). Indeed, therapists, even very experienced ones, tended to respond to a patient's hostility with counterhostility, coldness, distancing, and other forms of rejection. Based on these findings, the view developed that specific technical deficiencies on the part of the therapists exacerbated the problems that emerged in the therapeutic relationship. This suggested that psychotherapy could be improved by specifying principles and strategies geared toward the assessment and management of potential problems in the therapeutic relationship. TLDP, however, also aspires to the broader objective of helping patients whose difficulties in living, sometimes expressed in terms of symptoms of anxiety and depression, are the product of chronic maladaptations that are similar in form to the problems that emerge in the therapeutic relationship.

TLDP is not primarily addressed to the amelioration of presenting symptoms, although improvements in this domain are obviously expected. Rather, TLDP emphasizes changes in the maladaptive behavior patterns (character structure) that are presumed to underlie the patient's presenting difficulties. In addition, TLDP is not presented as a health care technology consisting of a set of techniques whose effectiveness can be evaluated apart from the practitioner employing them and the patient to whom they are applied (Butler & Strupp, 1986). Instead, TLDP should be viewed as a perspective, a way of thinking about patients and psychotherapy that is coherent and has direct implications for therapists' actions.

General Principles and Strategies of TLDP

The principles and strategies that comprise TLDP have been described comprehensively elsewhere (Strupp & Binder, 1984). What follows is a brief overview of important TLDP assumptions and concepts that will be necessary for an understanding of how affect is viewed theoretically and technically. For TLDP, psychotherapy is basically a set of interpersonal transactions. Thus, any full understanding of the therapeutic process, for either scientific or clinical objectives, requires an appreciation of the interpersonal context within which the phenomena occur. This characterization of psychotherapy articulates well with those theoretical perspectives that regard human personality as fundamentally an interpersonal construct (Sullivan, 1953). In this respect, human beings are considered interpersonal beings, conceived, reared, and living their lives in the context of interpersonal relationships (Kelley et al., 1983). There are several crucial derivatives of this perspective. First is the recognition that the most important realm of meaning for people, what is *most* meaningful to them, are interpersonal relationships; how they see others, how others see them, which influences how they see themselves. Thus, any given event or experience, including emotion, acquires or fails to acquire significance primarily in terms of the meaning attributed to the event or experience.

This meaning, in turn, is most productively understood in interpersonal terms.

Psychological problems are, therefore, best understood as occurring within an interpersonal matrix. Symptoms such as anxiety, depression, and somatic complaints result from self-defeating attempts to manage or cope with interpersonal or social situations, "real" or imagined. These maladaptive patterns are learned, usually in childhood as a response to certain familial situations, and usually involve problems of intimacy and autonomy. Thus, early experience of deprivation, traumatic experiences, and parental attitudes of hostility, rejection, indifference, or self-absorption can cripple a person's self-esteem along with his/her ability to love and trust others. Unable to obtain sufficient satisfaction from relationships with others and lacking adequate resources (or denying their existence) to mold the environment in accordance with legitimate wishes and needs, these people frequently feel stymied and unable to "connect" with other people. Such people often have unrealistic expectations of themselves or others and develop rigid patterns of dealing with life changes. Anxiety and depression accompany the resulting, pervasive sense of helplessness, frustration, and dissatisfaction. What everyone learns early in life is to avoid, as far as possible, experiences that reinstate painful affects aroused by memories (as well as misconstructions) of earlier experiences. If this means avoiding or otherwise restricting intimacy in interpersonal relationships, that is the price that will have to be paid. The maladaptive patterns that emerge in this push toward and pull away from close relations with other people can be seen as serving a defensive and self-protective function by shielding the person (however ineffectively) from the experience of painful affects, such as anxiety. Psychotherapy, within the model prescribed by TLDP, is fundamentally addressed to these rigid, self-defeating patterns of living, rather than simply to the symptoms that arise from these patterns.

In TLDP the therapeutic relationship is viewed as an important interpersonal relationship for the patient. That is, in therapy the patient confronts a relationship with a potential significant other, the therapist. Like other important relationships, the therapeutic relationship has certain parameters (boundaries, limits, and so forth) and serves certain needs for the participants. The patient, however, is someone who has a history of difficulty achieving satisfaction of his/her needs from existing significant relationships and so, has "unsuccessful" experiences with such relationships. Thus, when the patient enters therapy with the goal (or need) of improving functioning or alleviating suffering, he/she experiences essentially the same form of impediments to the success of *this* relationship (i.e., a successful therapy). As a result, the impediments or resistances to the therapeutic work on the part of patients are seen as manifestations of their difficulties in establishing a meaningful, collaborative, and successful relationship with the therapist and are not fundamentally different from problems establishing satisfying relationships outside therapy. The structure and purpose of the therapeutic contract inherently implies that one person (the patient) share, in a meaningful way, his/her most intimate thoughts, feelings, and experiences with another person (the therapist) who does not reciprocate with the sharing of the intimate details of his/her own life. The therapeutic situation, therefore, provides a unique social contract in which the "usual" rules of creating and maintaining an intimate relationship do not apply. The result is an interpersonal situation that places great demands on the patient's abilities to establish high levels of trust and openness. Thus, the therapeutic situation itself serves to cast the patient's difficulties with intimacy in bas-relief, making it an ideal structure for eliciting and observing issues of autonomy and intimacy.

TLDP and the Cyclical Maladaptive Pattern

The interpersonal problems described above can be more specifically delineated with the TLDP concept of "dynamic focus." Schacht, Binder, and Strupp (1984) created an explicit model of the dynamic focus, now called Cyclical Maladaptive Pattern (CMP). This is a working model of a central or salient pattern of interpersonal roles in which patients unconsciously cast themselves and others, and the resulting maladaptive interaction sequences, self-defeating expectations, and negative self-appraisals (for a complete description of the CMP procedure and rationale see Schacht et al., 1984). The CMP procedure involves the creation of a *narrative* that describes cyclical, maladaptive patterns in a consistent and coherent manner. The narrative idea is based on the assumption that the primary psychological mode of construing life experience is narration: the telling of a story to oneself and others (cf. Spence, 1982). In a story, experiences and actions become sequentially organized into more or less predictable patterns of situational feeling, perceiving, wishing, anticipating, and acting. Such stories render our lives comprehensible, but when the patterns lead to problems in living, they become the subject matter of psychotherapy.

The CMP takes the form of a prototypic or schematic interpersonal narrative which describes human *actions* embedded in a context of *interpersonal transactions* that are organized in *cyclical psychodynamic patterns*. These patterns, in turn, are a recurrent source of problems in living. The emphasis on action reflects a perspective that people are active agents in their respective scenarios, rather than passive victims of situations, illnesses, or impulses. Interpersonal transactions, then, define the meaningful context of these actions. That is, the actions in question are important because they refer to actions and reactions of the patient and significant others. These transactions are then organized into cyclical patterns reflecting the rigidity, chronic repetitiveness, and self-perpetuating nature of neurotic and characterological problems (cf. Wachtel, 1982). Finally, the cyclical patterns are viewed as recurrent. As such, they are relevant historically, play a crucial role in relationships with current significant others, and may be enacted within the therapeutic relationship (Butler & Binder, 1987).

The structure of the CMP narrative consists of four categories of actions that presuppose a framework of interrelations between the categories that are cyclical in nature. The four categories are as follows:

Acts of Self. These refer to actions of the self toward other people. The emphasis here is on what the patient actually does to, for, with, without, and in spite of another person. These actions can be overt, public ones ("I yelled at her"; "I told him to get out"; "I tried to help them"; "When I'm depressed, I withdraw"; etc.), or the actions can be private, internal ones ("I've always hated my mother"; "I just ignore her"; "I never tell him how I'm really feeling," etc.).

Expectations of Others' Reactions. This category refers to the imagined reactions of others to one's own actions. What the person expects of others is assumed to influence how he/she interprets the actions of others. It is further assumed that others' actions are systematically *misinterpreted* according to *preconceived sets.* This category attempts to describe these preconceived sets by eliciting the patient's wishes, fears, and fantasies with respect to others' reactions (e.g., "No matter what I do, he would never like me"; "If I ask her out she would only laugh at me," etc.).

Acts of Others toward Self. These are observed acts of others that are viewed as occurring in specific relation to the acts of self. These are often actions of others that appear to be evoked by the patient's own actions. As with the acts of self, acts of others may be public or private actions (e.g., "When I asked for the money, he thought I was lazy"). At this point it is important to emphasize the necessity of understanding the CMP as involving actions. If a patient reports, "When I try to talk with her about my feelings, she gets uncomfortable," the question should be, "How do you know she's uncomfortable? What does she *do*?" This clarification is important for understanding what information about the other person is perceived and interpreted by the patient as uncomfortable, angry, bored, disappointed, and so forth. It is the selective attention involved in what is perceived and the particular interpretation (or misinterpretation) of others' actions that reflects the patient's preconceived sets for construing social reality.

Acts of Self toward Self (Introject). This category of actions refers to how one treats oneself (self-controlling, self-punishing, self-congratulating, self-destroying, etc.). These actions are articulated in specific relation to the acts of self, expectations of others, and acts of others. The action notion embedded in this view of a patient's introject is an important component of the overall emphasis on the patient's active role in the cyclical pattern. Thus, if a patient says, "When she left me, I got depressed," the follow-up attempts to clarify what the patient *does* to himself to make him/herself depressed (e.g., "I tell myself I'm no good to anyone"; "I'm just unlovable," etc.).

The information from these four categories can be arranged into a narrative or story that captures the essence of the prototypic, maladaptive, cyclical interpersonal pattern. To illustrate a typical cyclical maladaptive pattern, consider the following hypothetical case. Imagine a depressed and withdrawn young man whose presentation is very helpless and passive. He indicates that he acts very shy around people, especially women. He does not say much and rarely makes eye contact. He states that he never gets angry with anyone. If someone offers to arrange a date or invites him to a social engagement, he always turns it down because it would undoubtedly be a disaster. This patient wishes that someone would see the loneliness and pain behind his shy presentation and convince him that he is wanted and special. He expects, however, that almost any effort on his part to draw attention to himself or assert himself is doomed to failure, because people will see his flaws and reject him. Furthermore, he observes that people in fact do seem to reject him. They may try to engage him, tell him to "loosen up, have a good time," but inevitably sooner or later they quit trying and don't come around any more. Most of the time people seem to ignore him or not even notice him.

The patient interprets these reactions, not as reasonable responses to his passivity, but as confirmation that he is worthless and flawed. He can only be a disappointment to anyone who tries to help. He berates himself for even hoping for a relationship and angrily tries to suppress desires for intimate relationships.

Thus, the cycle is complete. By seeing himself as a victim of his flaws in a world that refuses to care, he is locked in a maladaptive pattern from which there is no escape. This patient's passivity pulls for responses from other people that confirm his reasons for acting so passive and withdrawn.

Although patients are typically unaware of these patterns, they implicitly believe that the outcomes of such patterns are inevitable (Strupp & Binder, 1984). As the therapeutic transference evolves, it is these patterns that will be enacted with the therapist. The therapist's task, then, consists of identifying the CMP(s) as these evolve in the therapeutic relationship and helping the patient to understand, rather than act out, the problematic interpersonal scenarios. Therapeutic change is thus hypothesized to occur as a result of the patient's developing an *awareness* of his/her self-defeating patterns and the *experience* of a different outcome within the therapeutic relationship itself. In order to achieve this type of "corrective emotional experience" (cf. Alexander & French, 1946; Marmor, 1986), the therapist uses the role of participant observer, both to participate, to a limited extent, in the patient's problematic patterns and to reflect upon and restrict enactment of the unrealistic scenario. This effort will help the patient modify and correct the assumptions that underlie the CMP. If such ameliorative efforts are not taken, the therapist runs the risk of re-enacting the patient's "typical" scenario, which merely serves to confirm, in the eyes of the patient, the validity of his/her perceptions.

In the next two sections, we will focus on recent developments in the conceptualization of affect from the perspectives of modern psychodynamic theory and interpersonal theory, which have greatly influenced the manner in which affect is viewed in TLDP. We will then outline specifically the way in which affective experiences are represented in the CMP and present some examples of how these are handled technically.

THEORETICAL INFLUENCES

The Role of Affect in Modern Psychodynamic Theory

Much of the controversy in modern writings over the role of affect in dynamic psychotherapy can be traced to Freud's tendency to conceptualize affect using quasibiological metaphors. Freud's writings convey a view of affect as a biological quantity or entity that more or less "happens" to a person. Sulloway (1983) makes this clear when he describes Freud's "fundamental hypothesis of a displaceable 'quota of affect' undergoing 'discharge' and obeying the laws of psychic 'constancy'" (p. 91). And later, he describes Freud's theory of somatic conversion as a result of "accumulation of a traumatic and unabreacted quota of affect within the psyche" (Sulloway, 1983, p. 106). Consistent with this view of affect as a "thing" or quantity of energy, feelings are commonly talked about as being "mixed," "pent-up," "let out," or "held in." Affect becomes something to be controlled, discharged, reversed, or repressed.

As with concepts such as "instincts" and "libidinal impulses," Freud's uses of this metaphorical language in describing affect was intended to emphasize the universality of certain needs and experiences that are, or seem to be, biologically based. As psychoanalytic theory has continued to evolve since Freud, the utility of this biological metaphor has been strongly debated. This debate is beyond the scope of this chapter (see Eagle, 1984, for an interesting and thorough examination of these issues). What is important here is our general allegiance toward those who would minimize the use of the biological metaphors of fundamentally psychological phenomena (cf. Parisi, 1987). Consequently, for purposes of psychotherapy,[1] we have been influenced by Schafer's (1976) proposal to render affect or emotion as actions or modes of action. From this perspective, theoretical discussions of an affect (emotion or feeling) are discouraged in favor an "emotion-action or doing an action in an emotion-mode" (p. 271). Schafer proposes that emotion be considered "one of the things people do or one of the ways in which they do things" (p. 271). A full justification of this point of view is beyond the scope of this chapter. The reader is referred to Schafer's lucid work for a complete presentation of the utility of an "action language" for psychotherapy.

This conceptualization of emotion in action terms articulates particularly well with our overall emphasis on patients as active agents who contribute to and help sustain cyclical maladaptive patterns. And there are further implications of this perspective that are relevant to our view of affective experience in psychotherapy. Psychotherapy, for instance, does not address itself to "aggression" or its variations of anger, hostility or hate. Rather one is "acting in a hostile manner" or "acting angrily." As people and therapists, we *infer* the state of aggression, in ourselves and patients, from what we observe ourselves and our patients doing. Such inference involves perceptions of tensing muscles, clenching teeth, hitting, yelling, thinking of attack, saying one is angry, imagining acts of destruction, and so on. Such actions can be determined for other feelings, from "feeling guilty" to "feeling depressed." The latter Schafer describes as "simultaneously acting angrily, fearfully, self-punitively, even self-protectively or lovingly" (p. 349). In this sense, depression, like other affects, is not something one has or something that has happened to one, but something one does.

One important effect of such a view of emotions is that they are not cast as a special kind of human experience (internal energy or force), requiring special therapeutic handling. Rather affect is simply one type of action that can emerge as a problem for the person. Furthermore, as with all actions considered within a dynamic perspective, the action is considered to have meaning, to fit into the context of a particular patient's life in a way that can be comprehended.

The Role of Affect in Interpersonal Theory

Interpersonal theory readily offers a satisfactory approach to conceptualize the meaning of particular affective experiences for a given individual (cf. Butler & Strupp, 1986). This follows from the assumption in interpersonal theory that *"the most important class of situations for human behavior is that of other persons, in contrast to impersonal situations"* (Kiesler, 1982, p. 9, italics in original). Thus, if affects are to be defined for psychotherapy as a type of patient action, then the nature of these actions must be understood within the interpersonal context in which they emerge as problems. In therapeutic settings, affects gain attention because of some problem associated with their experience or expression. How people experience a given emotion depends, in this view, on perceptions of the interpersonal implications and consequences of experiencing and/or expressing that emotion. These perceptions can be based on misinterpretations or otherwise faulty perceptions, and the subsequent meaning(s) attributed to the affects is theorized to have critical implications for a person's self-image. Consistent with our view of psychological problems, unrealistic and uniformly negative interpretations of the interpersonal consequences of emotional material would be expected to contribute to psychological distress. In this sense, the problem is not the passive experience of certain emotions, but the distorted, maladaptive *meaning(s)* attributed to particular affective situations by the individual and his/her significant others.

This interpersonal emphasis has other relevant implications for a theoretical understanding of affect and psychotherapy. Defined in interpersonal terms, a patient's experience of emotion is seen as an integral component of that person's *interpersonal transactions*. As Kiesler (1982) has noted in his "Interpersonal Manifesto," such transactions reflect a reality of circular, rather than linear, causality; a bidirectional, simultaneous, mutual influence where the effect influences or alters the cause. In line with this view, affect is seen in terms of actions on the part of patients that have particular interpersonal consequences, implications, and meanings that serve to sustain cyclical patterns. Theoretically and practically, this view of affect is more coherent than a conception of problematic emotions that emerge from "within" the individual, and that press for expression in the environment causing distress, tension, and interpersonal problems. The vehicle for human transactions is communication, that involves messages on both linguistic and nonverbal channels. Often what we speak of as "affect" or emotion are those messages sent and received via nonverbal (and paraverbal) channels.

The problems addressed by psychotherapy, while couched in the language of symptoms and affective experiences (e.g., anxiety or depression), are best conceptualized by the psychotherapist as "problems in living" (Butler & Strupp, 1986; Kiesler, 1982; Strupp & Binder, 1984). These problems in living emerge in the recurrent transactions of a person with others, especially significant others, in his life. Problems in living have been defined by Kiesler (1982) as disordered, inappropriate, or inadequate interpersonal communications. These disordered communications result from the person neither attending to nor correcting self-defeating aspects of his/her communications to others. From this perspective, affect must be considered within the larger context of *how a person is in the world*; the integrated affective and cognitive processes that constitute that person's "style." Therefore, a particular affective experience (which might be described, for instance, with terms such as emotional, emotionless, anger, hostility, sadness, depression, etc.) is important to a psychotherapist because it is part of an integrated constellation of psychological processes that comprise the patient's interpersonal style. The interpersonal perspective views a person with psychological problems as having a "rigid" style of interacting with others such that the patient lacks the flexibility to respond appropriately to various interpersonal situations by drawing on a broad range of possible actions or reactions.

A very powerful notion, central to interpersonal theory and based on Sullivan's (1953) "theorem of reciprocal emotion," entails the assertion that all human transactions (including psychotherapy) obey certain "laws" specified by a reciprocal–circular causal model of interactions, as opposed, for instance, to Freud's unidirectional, predetermined, and intrapsychic linear model. Thus, the constricted, inflexible style of the patient does not simply occur in a vacuum, but emerges in interaction with the therapist. The reciprocal–circular model of interpersonal theory predicts that the therapist's response to the patient's style will be an important component of the resulting interaction. Constricted actions on the part of patients tend to "pull" for constricted reactions on the part of the therapist. For example, if the patient's style involves a very depressed and helpless stance, the natural "pull" may be for the therapist to want to "do something" to help, to cheer the patient up or to try valiantly to solve the current dilemma. The therapist's willingness to treat the patient as a competent, independent adult is overridden, limited, or constricted by the pull to treat the patient as dependent and incompetent.

Interpersonal theorists usually conceptualize such a "pull" as being *evoked* by the patient's behavior. A kind of interpersonal or social "pressure" develops for the therapist to provide the *complementary* response to the patient's style. The locus of such complementary communication is usually considered to be predominantly the nonverbal, emotional component of the communication between interactants (Kiesler, 1982). Complementary responses on the part of the therapist lead to a repetition of the patient's original actions, since they are interpreted as confirmation that such actions are necessary. This circular model of causation of psychological problems has led to a reconceptualization of Freud's ideas of transference and countertransference. No longer viewed as intrapsychic, self-generated behavior, transference and countertransference are viewed as occurring in a two-way phenomenological field (Chrzanowski, 1973). This position necessitates a revised concept of countertransference that goes beyond the traditional notion of the therapist's unique, intrapsychic conflicts to include the reasonable and socially expected responses to the patient's transference manifestation or interpersonal style. Indeed, that the patient experiences, and has come to expect, certain negative reactions ubiquitously throughout his/her interpersonal environment, is an essential assumption underlying the interpersonal view of neurotic and characterological problems.

Assessment/diagnostic procedures and treatments based on these principles have been devised by a number of interpersonal theorists (Benjamin, 1974, 1982, 1987; Kiesler, 1986; Wiggins, 1982).

Kiesler (1986) has summarized the fundamental assumption underlying all interpersonal intervention, namely that the patient's maladaptive transaction cycle must be disrupted. To do this, the therapist must respond to the patient's evoking style in a manner that is markedly different from that of others in the patient's life. "That is, the therapist must respond to the patient with something other than complementary responses" (p. 13). To do otherwise runs the risk of confirming or reinforcing the patient's maladaptive style. The therapist's next task is then to "metacommunicate" with the patient about the patient's evoking style and its self-defeating consequences both with the therapist and with significant others.

TLDP PERSPECTIVE ON AFFECTIVE EXPERIENCE

Affect and the Cyclical Maladaptive Pattern

TLDP integrates the views of affect outlined above by defining affect in terms of actions that comprise the person's style of interacting with other people. It is this style that tends to evoke a constricted range of responses from significant others, including the therapist, and thus serves to maintain the maladaptive patterns. Like other interpersonally relevant actions, problematic affects can be described, using the CMP procedure, as contributing to and sustaining a patient's maladaptive patterns.

Acts of Self. Here the patient's characteristic mode of handling (expression/nonexpression) of affective experience is addressed. The focus is on precise descriptions of what the patient *does vis-à-vis* a significant other in situations where emotion (love, sadness, anger, fear, etc.) is problematic. Does the patient inhibit expression totally? Is there excessive or inappropriate expression? Is there passive expression (e.g., passive aggression)? Whatever the patient's typical style of handling emotional experience, he/she will *do* the same things when emotions are experienced in the presence of the therapist.

Expectations of Others. A patient's particular mode of expression/ nonexpression will be mediated by expectations of the reactions of others. Will others find the patient's expression of emotion repulsive? Will expression of some emotions such as sadness or love be seen as weakness and ridiculed by others? Are others so hostile that the only "safe" response is to strike first? Expectations of such negative evaluations of others can be seen as the patient's rationale for adopting the preferred style.

Acts of Others. As outlined above, the significant other's response is "pulled for" by the patient's evoking style. However, rather than seeing this response as elicited by the patient's own style, he/she interprets these actions according to the preconceived sets that comprise the patient's expectations.

Introject. How the patient responds to the perceived consequences of an emotionally charged interpersonal scenario is seen as a critical link in the maintenance of the patient's style. For the CMP, this response involves the patient's treatment of himself. Thus, the patient may respond to a given scenario with self-disgust or self-loathing, thereby setting the stage for aggressive or withdrawn acts of self. Another characteristic way in which patients may respond to affective situations is by attempting to inhibit all affective experience and/or expression. These efforts at self-inhibition are intended to forestall further painful experiences by, for example, vowing (again) to never show emotion. Another possibility is for patients to ignore their own experience and deny any affective response. Such responses are seen as reinforcing the maladaptive pattern by directly influencing the acts of self, thus completing the cycle.

Technical Considerations

We began this chapter by defining TLDP as a perspective or way of thinking about psychotherapy and psychopathology, rather than a set of "techniques." Nevertheless, the TLDP model involves technical considerations that are derived from the theoretical foundation of TLDP. We prefer to stay away from specific descriptions of "techniques," which often reflect a particular theorist's personality style, in favor of describing general therapeutic strategies. These strategies are derived from the TLDP model, but the particular manner in which these strategies are implemented will depend on the personality and preferences of the particular therapist. Despite the individual styles of different therapists, the basic strategies of TLDP can be clearly stated and adherence to the model can be measured (Butler, Strupp, & Lane, 1987).

As already noted, the primary responsibility of the TLDP therapist is to point out, rather than act out the patient's maladaptive scenarios. Stated differently, the therapist must minimize negative complementarity when interacting with patients and metacommunicate to the patient about the nature of their interaction. While it is impossible for the therapist to avoid completely being drawn into the problematic interactions, he/she should be expected to recognize the emergence of such problems as they are occurring (or soon thereafter), to avoid the "pull" to provide the expected response, and instead, to relate these immediate events to the CMP. This activity requires intensive scrutiny of the moment-by-moment process of the therapeutic interaction. This process, in turn, is best facilitated by a sustained focus on what the patient is feeling in the here and now, the quality of the experience, and the meaning of the experience with respect to the patient's actions and fantasies about the therapist's and other's reactions. An attitude of nondefensive, empathic curiosity on the part of the therapist regarding the details of the patient's moment-by-moment experience is often the best way to avoid negative complementarity, which can be so destructive to the therapeutic work.

PATIENTS WITH PROBLEMS IN EMOTIONAL EXPRESSION

In order to illustrate the principles and strategies outlined above, we will now present vignettes from two cases. These cases have been selected as examples of two difficult types of affective problems therapists routinely encounter in their practice, the hostile or overly angry patient and the patient whose affect is particularly inaccessible.

The Hostile Patient

Patients who are overtly hostile and angry may represent one of the most difficult affective situations for therapists to handle, especially when the hostility is directed toward the therapist. Indeed, as previously described, one impetus for the creation of TLDP was our observation (Strupp, 1980d) that once hostility emerged in the relationship with the therapist, the potential for a positive outcome was drastically reduced. Overly aggressive and angry actions on the part of patients create a situation in which the therapist must resist an extremely strong pull to provide socially expected responses such as withdrawal or counterattack. Rather than viewing such anger as the result of acquired maladaptive patterns, the natural human reaction is to "take it personally." By doing so, however, the therapist becomes embroiled in the sequence of interpersonal transactions which sustain the patient's vicious cycle.

The Vignette. The patient is a 26-year-old divorced white woman who reported to our research clinic complaining of being depressed, anxious, and "hyper," which meant to her "angry." She indicated that her major problem is that others in her life, especially her mother and sisters, tell her she has a "negative attitude," which meant, at least in part, that she gets "defensive" or "obstinate" with people. She also said that she is lonely and has few heterosexual contacts since her divorce about a year ago. At intake she noted that, like her husband, many men are irresponsible and cannot be trusted or counted on.

By the fourth session, her therapist, a male clinical psychologist on staff at the Vanderbilt Center for Psychotherapy Research, had developed the following CMP:

Acts of Self. This patient's interpersonal stance involves the presentation of herself as tough, defiant, and hateful. She describes herself as having a "negative attitude," which means interpersonally that she is hostile and on the offensive, verbally and, sometimes, physically. Her verbal hostility involves being confrontative, challenging, and sarcastic. If she is not on the offensive, then she is vulnerable. She states that she does not "mean to be hateful," but her overriding concern is to be sure not to show any vulnerability.

Expectations of Others. She expects people to see her as a burden and reject her. She sees the world primarily as a source of rejection. The pain of these rejections is increased if it is accompanied by the humiliation of having exposed any vulnerability. She clearly expects people to respond to any show of vulnerability in a callous, judgmental, and rejecting way.

Acts of Others. She observes that significant others (especially her former husband, mother, and sisters) are critical and abusive. They have all lied to her, and "they take and give nothing in return." She also observes that people "misunderstand" her, that she wants to be liked. She is aware that, occasionally, people have been badly hurt by her aggressive actions (verbal and physical).

Introject. She takes these observations as confirmation of two beliefs. The first is that significant others will inevitably hurt her if she lets them. She must inhibit herself by denying any vulnerabilities (pain, sadness, tenderness, caring, etc.) to avoid being abused by others. She berates herself for any show of vulnerability; when she has not been tough, then she has been weak. Secondly, she despises herself. She has a "bad attitude" and hurts people, confirming that others are probably right, she *should* be rejected. In this conflict, she retreats from the world into a hostile, guarded shell, secretly hoping someone will understand her.

The following vignette is drawn from the sixth session. The therapist had canceled the previous week's session due to illness. The current meeting takes place at the regular time the following week. The session begins with the patient's recounting how, upon learning that the session was canceled the previous week, decided to go drinking with a girl friend that afternoon. Although the evening started out "fine," she became so drunk that she could not remember 2 hours. Exploration reveals that she has not been inebriated to this extent for a long time. The therapist asks if there might be any connection with his canceling the session and her getting drunk. Her denial, though not unexpected, prompts the therapist to explore the abruptness and emphasis with which she denies any connection. At one point she mumbles, "I'm not supposed to let you affect me that way." She immediately changes the subject to discuss some goldfish she bought. After a few moments, the therapist interjects:

THERAPIST: I feel like I'm behind.
PATIENT: Behind what?

T: Behind you. We got to a point a minute ago where you said, "Listen fella, you aren't going to hurt me, you know, there's no way you're going to get to a place where you matter enough that it's going to make any difference in my life . . ."

P: I don't mean it hateful, I'm just saying I'm not gonna let myself get so involved in you that I'm gonna get upset when you cancel an appointment, you know? People do it every day.

T: OK, well, then you went on and started talking about the goldfish and about . . .

P: I changed the subject.

T: How come you changed the subject then?

P: I don't know. I guess I thought you were gonna start in on me again, which you're getting ready to do now.

T: Start in on you?

P: Mm-hm.

T: You're smiling.

P: I'm just being a bitch today, I guess.

T: You feel like you're being a bitch now . . . giving me a hard time?

P: Why not? I hadn't gave you a hard time yet . . . Not that I won't.

T: Am I giving you a hard time?

P: Yeah, I don't think you're really trying to, you're just . . .

T: What am I trying to do?

P: I don't know, you're just digging and prying. Giving me a hard time, acting like my husband.

T: Yeah?

P: Repeating yourself over and over again. (*pause*) It's what he does. If he don't get what he wants, he repeats hisself.

T: When he finally gets it, what happens?

P: He shuts up.

T: He leaves you alone?

P: Right.

T: Mm.

P: Mm. (*mocking*) (*long pause*)

[*Comment*: Here the therapist has become embroiled in one of the patient's scenarios. The patient has interpreted the therapist's attempts at exploration as "digging and prying," and her aggressive, challenging, and otherwise provocative stance has culminated in an invitation to respond with negative complementarity as does her husband, by angrily submitting or possibly by counterattacking, perhaps by "pulling rank," implying, for instance, "I am the therapist and we will talk about these things, etc." The therapist's task here is to extricate himself from the scenario without either withdrawing or counterattacking.]

T: OK. (*chuckle*) Well, I don't know what to do now, so (*laugh*) what do you want to do?

P (*laughs*): I don't know.

T: Your husband harps on stuff?

P: Yeah. It's like, you know, you might as well not talk. Nothing you say makes any difference anyway, so why bother? I've acquired that over the years, you know. It's just when somebody keeps pressing something, it pisses me off. And I told you already twice how I felt, and you kept saying, "No, there's something more."

T: Well, what do you think we got to? Anything?

P: That I wasn't gonna let you affect me.

[*Comment*: Here the mood has been lightened somewhat and, most importantly, the therapist has declined to play out the scenario. In the face of her provocations, he has not attacked her but neither has he withdrawn in angry submission. As the session progresses, the patient becomes much less aggressive and more cooperative in the interaction. Exploration reveals that she is not going to become so involved in the therapy that she might be hurt. Later in the same session, the therapists attempts to relate what has happened to the CMP.]

T: OK, let me tell you how I'm seeing this.

P: OK.

T: It seems like you've been hurt a lot, an awful lot by people who . . .

P: I've trusted.

T: . . . you've . . . you trusted.

P: Yeah.

T: So when you say to me, "I'm not going to let you hurt me," part of what I hear is, "I'm not going to trust you so . . ."

P: So you can't hurt me.

T: So, part of what it seems is that there's like a crust around you that you've built up to keep people at a safe distance.

P: Well, it became necessary.

T: I don't doubt it, just in terms of what you've told me so far. So when I talk about getting inside that crust . . .

P: Well, if I let you in that crust, then I will feel closer to you and I may begin to care about what you think. I don't want to get emotional about what you think.

T: OK, because that'll hurt.

P: 'Cause that'll hurt, right.

T: But the problem is that what I get are messages from outside here, that there's sadness and loneliness on the inside there.

P: Yeah, I won't deny that, and mad too, you know? All kinds of f---g nasty things.

[*Comment*: Here the patient's "attitude problem" is referred to metaphorically as a "crust," which has both harsh connotations as well as protective ones. By objectifying her style in this way, it (the style) becomes an object which can be discussed and is somehow separate from her (implying that it can be discarded, changed, etc.). Later the therapist continues . . .]

T: . . . if someone [a man] does come along who's interested in you or something, then what are they going to see?

P: I don't know.

T: . . . maybe what they see is the chip on your shoulder or the crust or the negative attitude, and before anybody get's a chance to get very far they're gone. So I guess the thing now is, based on your life in the past, how are you going to be able to tell the good ones from the bad ones?

P: I don't know.

T: Or is there such a thing as somebody getting inside the crust and not hurting you? Is that even possible?

P: I doubt it, no. I've gotten to the point where I expect people to hurt me, you know?

In this vignette, the therapist was able to avoid the invitation to respond in a complementary or otherwise negative manner to the patient's evoking style. Rather than enacting the scenario, he attempted to use the patient–therapist interaction to highlight the existence and purpose of the patient's problematic style and relate this to the CMP. The patient seems to have responded as though the therapist had "passed a test" (see Weiss, 1986; Silberschatz, Fretter, & Curtis, 1986), and she gradually drops her aggressive, noncooperative stance and begins to collaborate in the therapeutic process. As she engages in this process, she begins to fill in aspects of the CMP categories for herself, as when she acknowledges that she "expects" people to hurt her.

The Intellectualizing Patient

In contrast to hostile patients, whose problems involve the overt expression of negative affect, are those patients who tend to have great difficulty experiencing or expressing *any* real affect. These patients are sometimes quite intelligent, verbally skilled, and comfortable with abstract language. The use, or overuse, of abstract thinking as a way of avoiding direct affective experience, commonly referred to as the defense mechanism of intellectualization, often creates problems for therapists. This is because, *on the surface*, the patient appears involved in "analyzing" his/her thoughts, feelings, and interpersonal relationships, while remaining affectively removed from the process. Without the spark of true affective involvement in the process of psychotherapy, the process runs the risk of simply being one more empty experience for the patient. This, of course, is an important part of the problems that these patients face.

As with the hostile patient, the therapist must guard against unwittingly responding in a complementary fashion to the patient's style. The intellectualizing style can be viewed as the patient's effort to detach him/herself from the interpersonal situation often involving a "walling off" of the self from the other person. In therapy, the pull for the therapist is to neglect the patient's emotional life by ignoring subtle signs of emotional response. Indeed, this complementary response cycle, namely the mutual avoidance of affective material, is what the patient has learned to expect from his/her social environment and is taken as implied confirmation of the belief that affect must be stifled. It is this interpersonal sequence, occurring with significant others, which contributes to a general sense of emptiness and isolation.

The therapist can avoid the pull to join the patient in this sequence by focusing on the automatic (or unconscious) strategies the patient uses to insulate him/herself and the therapist from emotional material. This involves exploration of both the way(s) in which the patient inhibits experience and expression of emotion and the expectations of the interpersonal consequences of experiencing and expressing affect (e.g., ridicule, rejection, etc.). Thus, the goals of the therapist's interventions are twofold: first to de-automatize the strategies by which the patient inhibits affect and secondly, to question the interpersonal assumptions/expectations that underlie these strategies. Although the first stages of this process often involve an increase in the patient's intellectual awareness of his/her defensive maneuvers for avoiding feelings, the therapist must be certain not to avoid affectively charged material. As this work proceeds, the patient's fear of the consequences of giving expression to his/her emotional side can give way to greater trust. As this trust increases, the patient may eventually risk the experience of affect in the therapeutic situation. At this point, the therapist must be careful to acknowledge and tolerate the fact of the expression. To do otherwise runs the risk of confirming the patient's old expectations that such expression is dangerous, wrong, and so on.

The Vignette. The patient is an intelligent and articulate, 38-year-old married man. He is self-employed as a free-lance writer and works alone most of the time. His presenting complaint is a sense of isolation and an inability to have "deep" and "meaningful" interpersonal relationships. He describes himself as a "workaholic" who has no friends and feels close to no one, including his wife and child. The relationship with his wife is described as a "sham," because he believes that there is "a lot" that he and his wife do not know about each other. His goal is "honesty" in the marital relationship.

The following vignette is taken from the seventh hour with a male clinical psychologist on staff at the Center for Psychotherapy Research. At this point, the patient has been exploring his relationship with his father, whom he describes as withdrawn and critical.

T: The way you describe your father . . . is . . . that he is prototypic of the other person [who] doesn't want to be bothered by your feelings, whatever they are, and maybe he doesn't even like you. Look, you're a little kid growing up and here you have this imposing figure, your father. And you're bursting with all kinds of things that you want to say and tell, and reactions you want from your father, and he doesn't seem to want to listen or give anything. The obvious conclusion is he doesn't want to be bothered with you, doesn't like you, you're not worth bothering him. (*pause*) And, you know, what I'm suggesting is more than just speculation, because, look what you experienced with me today. That I'm reserved, and that must mean I don't want to be bothered by your feelings, and maybe I don't even like you.

P: Yeah, I'd go along with that. You know, since the last time we talked, I had been trying for 2 weeks to just remember my childhood. I'd sit back and just try to remember anything about my childhood. I'd think back to places that we had lived, you know, houses I could remember, just trying to think what was my father like. What kind of relationship did I have with him. And I couldn't come up with anything. I must've done this, uh, ten times since the last time we met. I just couldn't come up with anything. . . . Yesterday, I took a nap, and I had a—it wasn't really a dream exactly, but I remembered my fifth-grade teacher. It was as if I was just crying and crying, remembering this guy, because he was such an opposite from what my father was. He seemed so human, so approachable, uh, he seemed to take such a concern with me. Uh, and, uh, I was just remembering him, his face, and it was just as if I was crying and crying. I wasn't really crying 'cause I was asleep, but when I woke up from that and remembered it, I realized that I had finally remembered something from my childhood that was really significant to me, namely this other man who, uh, who really did seem to care about me more than my f-fa-fa-father did.

T: I noticed you—you stuttered there where your father's—well, not your father's name, but—the word.

P: Mm-hm.

T: Is that meaningful?

P: I think it means that for some reason, uh, saying that this man, my fifth-grade teacher cared more about me than my father did was something that I shouldn't have been saying. And therefore I had to struggle to say it, uh, because it seems like a terrible thing to say.

T: You felt that it was an indictment of your father that's not fair to make?

P: Not that it wasn't fair, necessarily. But just that it seemed like a bad thing to say, uh, not a nice thing to say, somehow, about him whether it was fair or not.

T: In the dream, you said you were crying and crying. Do you remember the feeling associated with the crying?

P: Yes, it was almost a feeling of—of having lost someone that you love. I just kept seeing his face, and he was like talking, even though I couldn't hear what he was saying. He just had such a friendly, warm, approachable, uh, demeanor, it was like I was just longing to be with him.

T: So it's like a profound sadness.

P: Even grief would even more be it, because it was like (*sigh*), um, (*sigh*) I knew that this was just an image of this man and therefore, it was just an image of something that I had for a brief time and then—and then I lost it.

T: As you're recalling it now, does it stir up any feelings now?

[*Comment*: The therapist has picked up on the significant "clue" of feelings presented by the patient when he notes the stuttering. The patient follows up on this in his usual intellectual way, so the therapist gently pushes for more expression of feeling by asking what feelings are associated with the crying in the dream. The patient's answer, while revealing, is intellectualized. Therefore, the therapist helps him to label the feeling (i.e., sadness). Gradually, the therapist brings the feeling (or the potential for feeling) into the here and now of the therapy session.]

P: Yeah, somewhat the feeling of wishing that I could have a relationship like that and also be a person like that, or just have that quality. I think in some ways he personifies to me, uh what is lacking in my life.

[*Comment*: The patient's response to inquiries regarding immediate affect is to deflect the conversation to a more abstract topic. The therapist attempts to bring the focus back to feelings.]

T: Is there any of the sadness right now?

P: Yeah, though just when I started describing it, I lost a bit of it. If I think about it, if I just think about his face as I was imagining it, uh, I can bring up that feeling . . . of longing, and uh, grieving, that I sort of have to go back to the fifth grade to find that. And this sort of sense of—of empty years . . .

T: Even as you're feeling some of it now, you—you're—from the outside, you're very successfully keeping it well hidden inside.

[*Comment*: Here the therapist uses his own perceptions of the patient to introduce the idea that the patient is defending against the actual expression of the feelings.]

P: I'm sorry. I'm not—I'm not being real successful in getting into it.

T: Maybe, as you said, even as you start talking about it, it fades.

P: Mm-hm.

T: Which is kind of striking because, you know, typically as [people] talk about feelings, they become clearer. In the context of what we've been talking about today, I wonder if there's a part of you that feels that even as we're talking about assumptions about what you can share with other people, that as you begin to talk about feelings with, in this case, me, this part of you feels you've got to stifle them, that I won't, um, I don't want to be burdened with it.

P: I don't know if that's it or not. This feels like it's a very deep thing. It's very hard for me to stay in touch with it because of that. As you were talking, I started to get more in touch, and now as I start talking, I'm losing it again.

[*Comment*: This process, of the patient beginning to notice and report moment-by-moment experiences is very important. Although no rush of affect is in sight, the patient's ability to observe and monitor his defenses is an important first step to change.]

T: It sounds as though you can't share it. As you begin to get closer to sharing these very personal feelings with me, you've got to stifle them. It's in such contrast to that dream, where you so much want to be close and to share feelings with a man—you know—the fifth-grade teacher . . .

P: Mm-hm.

T: . . . your father and me. I mean, you have the dream a day before . . .

P: Mm-hm.

T: . . . before we're going to be together. (*pause*) I mean, it sounds like you very much want us to be closer, but the more directly we talk about it, the more the feelings fade.

P (*sigh*): Um . . . (*pause*)

T: There, by the way, is also something I think would be real important to look for in other relationships. The more you want to be closer to somebody, the more the feeling of it gets stifled. Your wife, your child, other people . . . (*long pause*)

P: All I can say is, Yeah. I, uh, feel a bit dumbstruck, you know, by the sort of strange, quirky nature of myself . . .

Conclusion

In this vignette, as in the preceding one, the therapist has attempted to deal with the patient's affective experience by attending to a few technical strategies. In both vignettes, the therapists attempted to (1) avoid the potential traps set by their patient's evoking style, (2) draw the patient's attention to the nature of this style and the manner in which it had manifested itself in the relationship with the therapist, and (3) relate it to a larger picture of the patient's problems with significant others. Although the styles of these two patients are quite different, the stance of the therapist in each case is fundamentally the same. Actually, despite the apparent differences between these patients, it is important to note that, for hostile patients, feelings other than hostility (especially more "vulnerable" feelings such as tenderness and love) are often very difficult to experience and express. The observed hostility can often be seen as a reaction against certain feelings that are associated with vulnerability. In the example of the hostile patient presented above, the angry reaction arose in the context of the suggestion that the patient might care about (be saddened by?) the canceled session. Here, the anger is part of the strategy used by the patient to inhibit other, potentially more threatening feelings. Thus, with problems reflecting both the overexpression and underexpression of affect, the therapist's tasks remain the same.

The therapist's tasks also remain fundamentally the same when considering the handling of those affective experiences that arise in response to the time-limited nature of TLDP. The significance of the *termination phase* of therapy has been particularly illuminated by the short-term psychodynamic theorists. For both the patient and therapist, the process of termination in psychotherapy stimulates conflicts around issues of separation and loss (Mann, 1973). The termination of the therapeutic relationship typically evokes memories of earlier separations and the associated painful affects, such as guilt, grief, rage, disappointment, sadness. The reality of an impending end to the therapeutic enterprise may elicit strong feelings about the therapist along with equally strong pressure to defend against the experience and expression of these feelings. Thus, in principle, the termination phase is considered merely one more context in which the patient's problematic styles for coping with affect can be observed and pointed out to the patient. Although the termination phase of TLDP has issues uniquely its own, these cannot be isolated from the concerns that have been the focus of attention throughout the treatment. The TLDP therapist strives to remain alert to the patient's reactions to the time limits of the therapy and brings these to the patient's attention as they are detected. As always, the therapist attempts to make sense of the patient's communications, including the affective component, in terms of the CMP.

Thus, rather than a distinctly different phase of therapy, the termination phase simply presents one more opportunity for the therapist to help promote the patient's understanding and self-awareness.

THEORETICAL AND RESEARCH CONSIDERATIONS

The TLDP perspective on affect outlined above carries with it certain assumptions about the nature of affective experience. Of course, a term such as "affect" covers a very large area of psychological and physiological phenomena. Indeed, emotions may be considered a relevant aspect of any conceivable human experience. Efforts to explain "affect" must, therefore, take into account intricate interactions of psychological and physiological systems occurring in a wide variety of situations and conditions. Injections of hormones or drugs or electrical stimulation of the brain can elicit emotional reactions just as being fired from one's job or meeting a dangerous animal in the forest can cause emotional responses. Given the extreme complexity and pervasiveness of affective experience, it is unlikely that adequate explanations of such experiences will be forthcoming without an appreciation of the context in which a particular emotional reaction is being considered. By disregarding the context of an emotional experience or set of experiences, one is left with a confusing array of isolated instances of emotional response. Artificially removing affective experience from meaningful contexts will most likely lead only to inconclusive disputes in the literature, such as the recent attempts to establish the "primacy" of affect or cognition (e.g., Zajonc, 1984; Lazarus, 1984).

In this chapter we have considered affect in the context of psychotherapy. When affective experience arises as an issue in this context, it presumably does so because the patient, the therapist, or both, consider it relevant to some problem in living that the patient is trying to resolve. As we have made clear, it is the particular constellation of the patient's interpersonal concerns that defines the problematic nature of specific affective experiences. As far as psychotherapy is concerned, affective experience by itself is rarely a problem. Sadness, grief, pride, guilt, jealousy, shame, joy, sexual arousal, anger, curiosity, and other affective reactions are not inherently problematic experiences. Such feelings are universal, and the simple fact of the experience is rarely cause for seeking therapy. Rather, the clinical problem arises from the manner in which these experiences tend to be interpreted. This interpretation often involves the labeling of an affective experience as "bad," "terrible," "sick," "disgusting," and so forth. When asked to extend these labels, patients will invariably relate the undesirability of affective experiences to their fantasies about others' reactions to their feelings; a kind of "if . . . then . . ." sequence of interpersonal implications. As an example, the hostile patient discussed above seemed to believe that "if I am hostile, then people will be hurt proving I deserve to be rejected" (to have or express angry feelings is to be "bad"). This interpersonal implication conflicted with her sense that "if I care about you (have tender, enjoyable feelings), then I will get hurt" (to have pleasant feeling is also "bad"). These problematic interpretations or meanings of emotional experience are always linked to interpersonal concerns.[2]

The idea of a fundamental link between affective experience and interpersonal concerns is well illustrated in Sullivan's (1953) writings on the development of personality structures in the infant. Sullivan proposed that the earliest affective experiences of the infant are tied to mixtures of two more or less undifferentiated, biological states that he called *euphoria* (equilibrium or well-being) and *tension* (need state). The need states mobilize *actions* that are capable of eliciting *responses* from significant others, usually the mother. These responses are essential for the infant's survival and serve to maintain or re-establish the infant's equilibrium. Another fundamental affective experience, anxiety, is said to be different from tension associated with the need state because it is not the result of biological needs. Instead, anxiety is *induced* in the infant through interaction with an anxious mother. This transmission of the experience of anxiety is made possible by the "empathic linkage" (p. 43), which serves both to connect the infant with the human community and to detect threats to that connection. Relief from the anxious state is experienced as "interpersonal security" (p. 42), rather than satisfaction of a need. Thus, the infant's first, rudimentary experiences of emotion are, in fact, part and parcel of the child's first interpersonal transactions. Furthermore, since these communications involve sequences of actions, responses, and reactions on the part of the infant and significant others, a circular process of interpersonal feedback and subsequent modification of actions and responses is initiated. This process represents the beginnings of the interpersonal patterns that will eventually result in the child's socialization into the human community.

From these building blocks Sullivan constructed a theory of personality development that presupposes a profound integration of affective experience and interpersonal communication. As the child matures, consistent patterns of interaction develop that will ultimately result in a relatively stable personality style. This style incorporates, monitors, manages, and communicates affective experience based on the individual's developmental history, that is, his/her history of interpersonal interactions.

By linking affective experience, personality development and interpersonal communication in this manner, we are led to the conclusion that affective experience can be conceptualized as a two-person process. A person's experience of particular affective states is inseparable from his/her perceptions, wishes, fantasies, and expectations of other people. In the therapy session, the patient's experience of affect occurs in the presence of a therapist. The patient's fantasies about the therapist's response to the emotion influences the experience of the affect. This is nicely illustrated by the intellectualizing patient, described above, when the feelings about the father/teacher diminish in the course of sharing them with the therapist, who, like his father, will not want to be bothered. Thus, in order to study the patient's affective experience in psychotherapy, one must study sets of interpersonal events (transactions) between the patient and therapist.

Our interest, as therapists and researchers, is in the observed interpersonal interactions that comprise the therapeutic process. Since the patient is impelled to re-enact cyclical maladaptive patterns with the therapist, we can observe, firsthand, the patient's affective problems. Through such observations, we can begin to establish a "catalog" of problematic affective situations that arise in psychotherapy and begin to describe and explain consistent patterns of interactions associated with various affective problems.

Such investigations will require detailed analyses of the transactions between patients and therapists. An example of a relatively new methodology, utilized at the Vanderbilt Center for Psychotherapy Research, is Lorna Smith Benjamin's (1974, 1982) Structural Analysis of Social Behavior (SASB) method. SASB is a detailed, conceptually rigorous, and empirically validated measure of moment-by-moment patient–therapist interactions, based on the circumplex model of interpersonal transactions. This model permits interpersonal behaviors to be described as the intersection of two vectors, one representing the degree of affiliation–disaffiliation and the other representing the degree of independence–interdependence (control). Among other uses, SASB permits the researcher to define operationally specific transactions as complementary and to determine whether the complementarity observed is positive or negative.

Preliminary efforts to utilize this technology (Henry, Schacht, & Strupp, 1986) have shown that, compared with poor outcome cases, good outcome cases have greater positive complementarity, less negative complementarity, and greater total complementarity. Efforts to replicate these findings are currently under way at our Center. Such findings suggest that the SASB technology, along with other measures of therapy process, may soon permit researchers both to identify key emotional transactions between the therapist and patient and describe the crucial aspects of the therapist's response. It is our expectation that such methodological advances will foster a new understanding of the role of affective experiences in psychotherapy process.

SUMMARY

We have attempted to describe the manner in which the TLDP model of psychotherapy addresses the role of affect in psychodynamic psychotherapy. Consistent with recent contributions to the psychoanalytic and inter-personal literature, TLDP does not address "affect" as an entity. Rather, a patient's experience of affect must be considered within the context of the patient's overall personality organization, the meaning of the affect *vis-à-vis* significant others, and the intended role of the other person, which in the consulting room is the therapist. Accordingly, affect is considered an action or action mode to be viewed as part of a cyclical maladaptive pattern sequence. This sequence represents the repetitive, self-sustaining nature of the patient's neurotic and characterological problems. The therapist's role is to point out rather than act out this maladaptive pattern, thereby providing both increased awareness of the patient's role in the problematic patterns as well as the experience of disconfirming the inter-personal expectations that keep the cycle in motion. Two cases, represent-ing different types of emotional difficulties are presented, that of a hostile patient and one whose emotional experience is relatively inaccessible.

Theoretically, the patient's experience of affect in psychotherapy and his/her attempts to cope with these experiences are viewed as integral to the patient's personality style. Furthermore, these characteristic ways of expressing and managing emotions are fundamentally interpersonal in nature. The view of affective experience as an interpersonal, two-person process, permits research efforts to be directed toward the delineation and description of consistent patterns of patient–therapist interactions asso-ciated with various affective problems. Such efforts may be expected to lead to greater understanding of the influence (both positive and negative) of therapists' responses.

ACKNOWLEDGMENTS

This work was supported in part by National Institute of Mental Health Research Grant MH-20369, Hans H. Strupp, principal investigator. We wish to thank Jeffrey L. Binder and Thomas E. Schacht for their helpful comments on an early draft of this chapter.

NOTES

1. We limit our argument to psychotherapy as opposed to, for instance, develop-mental or experimental considerations of affect, simply because we do not con-sider our conceptualization of affect as *necessarily* relevant to other efforts toward understanding and investigating this large area of human experience.

2. Clinically we know that successfully treated patients do not experience an absence of sadness, guilt, shame, and so on. Instead, such feelings somehow seem less important, and therefore, less troublesome. Our position holds that the

meaning of the emotional experience has changed, rather than any change in the emotion itself.

REFERENCES

Alexander, F., & French, T. M. (1947). *Psychoanalytic therapy: Principles and applications.* Ronald Press.

Anchin, J. C., & Kiesler, D. J. (1982). *Handbook of interpersonal psychotherapy.* New York: Pergamon.

Beck, A. T., Rush, A. J., Shaw, B. F., & Emery, G. (1979). *Cognitive therapy of depression.* New York: Guilford.

Benjamin, L. S. (1974). Structural Analysis of Social Behavior. *Psychological Review, 81,* 392–425.

Benjamin, L. S. (1982). Use of Structural Analysis of Social Behavior to guide intervention in therapy. In J. C. Anchin & D. J. Kiesler (Eds.), *Handbook of interpersonal psychotherapy.* New York: Pergamon Press.

Benjamin, L. S. (1987). Use of the SASB dimensional model to develop treatment plans for personality disorders. I: Narcissism. *Journal of Personality Disorders, 1*(1), 43–70.

Bergin, A. E., & Strupp, H. H. (1972). *Changing frontiers in the science of psychotherapy.* Chicago: Aldine-Atherton.

Breuer, J., & Freud, S. (1895). *Studies on hysteria.* New York: Basic Books.

Butler, S. F., & Binder, J. L. (1987). Cyclical psychodynamics and the triangle of insight: An integration. *Psychiatry, 50,* 218–231.

Butler, S. F., & Strupp, H. H. (1986). Specific and nonspecific factors in psychotherapy: A problematic paradigm for psychotherapy research. *Psychotherapy, 23,* 30–40.

Butler, S. F., Strupp, H. H., & Lane, T. W. (1987, June). *The Time-Limited Dynamic Psychotherapy Therapeutic Strategies Scale: Development of an Adherence measure.* Paper presented at a meeting of the Society for Psychotherapy Research in Ulm, West Germany.

Chrzanowski, G. (1973). Implications of interpersonal theory. In E. G. Witenberg (Ed.), *Interpersonal explorations in psychoanalysis.* New York: Basic Books.

Eagle, M. N. (1984). *Recent developments in psychoanalysis: A critical evaluation.* McGraw-Hill.

Henry, W. P., Schacht, T. E., & Strupp, H. H. (1986). Structural Analysis of Social Behavior: Application to a study of interpersonal process of differential therapeutic outcome. *Journal of Consulting and Clinical Psychology, 54,* 27–31.

Kelley, H. H., Berscheid, E., Christensen, A., Harvey, J. H., Huston, T. L., Levinger, G., McClintock, E., Peplau, L. A., & Peterson, D. R. (1983). *Close relationships.* New York: W. H. Freeman.

Kiesler, D. J. (1986). Interpersonal methods of diagnosis and treatment. *Psychiatry, 1*(4), 1–23.

Klerman, G. L., Rounsaville, B., Chevron, E., Neu, C., & Weissman, M. M. (1984). *Interpersonal psychotherapy of depression (IPT).* New York: Basic Books.

Lazarus, R. S. (1984). On the primacy of cognition. *American Psychologist, 39*(2), 124-129.

Luborsky, L. (1984). *Principles of psychoanalytic psychotherapy: A manual for supportive expressive treatment.* New York: Basic Books.

Mann, J. (1973). *Time-limited psychotherapy.* Cambridge, MA: Harvard University Press.

Marmor, J. (1986). The corrective emotional experience revisited. *International Journal of Short-Term Psychotherapy, 1,* 43-47.

Parisi, T. (1987). Why Freud failed: Some implications for neurophysiology and sociobiology. *American Psychologist, 42*(3), 235-245.

Schacht, T. E., Binder, J. L., & Strupp, H. H. (1984). The dynamic focus. In H. H. Strupp & J. L. Binder, *Psychotherapy in a new key.* New York: Basic Books.

Schafer, R. (1976). *A new language for psychoanalysis.* New Haven, CT: Yale University Press.

Silberschatz, G., Fretter, P. B., & Curtis, J. T. (1986). How do interpretations influence the process of psychotherapy? *Journal of Consulting and Clinical Psychology, 54,* 646-652.

Spence, D. P. (1982). *Historical truth and narrative truth.* New York: W. W. Norton.

Strachey, J. (1943). The nature of the therapeutic action of psychoanalysis. *International Journal of Psycho-Analysis, 15,* 117-126.

Strupp, H. H. (1967). *An introduction to Freud and modern psychoanalysis.* New York: Barron.

Strupp, H. H. (1980a). Success and failure in time-limited psychotherapy: A systematic comparison of two cases—comparison 1. *Archives of General Psychiatry, 37,* 595-603.

Strupp, H. H. (1980b). Success and failure in time-limited psychotherapy: A systematic comparison of two cases—comparison 2. *Archives of General Psychiatry, 37,* 708-716.

Strupp, H. H. (1980c). Success and failure in time-limited psychotherapy: A systematic comparison of two cases—comparison 3. *Archives of General Psychiatry, 37,* 831-841.

Strupp, H. H. (1980d). Success and failure in time-limited psychotherapy: A systematic comparison of two cases—comparison 4. *Archives of General Psychiatry, 37,* 947-954.

Strupp, H. H., & Bergin, A. E. (1969). Some empirical and conceptual bases for coordinated research in psychotherapy. *International Journal of Psychiatry, 7,* 18-90.

Strupp, H. H., & Binder, J. (1984). *Psychotherapy in a new key: A guide to Time-Limited Dynamic Psychotherapy.* New York: Basic Books.

Sullivan, H. S. (1953). *The interpersonal theory of psychiatry.* New York: W. W. Norton.

Sulloway, F. J. (1983). *Freud, biologist of the mind: Beyond the psychoanalytic legend.* New York: Basic Books.

Wachtel, P. (1982). Vicious circles: The self and the rhetoric of emerging and unfolding. *Contemporary Psychoanalysis, 18,* 259-272.

Weiss, J. (1986). Part I: Theory and clinical observations. In J. Weiss, H. Sampson,

& the Mount Zion Psychotherapy Research Group, *The psychoanalytic process: Theory, clinical observations, and empirical research*. New York: Guilford.

Wiggins, J. S. (1982). Circumplex models of interpersonal behavior in clinical psychology. In P. C. Kendall & J. K. Butcher (Eds.), *Handbook of research methods in clinical psychology*. New York: Wiley.

Zajonc, R. B. (1984). On the primacy of affect. *American Psychologist, 39*(2), 117–123.

5

Affects in Psychopathology and Psychotherapy

GEORGE SILBERSCHATZ
HAROLD SAMPSON
Mount Zion Hospital
University of California Medical Center

INTRODUCTION

This chapter examines the role of affects in psychopathology and in psychotherapy from the perspective of "control-mastery theory,"[1] a cognitively oriented psychoanalytic theory developed by Weiss (1971, 1986) and empirically tested by the Mount Zion Psychotherapy Research Group (Weiss, Sampson, & the Mount Zion Psychotherapy Research Group, 1986; for an overview of this research, see Silberschatz, Curtis, Sampson, & Weiss, in press). We will briefly describe Weiss's theory, focusing on the adaptive nature of affects. We will then discuss why affects may be inaccessible, and how such affects may be recovered in psychotherapy. In this context, we shall note how a patient's unconscious guilt may play a significant role in making his affective life inaccessible to him/her, and how overcoming this guilt may make it possible to recover his/her affects. Finally, using transcripts of a brief psychodynamic psychotherapy, we will present a case of a patient who sought treatment because of difficulty experiencing any kind of emotion and illustrate how unconscious guilt (based on certain pathogenic beliefs developed during the patient's childhood) had prevented him from having access to his emotional life.

ADAPTATION AND AFFECT

The control-mastery theory assumes that, from infancy, human mental life is regulated by efforts to adapt to reality (Weiss, 1986, 1989; see also Sampson, 1989). As part of this adaptive effort, the infant actively seeks reliable knowledge about reality, which includes him/herself, his/her interpersonal world, and the moral and ethical assumptions of his/her world (Weiss, 1989). The infant urgently needs this knowledge as a guide to behavior, and acquires it through experiences. This acquired knowledge is represented intraspsychically by beliefs—unconscious as well as conscious—about oneself and the world.

Affects are an innate part of a person's appraisal system and hence represent a central aspect of one's adaptive capacities. Affective responses may be seen as internal cues (signals) that help a person understand him/herself, relationships, and reality. Indeed, they provide crucial guides to one's overall assessment and experience of the world (i.e., is it pleasurable or frustrating, frightening or interesting, exciting or depressing).

A person's beliefs about reality (unconscious as well as conscious beliefs) ordinarily determine to a large extent one's affects. For example, a person who believes that he/she is in a dangerous situation is likely to feel anxious; a person who believes that he/she has been rejected by someone who is important is likely to feel sad; a person who believes that he/she has been unfairly criticized may feel anger. In other words, affects are ordinarily reactions to a person's appraisals of (i.e., beliefs about) one's reality; they serve as guides to potential courses of action and as motivators for action.

Emotional reactions and cognitive appraisals are typically intertwined in a person's ongoing appraisal of his/her reality. For example, a jogger confronted by a big dog running toward him may immediately feel frightened. His instantaneous affective reaction is based on a belief that the situation is potentially dangerous. The affective reaction alerts the runner and prepares him to take action. Fright may decisively shape his subsequent appraisals of the danger situation; however, his appraisal may be substantially modified by later perceptions. The jogger may, for instance, notice that the dog's tail is wagging, the dog is a golden retriever (a usually friendly breed), and the dog appears to be very playful. Because of his altered appraisal of the situation, his fear will subside.

Our conception of affect is consistent with an evolving cognitive view of emotions evident in many recent psychoanalytic contributions to affect theory that emphasize the continuity between affect and cognition (e.g., Basch, 1976; Brenner, 1974; Dahl, 1979; Emde, 1980; Lewin, 1965; Schur, 1969). Emotion is not regarded as the antithesis of thought or reason; rather, "affective reactions are part and parcel of the cognitive process" (Basch, 1976, p. 771). For example, in Dahl's (1979) model (see Chapter 6, this volume), anxiety, depression, contentment, joy (and other "me" emotions) represent an appraisal of the status of one's goals or enterprises: "Positive me" feelings convey a signal or message that important wishes are being satisfied, while "negative me" feelings indicate that wishes are not being satisfied.

One common element in these recent psychoanalytic theories is that affects are an important source of adaptive information. Many emotion theorists working outside of a psychoanalytic framework have advocated a similar view (e.g., Arnold, 1970; Greenberg & Safran, 1987; Lazarus, 1984; Leventhal, 1984; Plutchik, 1980). In their recent review paper on the role of emotions in psychotherapy, Greenberg and Safran (1989) pointed out that the distinctions that have often been made between affect and cognition are breaking down and being replaced by information-processing models that integrate cognition and emotion. They noted that affective responses are often an important aid to problem solving and that it is therefore highly adaptive for a person to be able to access disavowed (i.e., repressed) emotions:

> Organisms that ignore their own affective feedback are not well situated to behave adaptively. Acknowledging affective responses that were previously disallowed makes certain reactions and moods more understandable and acknowledging disclaimed tendencies provides new impetus for action and need satisfaction. (p. 24)

AFFECTS IN PSYCHOPATHOLOGY

According to Weiss (1986), psychopathology stems ultimately from certain beliefs that impair functioning. Weiss refers to these as *pathogenic beliefs*. Pathogenic beliefs are beliefs about oneself and the world that are inferred from experience—typically, from traumatic experiences in childhood. Pathogenic beliefs warn the person who adheres to them about the dangerous consequences of pursuing certain important goals or experiencing certain ideas, wishes, or affects. For example, a child who noticed that his mother became depressed shortly after he began school and started to develop relationships outside of the home, developed the unconscious pathogenic belief that his independence caused his mother's depression. In obedience to this belief he renounced strivings toward independence and remained emotionally dependent upon his mother.

Pathogenic beliefs may impair emotional functioning. In some instances, a pathogenic belief may make a person unable to experience certain affects. For example, a patient whose father was chronically ill throughout the patient's childhood, warded off powerful feelings of anger, sadness, and depression because he was reluctant to burden his preoccupied mother with his feelings. In other cases, pathogenic beliefs may compel a person to experience powerful affects that produce distortions of current reality and impede adaptation.

Pathogenic Beliefs and Inaccessible Affects

In general, a person may lack access to certain affects because he/she believes it would be dangerous for him/her to experience them. In certain instances, a person may believe that he/she is not entitled to virtually any affect. For example, a woman who grew up with a schizophrenic brother did not feel entitled to almost any strong feelings because she feared that such feelings would burden her beleaguered and overwhelmed parents.

It is maladaptive to be cut off from one's emotional responses because these responses provide crucial information of how one experiences and appraises important situations. Therefore, gaining access to previously inaccessible emotions can be an important step in correcting distorted (maladaptive) views of oneself and of important relationships. Weiss (1989) described a case of a patient who initially was not aware of mistreatment by his parents during his childhood. During his psychoanalysis, his first awareness of such mistreatment was becoming conscious of intense angry feelings toward both parents. This affect was followed by memories of humiliations by his mother and rejections by his father. The patient's becoming conscious of his previously repressed anger toward his parents was an important step in his recovery of key childhood memories and in his changing earlier beliefs about himself and his parents. Greenberg and Safran made a similar point in suggesting that the "evocation of emotional experience makes previously inaccessible beliefs available to consciousness" (1989, p. 24).

Pathogenic Beliefs and Dysfunctional Affects

Although emotional responses are part of a person's appraisal system, and hence crucial to adaptation, powerful affects (based on pathogenic beliefs) may in certain instances disrupt effective problem solving and impede successful adaptation. For example, a person who was ignored and disregarded by his parents in his childhood developed the belief that he was worthless, a "nothing." As an adult, he experienced the slightest instance of nonrecognition by his spouse or his boss as an unbearable insult confirming his worthlessness. He reacted by intense anger and urges toward violent attack against the person who had offended him. His anger was adaptive in the sense that it was a way of fighting back against the belief that he deserved to be disregarded; however, the rage distorted his perception of current situations, and was an inappropriate reaction to these situations. It also impaired his capacity to form a realistic judgment about useful courses of action. The solution to his problem did not lie in becoming more aware of his anger; rather it involved overcoming the underlying pathogenic belief so that he could react more appropriately and effectively to contemporary situations.

In a second example, the patient suffered from the unconscious pathogenic belief that it would be a betrayal of her mother to have a better marriage and family life than her mother. The patient's mother had ruined her marriage and family life by her constant outbursts of rage that alienated her from her husband and children. The patient, in obedience to her pathogenic belief, constantly flared up toward her husband and children, thereby spoiling her relationship to them. The solution to this patient's problem was not an increased awareness of anger or insight into its ostensible contemporary sources. Rather, the solution required that she become aware of her unconscious identification with her mother and overcome the pathogenic belief (i.e., that she should not be happier or better off than her mother) that gave rise to this identification. As the patient overcame her pathogenic belief she no longer had to be an angry person who spoiled intimate relationships as her mother had done.

HOW PREVIOUSLY INACCESSIBLE AFFECTS
BECOME CONSCIOUS IN PSYCHOTHERAPY

The patient's problems may arise from the all too ready emergence of dysfunctional affects, as just discussed, or from the inaccessibility of affects that are defended against. We shall take up here the broad issue of how a patient in psychotherapy becomes conscious of previously inaccessible affects. In doing so, we shall focus on underlying processes that determine whether an inaccessible affect may become available to the patient.

A central question for all uncovering therapies is: How do previously warded-off feelings or ideas become conscious? The control–mastery theory emphasizes that a person exerts considerable control over one's conscious and unconscious mental life, and that perceptions of danger and safety (derived from beliefs about reality) play a central role in explaining human motivation and behavior (Weiss, 1971, 1986). The theory postulates three broad principles concerning the emergence of previously repressed material: (1) a patient may *unconsciously decide* to bring previously warded-off feelings into awareness; (2) the patient's decision is based on whether he/she feels he can do so safely; (3) the patient brings previously warded-off mental contents into consciousness as part of an effort to master problems and conflicts and not to gratify infantile wishes.

Weiss (1971) identified three processes in psychotherapy that may influence a person's perception of safety or danger: external circumstances, degree of control over defenses, and the therapeutic relationship. The phenomenon of "crying at the happy ending" (Weiss, 1952, 1986) is an example of how an external change may make it safe for a person to experience previously warded-off affects. A person watching a movie of a love story may experience little emotion while the lovers quarrel, but is moved to tears at the happy ending when they are reunited. According to Weiss's explanation (1986), the moviegoer identifies unconsciously with one of the lovers. When the lovers are separated, the viewer is in danger of feeling intensely sad and consequently intensifies his/her defenses against sadness. When the lovers reunite, the moviegoer no longer has reason to feel sad. He/she unconsciously decides that it is safe to experience sadness (since it is now less of a threat) and lifts his/her defenses against the previously warded-off sadness. Patients in psychotherapy similarly make unconscious decisions to experience previously warded-off feelings when they feel that it is safe to do so (Weiss, 1986; for empirical research supporting this view, see Gassner, Sampson, Brumer, & Weiss, 1986).

Another example of how an external event may make it safe for a person to bring forth previously repressed painful affects is Weiss's vignette of Dr. N (Weiss, 1986, p. 10). In her second marriage, Dr. N was intensely moved by the birth of her son. Shortly after her son's birth, she wept profusely and retrieved memories of a son from her first marriage who had died several years earlier. Prior to the birth, she had no memories of her dead son (in fact, she had not recognized his picture in a family album). However, after the birth of her second son, she was able to recall and experience both how happy she had been with him and how devastated she was by his death. Weiss's explanation of Dr. N's bringing forth previously warded-off memories and affects parallels his description of the moviegoer's crying at the happy ending: Dr. N had repressed her sadness (and any memory of the dead son) because she was in danger of feeling overwhelmed by feelings of grief and loss. The birth of her second son is analogous to the happy ending in the movie. She was overjoyed by the birth, experienced it as partly making up for her earlier devastating loss, and consequently felt that she could now tolerate and face her sadness without feeling devastated and overwhelmed.

A second factor that may increase a person's sense of safety and facilitate the emergence of warded-off affects is a change in defensive structures, or what Weiss (1967) termed the integration of defenses. A person who has little control over a defense is likely to feel endangered by the affects, ideas, or memories that the defense is warding off. If a person is able to develop control over one's defenses (e.g., through successful therapeutic work) then he/she can use the defense to regulate the emergence of unconscious contents: "The patient's capacity to regulate the warded-off mental content makes it safe for him to experience it, because he can control the experience, turning away from it at will if it becomes too painful or threatening. In this way, the patient can dose the new experience (the warded-off content), and can reassess the danger associated with it" (Sampson, Weiss, Mlodnosky, & Hause, 1972, p. 525).

Sampson, Weiss, et al. carried out an empirical study of a psychoanalytic case that investigated the relationship between a patient's developing greater control over his defenses (in this particular case, the defense of undoing) and the emergence of previously warded-off affects. A strong, statistically significant relationship was found between the patient's developing control over undoing and his capacity to tolerate previously repressed affects. These results support the hypothesis that the patient's increased capacity to control his defenses made it possible to regulate previously warded-off emotion and, hence, made it safe to experience the affect. In a study of a different psychoanalysis (the case of Mrs. C; see Weiss, Gassner, & Bush, 1986, for a description), Horowitz, Sampson, Siegelman, Weiss, and Goodfriend (1978) investigated the relationship between the patient's ability to distance herself from others (referred to as Type D behaviors and feelings) and her ability to express positive, loving feelings and to be close to others (Type C feelings). Mrs. C sought psychoanalysis because of a chronic inability to feel close to her husband and to enjoy sexual relations with him. Horowitz et al. suggested that Mrs. C's difficulty feeling close to others was related to her inability to distance herself from others. They reasoned that if Mrs. C lacked the capacity to distance herself, then intimacy could be experienced as dangerous because she would not be able to disengage from closeness when she wanted to and would thus run the risk of feeling stuck or entrapped. They hypothesized that once Mrs. C gained the capacity to distance herself, she would have more confidence in her ability to regulate intimacy and consequently feelings of closeness would not be as threatening. Indeed, they found that progress in Type C feelings followed progress in expressing Type D feelings. As Mrs. C became more comfortable disagreeing with others and expressing critical feelings, she progressively felt less vulnerable. As a result, she could allow herself to experience feelings of closeness, affection, and intimacy.

The third factor influencing a patient's feeling of safety is the therapeutic relationship. Just as a change in external circumstances or in the degree of control over defenses can make it safe for a person to experience previously warded-off affects, so too may a change in a patient's relationship with the therapist. An important part of a patient's effort to solve problems and conflicts in therapy is bringing warded-off mental contents (wishes, affects, memories, experiences) into consciousness.

> The patient must do a great deal of work to overcome the internal danger he would face were he to experience a mental content he had warded off by defense. He does this work by attempting to create with the analyst a relationship that would protect him from this danger. An important part of this work is the patient's testing the analyst to assure himself that were he to bring the warded-off mental content to prominence or to consciousness, the analyst could be relied upon to respond in a way that would afford protection against the danger. (Sampson, 1976, p. 257)

A patient may test the therapist in order to assess the safety of bringing repressed affects or ideas into the therapeutic work (Weiss, 1971, 1986). For example, in the case of Mrs. C (referred to above) the patient tested the therapist by tentatively disagreeing with him and expressing critical feelings toward him (the patient's father had been unable to tolerate any criticism and would react to such feelings by either becoming enraged or by withdrawing and sulking). When the therapist responded to these tests by encouraging the patient to say more about her critical feelings or by pointing out her discomfort in criticizing him, the patient felt reassured (increased sense of safety) and frequently brought up previously warded-off memories and affects. Research studies have shown that when a therapist's behaviors and interpretations increase the patient's sense of safety ("pass the patient's tests"), the patient shows immediate improvement. For instance, in an empirical study of a psychoanalysis, Silberschatz (1986) found a significant correlation between the degree to which the therapist passed the patient's tests and changes in the patient's level of experiencing and expression of affects. Similar results have been found in other studies (e.g., Bush & Gassner, 1986; Fretter, 1984; Silberschatz, Fretter, & Curtis, 1986; for a review of this research, see Silberschatz, Curtis, & Nathans, 1989; Silberschatz et al., in press).

The concept of pathogenic beliefs helps explain why these three factors (external changes, defensive control, and the therapeutic relationship) all may lead to increased safety and accessibility of warded-off mental contents. A person's assessment of safety and danger is strongly influenced by his/her unconscious pathogenic beliefs. Thus, any experience or interaction that disconfirms a pathogenic belief will increase a person's sense of safety and thereby allow him/her to lift repression against warded-off affects, ideas, and memories.

In the phenomenon of crying at the happy ending, a change in external events may help a person to disconfirm pathogenic beliefs. For instance, Weiss (1986) suggested that Dr. N (who, following the birth of her second son, recalled previously repressed memories of her first son's

death) unconsciously experienced the death of her first son as a punishment and developed the pathogenic belief that she did not deserve to have
a son. The birth of her second son helped her to disconfirm the belief that
she was undeserving and thereby allowed her to feel less endangered by the
previously warded-off memories of her first son's death. Once this belief
was disconfirmed, she could recall the death of her son and experience it
not as a punishment but as a tragic and undeserved loss.

Similarly, a patient in psychotherapy works to disconfirm pathogenic
beliefs by testing them in relation to the therapist and by using the
therapist's interpretations to understand and ultimately disconfirm these
beliefs. As the patient disconfirms pathogenic beliefs, he/she becomes less
frightened of the dangers they foretell. Consequently, the patient may
decide (unconsciously) that he/she can safely experience certain previously warded-off contents and that it is safe to bring them into consciousness.

PATHOGENIC BELIEFS, FEELINGS OF GUILT,
AND THE ACCESSIBILITY OF AFFECT

Traumatic childhood experiences lead to pathogenic beliefs that may
block access to one's emotional life. Beliefs of being punished for expressing affect (e.g., anger, rivalry) or fears of being overwhelmed by the
intensity of emotion (e.g., sadness) are widely understood obstacles to
affective expression. We will briefly discuss a less recognized though significant factor for warding off emotions: pathogenic beliefs associated with
unconscious guilt (for a thorough discussion of the role of unconscious
guilt in psychopathology, see Bush, 1989; Friedman, 1985; Weiss, 1986,
pp. 43-67).

The control-mastery theory emphasizes a person's fear of hurting
others as the source of both rational and irrational guilt feelings. Bush
(1989) defined irrational guilt as an acutely distressing feeling stemming
from

> distorted unconscious beliefs about having done something bad in the
> fundamental sense of doing something hurtful or being disloyal to
> another person towards whom one feels a special sense of attachment or
> responsibility, such as a parent, sibling, or child. (p. 98)

Two major types of unconscious guilt feelings leading to psychopathology
are stressed in control-mastery theory (Weiss et al., 1986): separation
guilt and survivor guilt. Separation guilt stems from a pathogenic belief
that becoming independent of a parent will hurt the parent (Modell, 1965;

Weiss, 1986). Modell has noted that for people who suffer from this type of guilt, separation from mother is unconsciously perceived as killing her. Similarly, Loewald (1979) has suggested that many patients unconsciously experience becoming autonomous from their parents as tantamount to parricide.

The concept of survivor guilt is based on Niederland's (1981) psychotherapeutic work with survivors of the Holocaust. He conceptualized it as a powerful, often unconscious feeling of guilt, together with unconscious fears of punishment, for having survived a calamity in which others suffered or perished. The concept of survivor guilt has been further elaborated (e.g., Bush, 1989; Friedman, 1985; Modell, 1965, 1971; Weiss, 1986) to include experiences of guilt by people who believe that they have better lives than their family members or loved ones. For instance, Modell (1971) noted that survivor guilt is "not confined to particular diagnostic groups, but represents a fundamental human conflict" (p. 340) and thus has universal significance. Unlike Freud's model of unconscious guilt, which emphasizes sexual or aggressive wishes as its fundamental source, survivor guilt originates from a person's love for his/her family and from the false conviction that one has inadvertently harmed a love object—for instance, by getting more of the good things in life than a loved one has received.

This conceptualization of pathological guilt clearly highlights the interconnection between pathogenic beliefs and the affective experience of guilt. In his review of theories of guilt, Friedman (1985), building on Hoffman's work on altruism and empathy (1982, 1984), identified three components of guilt: affective, cognitive, and motivational.

> The affective component of guilt is a combination of empathic distress, the content of which will vary across situations, plus a common feeling, difficult to capture in words, but perhaps best described by Melanie Klein's term, depressive anxiety. The cognitive content of guilt is the belief that one's plans, thoughts, or actions are damaging to a person for whom one feels responsible. The motivational component consists of a plan either to avoid an intended action, to make reparation, or to defend against the guilt. (Friedman, 1985, p. 529)

CLINICAL ILLUSTRATION

We turn now to a psychotherapy case to illustrate how the disconfirmation of pathogenic beliefs that give rise to guilt feelings may contribute to the emergence of warded-off affects and memories (parts of the case description are taken from Silberschatz & Curtis, 1986). The patient, Mr. M, was a 25-year-old, single college graduate who sought therapy because he was unable to experience emotions strongly, "be they happiness, affection, or whatever." He had few interpersonal relationships, had a lifelong problem with sexual impotence, and was distressed about recurring sexual fantasies of being tied down or of tying a woman down. Although he had completed a year of graduate school, he felt very dissatisfied with and hopelessly stuck in a low-level job. Overall, he felt depressed, uninterested in anything, lonely, directionless, and in doubt whether it was worthwhile to go on living. He was very doubtful that therapy could actually help him.

Mr. M was the third of four children born in a small Midwestern city to very strict Roman Catholic parents. His father had remained in a low-level job throughout his career. Moreover, the father had had serious health problems since the patient's childhood but had never sought medical help. The father suffered from chronic emphysema, yet he refused to stop or cut down on his smoking. Similarly, the father refused for years to consult a dentist, and when he finally did so, his condition was so poor that all of his teeth had to be removed. The patient characterized his father as extremely passive, joyless, unable to "stick up for his rights," and as someone who was "hopelessly stuck."

The patient said little about his mother at intake, except to note that she was a kind, though "excitable" woman who sometimes took tranquilizers. He viewed her as a very weak woman who complied with her husband's drab life-style. Mr. M made clear that he disliked the dull, joyless, extremely sedentary life that both of his parents led: "When they were in their 40s, they lived their lives as if they were in their 70s." They did very little as individuals or as a family. The father came home from his low-level job and sat around passively or slept. The patient referred to his father as "dead at night."

Mr. M's primary pathogenic belief was that he was responsible for the unhappiness of both parents and, most manifestly, for the unhappiness of his father. Because he felt irrationally responsible for his father, the patient felt deeply frustrated by his inability to do anything useful for him. Throughout his life, the patient's own initiative had been squelched in various ways: by identification out of guilt with his passive parents, by the discouraging failure of any action he took actually to change his parents' situation, and by his belief that both parents were hurt by any initiative, independence, or happiness that the patient displayed.

The patient worked to disconfirm his pathogenic beliefs by testing them in relation to the therapist. For instance, he gave the therapist responsibility for his suffering and unhappiness as he had felt responsible for his parents' suffering and unhappiness. If the therapist did not feel irrationally responsible for him, this would reduce to some extent the patient's own belief that he was responsible for his parents. The patient also tested whether the therapist would feel helpless and discouraged by the patient's doubts, criticisms, and alck of responsiveness as he himself had been discouraged by his parents' behavior. These tests, which took place repeatedly over many sessions, were an integral part of the therapeutic process. As Mr. M began to disconfirm certain pathogenic beliefs (particularly beliefs connected to his omnipotence and irrational guilt) he felt less need to identify with his parents' beleaguerment and grimness. He then started to become aware of powerful, previously inaccessible affects—initially, feelings of sadness and anger toward his parents and subsequently, feelings of enthusiasm, affection, and pleasure.

In the following (disguised) excerpt, taken from the beginning of the 16th session, the patient describes newly emerging affects about himself and his family. This excerpt follows an interchange with the therapist regarding the patient's being behind in paying his bill. The therapist commented that the patient may feel guilty about doing something (keeping current with his bill) that his father was unable to do (father was frequently behind on bills, especially health care bills).

PATIENT: It just appears that some things were too big for him. I mean, not too big but too uh, too frightening and took too much, I don't know what you say, effort or maybe courage for him and my mother to face directly. So I get the feeling that I didn't face them at all. The obvious one that I've just kept saying over and over again is just that as his health continued to decline back in the days when something could have been done about it, nothing was done about it, and gradually what happened was unhealthy and uncomfortable situations that would be obvious to someone else, to an outsider, that would be obviously in need of correction, in need of some kind of attention, (sigh) were just tolerated. (silence) And I get the feeling that at least as far as I can tell, I am the one that is most annoyed at our family. My mother is, she must have lived with some kind of anxiety for a long time. She was always kind of nervous, but say ten years ago when, uh, when my father began to grow more uncomfortable, and as he continued to go to the doctor without any, without much sign of benefit, I, she must have felt some kind of anger and some kind of rage that he wasn't saying more to the doctor and that more wasn't being done. What she feels now is just, uh, resignation and, uh, she has told me on more than one occasion she just takes each day as it comes. As far as my brothers and sisters, I don't think any of them feel the way that I do. I think they're just, uh, I don't think any of them are hostile, I think they're just tired of the way things have been for so long. And I think, and I know everybody is sorry to see my father as uncomfortable as he is, but I think I'm the only one that's angry.

THERAPIST: You've implied that at various times, and seem to feel now that you shouldn't be.

P: Yeah. That's, that's, I think it depends on how I feel that day. If I'm feeling uh, if I'm feeling well, fairly comfortable and hopeful and optimistic and uh, I don't feel at odds with any particular thing in my life. (*sigh*) I don't, well I think I feel the anger but, uh, I'm not totally aware of it, and if I think, as I tend to think a lot, when I think about how, how the family ended up, how my folks ended up, I think, well that's too bad, it's too bad that it ended up that way. It's too bad that anybody has to live that way for so long, under such strained conditions, which you can't do anything about now. And I know it's days where I'm just sick of going to work or, uh, or another bill has come that I have to pay (*sigh*) that I'll get angry that I'm stuck or that I've been stuck, that I haven't made my life any different than it was, at least more comfortable, and almost always on days when I'm that, uh, when I'm that keyed up, I almost inevitably end up thinking about my father and myself and about the times that he did things that made me want to scream, even annoyed at myself. (*sigh*) I don't feel like I was pushed around but I just feel like I was so weak all the time, so weak and so afraid, afraid to say anything to him, afraid to, just to stand up against him.

T: Seems like you thought that you should've done more, that you felt some sort of responsibility.

P: Well, in some ways I feel, (*sigh*) I feel like all of us could have bugged him more to seek a better doctor than we had. But we didn't because nobody ever said to my father—my father never did anything he didn't want to do, and the family uh, struc—, the environment was not the kind that you might see on a TV show or the kind that Dr. Joyce Brothers might recommend where everybody gets together around the table and discusses problems bothering the family and makes suggestions. It wasn't like that. Things weren't going, on more than one occasion my father got up from the dinner table and just walked away because he didn't like what was being asked of him. (*sigh*) But more, (*pause*) the regret I feel and the feeling that I could have done more or taken more responsibility is not for him but for my own life. (*sigh*) And I did, I did do a lot of things that I didn't like doing or wasn't comfortable doing, uh, but I was, but I was always scared to take some other kind of step, to go in some other direction that nobody else was going in, such as staying out of school or, (*sigh*) or going to different schools when I didn't know what I was going to (*sigh*) or perhaps trying to mix with some other people than the people I used to hang out with that weren't always so much fun to be with. (*sigh*) And yet when I do something that I think is, is, uh, breaking away or going in another direction, I don't usually feel good about it.

This vignette illustrates the initial emergence of feelings of sadness and anger in a patient who came to treatment complaining of an inability to experience any emotions. In earlier sessions, as noted above, the patient had begun to disconfirm his pathogenic belief that he was responsible for his father's suffering by testing this belief in relation to the therapist. As the patient began to feel less irrational sense of responsibility, he could allow himself to become more separate from his father and his father's suffering, and thereby he could feel both greater sadness for him and for the family's suffering and anger at his father's inability to change. The therapist's interpretations just prior to the transcribed excerpt focused on the patient's identification with his father—expressed by keeping himself small and ineffective—because of guilt about doing better than father. The patient's subsequent anger at his father was an important step in allowing him to be different from his father; for example, to be more active, less resigned to fate, more able to use help, more alive. Indeed, in subsequent hours, the patient began to take more initiative, to show more enthusiasm, and even to begin to feel some pleasure and emotional involvement. The patient continued these changes after therapy. At the follow-up interview 1 year after termination of this brief (20-session) treatment, further progress was evident. The patient had started a relationship with a woman toward whom he felt affectionate, and he was able to enjoy sexual intercourse with her. The independent clinical evaluator who interviewed Mr. M at the 1-year follow-up was impressed with his strong, positive feelings toward this woman, his hopefulness and aliveness. This contrasted sharply to the initial, pretherapy interview in which the patient complained of an inability to feel emotions or to be interested in anything.

CONCLUSION

A person's affects are typically determined by his/her conscious and unconscious beliefs about reality; for instance, one is likely to feel anxious if he/she believes him/herself endangered, angry or frightened if he/she believes him/herself attacked, elated if he/she believes him/herself triumphant. The affective response is itself a vital source of information in appraising reality as well as a motivator of corrective action. Affects thus play a crucial role in adaptation. Certain pathogenic beliefs (Weiss, 1986) may interfere with the adaptive function of affects. Such pathogenic beliefs may either cause a person to experience affects that are inappropriate to the present situation or prevent a person from experiencing certain emotions, thereby depriving him/her of essential information about his/her reality. Successful psychotherapy helps the patient to disconfirm the pathogenic beliefs leading to these problems.

We have examined how a patient in psychotherapy may disconfirm pathogenic beliefs and gain access to previously inaccessible affects. An instructive paradigm of how this happens is the phenomenon of "crying at the happy ending," in which a change in external circumstances (a happy ending) disconfirms a pathogenic belief and thereby makes it safe to experience previously inaccessible affect (sadness). In psychotherapy, patients change their pathogenic beliefs by testing them in relation to the therapist and by using therapist interpretations to disconfirm these beliefs. As pathogenic beliefs are disconfirmed, the patient feels an increased sense of safety and may begin to experience previously inaccessible affects.

NOTE

1. The theory is referred to as the control–mastery theory because Weiss postulates that patients have *control* over their unconscious mental functioning and come to therapy to *master* their problems.

REFERENCES

Arnold, M. B. (1970). *Feelings and emotions.* New York: Academic Press.

Basch, M. F. (1976). The concept of affect: A re-examination. *Journal of the American Psychoanalytic Association, 24,* 759-777.

Brenner, C. (1974). On the nature and development of affects: A unified theory. *Psychoanalytic Quarterly, 43,* 532-556.

Bush, M. (1989). The role of unconscious guilt in psychopathology and psychotherapy. *Bulletin of the Menninger Clinic, 53,* 97-107.

Bush, M., & Gassner, S. (1986). The immediate effect of the analyst's termination interventions on the patient's resistance to termination. In J. Weiss, H. Sampson, & the Mount Zion Psychotherapy Research Group, *The psychoanalytic process: Theory, clinical observations, and empirical research* (pp. 299-322). New York: Guilford.

Dahl, H. (1979). The appetite hypothesis of emotions: A new psychoanalytic model of motivation. In C. E. Izard (Ed.), *Emotions in personality and psychopathology* (pp. 199-225). New York: Plenum.

Emde, R. (1980). Toward a psychoanalytic theory of affect. In S. I. Greenspan & G. H. Pollock (Eds.), *The course of life: Psychoanalytic contributions toward understanding personality development.* Rockville, MD: National Institute of Mental Health.

Fretter, P. B. (1984). The immediate effects of transference interpretations on patients' progress in brief, psychodynamic psychotherapy. *Dissertation Abstracts International, 46,* 1415-A. (University Microfilms No. 85-12, 112)

Friedman, M. (1985). Toward a reconceptualization of guilt. *Contemporary Psychoanalysis, 21,* 501-547.

Gassner, S., Sampson, H., Brumer, S., & Weiss, J. (1986). The emergence of warded-off contents. In J. Weiss, H. Sampson, & the Mount Zion Psychotherapy Research Group, *The psychoanalytic process: Theory, clinical observations, and empirical research* (pp. 171-186). New York: Guilford

Greenberg, L. S., & Safran, J. D. (1987). *Emotion in psychotherapy: Affect, cognition, and the process of change.* New York: Guilford.

Greenberg, L. S., & Safran, J. D. (1989). Emotion in psychotherapy. *American Psychologist, 44,* 19-29.

Hoffman, M. L. (1982). Development of prosocial motivation: Empathy and guilt. In N. Eisenberg (Ed.), *The development of prosocial behavior*. New York: Academic Press.

Hoffman, M. L. (1984). Interaction of affect and cognition in empathy. In C. Izard, J. Kagan, & R. Zajonc (Eds.), *Emotions, cognition and behavior*. New York: Cambridge University Press.

Horowitz, L. M., Sampson, H., Siegelman, E. Y., Weiss, J., & Goodfriend, S. (1978). Cohesive and dispersal behaviors: Two classes of concomitant change in psychotherapy. *Journal of Consulting and Clinical Psychology, 46*, 556–564.

Lazarus, R. S. (1984). On the primacy of cognition. *American Psychologist, 39*, 124–129.

Leventhal, H. (1984). A perceptual-motor theory of emotion. In L. Berkowitz (Ed.), *Advances in experimental social psychology* (pp. 117–182). New York: Academic Press.

Lewin, B. D. (1965). Reflections on affect. In M. Schur (Ed.), *Drives, affects, and behavior* (pp. 23–37). New York: International Universities Press.

Loewald, H. (1979). The waning of the Oedipus complex. *Journal of the American Psychoanalytic Association, 27*, 751–775.

Modell, A. (1965). On having the right to a life: An aspect of the superego's development. *International Journal of Psycho-Analysis, 46*, 323–331.

Modell, A. (1971). The origin of certain forms of pre-Oedipal guilt and the implications for a psychoanalytic theory of affects. *International Journal of Psycho-Analysis, 52*, 337–346.

Niederland, W. G. (1981). The survivor syndrome: Further observations and dimensions. *Journal of the American Psychoanalytic Association, 29*, 413–426.

Plutchik, R. (1980). *Emotion: A psychoevolutionary synthesis*. New York: Harper & Row.

Sampson, H. (1976). A critique of certain traditional concepts in the psychoanalytic theory of therapy. *Bulletin of the Menninger Clinic, 40*, 255–262.

Sampson, H. (1989). *The problem of adaptation to reality in psychoanalytic theory*. Paper presented to the American Psychoanalytic Association meeting, San Francisco.

Sampson, H., Weiss, J., Mlodnosky, L., & Hause, E. (1972). Defense analysis and the emergence of warded-off mental contents: An empirical study. *Archives of General Psychiatry, 26*, 524–532.

Schur, M. (1969). Affects and cognition. *International Journal of Psycho-Analysis, 50*, 647–653.

Silberschatz, G. (1986). Testing pathogenic beliefs. In J. Weiss, H. Sampson, & the Mount Zion Psychotherapy Research Group, *The psychoanalytic process: Theory, clinical observations, and empirical research* (pp. 256–266). New York: Guilford.

Silberschatz, G., & Curtis, J. T. (1986). Clinical implications of research on brief dynamic psychotherapy: II. How the therapist helps or hinders therapeutic progress. *Psychoanalytic Psychology, 3*, 27–37.

Silberschatz, G., Curtis, J. T., & Nathans, S. (1989). Using the patient's plan to assess progress in psychotherapy. *Psychotherapy, 26*, 40-46.

Silberschatz, G., Curtis, J. T., Sampson, H., & Weiss, J. (in press). Research on the process of change in psychotherapy: The approach of the Mount Zion Psychotherapy Research Group. In L. Beutler & M. Crago (Eds.), *International psychotherapy research programs.* Washington, DC: American Psychological Association.

Silberschatz, G., Fretter, P. B., & Curtis, J. T. (1986). How do interpretations influence the process of psychotherapy? *Journal of Consulting and Clinical Psychology, 54*, 646-652.

Weiss, J. (1952). Crying at the happy ending. *Psychoanalytic Review, 39*, 338.

Weiss, J. (1967). The integration of defenses. *International Journal of Psycho-Analysis, 48*, 520-524.

Weiss, J. (1971). The emergence of new themes: A contribution to the psychoanalytic theory of therapy. *International Journal of Psycho-Analysis, 52*, 459-467.

Weiss, J. (1986). I. Theory and clinical observations. In J. Weiss, H. Sampson, & the Mount Zion Psychotherapy Research Group, *The psychoanalytic process: Theory, clinical observations, and empirical research* (pp. 3-138). New York: Guilford.

Weiss, J. (1989). *The centrality of adaptation.* Paper presented to the American Psychoanalytic Association meeting, San Francisco.

Weiss, J. Gassner, S., & Bush, M. (1986). Mrs. C. In J. Weiss, H. Sampson, & the Mount Zion Psychotherapy Research Group, *The psychoanalytic process: Theory, clinical observations, and empirical research* (pp. 155-162). New York: Guilford.

Weiss, J., Sampson, H., & the Mount Zion Psychotherapy Research Group. (1986). *The psychoanalytic process: Theory, clinical observations, and empirical research.* New York: Guilford.

6

The Key to Understanding Change: Emotions as Appetitive Wishes and Beliefs about Their Fulfillment

HARTVIG DAHL
State University of New York Health Science Center at Brooklyn

INTRODUCTION

When Greenberg and Safran reviewed the "psychotherapy literature on the role of emotion in psychological functioning" for a theory to guide research on change they concluded that "one of the most noteworthy aspects of this literature is the absence of a systematic model of emotion" (Greenberg & Safran, 1987, p. 9).

Since they devoted nearly two pages to a careful and accurate description of just such a systematic model of emotion that I had published as "a new psychoanalytic model of motivation," their conclusion is puzzling. But since I share their belief that a coherent theory is essential to guide research into the role of emotions in therapeutic change I shall first very briefly summarize a revised version of my own theory.[1] Second, I will state two fundamental guiding propositions, or more accurately, hypotheses about therapeutic change to be tested by examining change events, and third, I will focus in some detail on two particularly dramatic change events that occurred during a 6-year tape-recorded psychoanalysis.

A BRIEF SUMMARY OF THE THEORY OF EMOTIONS

The theory was originally part of a more general "psychoanalytic model of motivation" called "the appetite hypothesis" of emotions, which is a "biopsychosocial" model. It tries to account for the profound *motivational* properties of emotions and their *cognitive* functions as well as the fact that there are different classes of emotions with radically different functions. I take it as a given that emotions evolved as a primary means for our mammalian ancestors to communicate with and understand the intentions of other members of their own species. In this sense they constitute a basic information-processing (i.e., cognitive) system highly conducive to differential survival rates. Moreover, emotions are the first language of every human infant before symbolic language is acquired. The common-sense knowledge that each of us has of our own and others' emotions is fundamental to all of our interactions with other humans and is widely shared across races and cultures (cf. Ekman, 1973; Izard, 1971; Tzeng, Hoosain, & Osgood, 1987).

The present version of this theory is based upon three fundamental propositions: (1) a three-dimensional classification scheme of emotions, (2) the cognitive concepts of *wishes* and *beliefs*[2], and (3) the biologically rooted concept of *appetites*.

A Three-Dimensional Classification Scheme for Emotions

I have adapted a three-dimensional scheme from de Rivera's (1962) "decision" theory of emotions, in part because his first three dimensions were so similar to Freud's (1915–1957) three "polarities" basic to mental life: Subject–Object, Pleasure–Unpleasure, and Active–Passive. The three dimensions are:

Orientation	[IT–ME]
Valence	[ATTRACTION/REPULSION–POSITIVE/NEGATIVE]
Activity	[TO/FROM–ACTIVE/PASSIVE]

A classificatory tree showing the results of the intersections of these dimensions is illustrated in Figure 6.1, together with typical examples of empirically derived emotion labels for each of the eight categories.[3]

If such a scheme has any validity, it surely implies that people have some kind of internal representation of these dimensions and ought to be able to use them to classify emotions. Indeed, Stengel and I (Dahl & Stengel, 1978) replicated and extended de Rivera's empirical classification, using the above three dimensions. Given abstract definitions of each dimension, 58 judges were able to classify 400 emotion words with alpha coefficient reliabilities from .95, to >.99. Intercorrelations among the dimensions were nil, indicating the empirical independence of the dimensions, and the judges' ages and sex were uncorrelated with their choices.[4] Thus, despite the fact that each person has direct access only to his own particular emotional states and in principle cannot have such access to

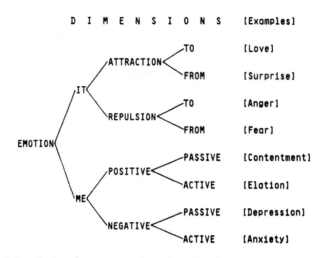

FIGURE 6.1.   A classification tree based on the three dimensions—orientation, valence, and activity—yielding eight major categories of emotions. Example labels are taken from the empirical results in Dahl and Stengel (1978).

another's comparable states, and despite the fact that each person has his/her own unique set of memories derived from one's own developmental interactions, it seems necessary to assume substantial shared experiential referents in order to account for the judges' agreement.[5]

Although this classification included all of the emotions that others have regarded as fundamental based on a variety of criteria,[6] quite unexpectedly it also provided a principled distinction for what now appear to be two major *functional* classes of emotions, IT and ME. Schwartz and Trabasso (1984) demonstrated the psychological reality of the IT-ME distinction in a study that showed that 6-year-olds understand the classificatory dimensions as well as the implicit wishes and beliefs associated with the IT and ME emotions. I shall return to this distinction shortly, but first some definitions.

Basic Definitions and Characteristics

Wish, Pleasure, and Unpleasure

The theory of emotions as wishes and beliefs rests firmly on a definition of a *wish* as *an attempt to achieve perceptual identity and/or symbolic equivalence with a previous experience of satisfaction.*[7] *Pleasure*, in this model, is the satisfaction of a wish, and *unpleasure* is the nonsatisfaction of a wish. These definitions have several decisive implications, some obvious, some not quite so. One implication is that certain basic initial experiences of satisfaction are phylogenetically adapted; that is, they are wired in by evolution. As Deutsch and Deutsch (1966) put it:

> It is the taste of water, the feeling of satiety, the sensations from the genitalia that an animal finds rewarding. The connection of these sensations with need reduction is not one which is made by each individual animal. Such a connection . . . has been made by the process of natural selection. Only those animals which have found certain sensations rewarding have survived. Learning . . . has already occurred in the species; the individual need not recapitulate it. (pp. 143–144)

Second, memory is required to record the experiences. Third, memories, when activated by any means, serve as a goal, which is to repeat the same experience of satisfaction (pleasure), that is, to achieve *perceptual identity*. Indeed Freud (1900–1953) postulated that the initial activation might be an hallucinatory fulfillment, that is, activation of the memory to hallucinatory intensity. Implausible as this may appear, Helen Keller (see Dahl, 1965) vividly described just such hallucinatory memories of previous experiences of satisfaction (e.g., the taste of ice cream) during the period before she acquired language at about the age of 6. The activation of memories is the attempt to achieve perceptual identity; until then the wish remains latent, that is, potential or descriptively and/or dynamically unconscious.[8] Fourth, the inclusion of symbolic equivalence allows for the human capacity for finding and satisfying alternate wishes as substitutes for primary experiences of satisfaction.

Finally, lest we be limited to highly restricted and stereotyped behavior, it is necessary to assume, with good evidence to support the assumption (e.g., Nachman, Stern, & Best, 1986; Sroufe & Waters, 1976; Wolff, 1966), that novel experiences, for all their variety, are perceptually identical in their property of unexpectedness and the aroused emotion of mild surprise; novelty *qua* novelty is an intrinsic experience of satisfaction. Thus we end up with a really interesting creature, one with built-in opposing tendencies: on the one hand to repeat the same old experiences of satisfaction, but on the other to enlarge its repertoire, to satisfy its curiosity and expand its range of experiences.

Appetite

There are four essential structural components of an *appetite*:

1. A perception of a specific internal (partly bodily) state (e.g., thirst or genital sensations),
2. An implicit wish to reinstate (achieve perceptual identity with) a previous experience of satisfaction (e.g., the taste of water or the sensations from copulation),

3. A consummatory act (e.g., drinking water or copulation),
4. A reafferent perception of the feedback from the consummatory act (e.g., the taste of water or the genital sensations and their motor accompaniments, which eventually terminate the act).

Lorenz (1965) emphasized the learning that takes place in the context of appetitive behavior via "the reafference which the organism produces for itself by performing the consummatory act in the adequate consummatory situation" (p. 88). This is the feedback that satisfies the wish. As I wrote (Dahl, 1978, p. 389), "Using the model of infant feeding, we can say that the infant's consummatory act of sucking teaches it that the incoming fluid satisfies its appetites of hunger and thirst because that is the way the infant is built." And, I would now stress, it is built by natural selection in the course of evolution.

Appetites also have a number of conspicuous properties. Most importantly they function as *instructions*. Initially there are objects that are specifically necessary for their satisfaction; however, in the absence of the specific objects substitutes may suffice. When satifaction is possible there is a strong tendency to self-stimulation of the appetite, and there is a tendency to expand the range and refine the discrimination of experiences that will satisfy, in other words a tendency to acquire new "tastes."

Emotion

According to this theory *emotions* are a special class of appetites, exhibiting the same structure and the above properties of somatic appetites. They function as *wishes* and *beliefs* in an evolutionarily given (i.e., phylogenetically adapted) nonverbal feedback information system. For the animal without symbolic language (which includes our evolutionary ancestors and every human before he/she acquires such symbolic language) emotions are the primary "intelligence" system for surviving in a complex world of diverse dangers and rewards. They enable conspecifics to display their intentions and to recognize each other's intentions.

An essential difference between emotions and somatic appetites lies in the fact that two major classes of emotions, the IT and the ME emotions, are specialized to fulfill different structural components of appetites. The IT emotions include the functions of the first three structural components: (1) the perception of a specific intentional state, (2) an implicit wish toward an object, and (3) a consummatory act, while the ME emotions function as the fourth structural component of an appetite, namely, (4) the reafferent perception of the feedback information about satisfaction or nonsatisfaction accompanying the consummatory act. Thus we have the following definitions and examples:

IT emotions have objects, function as appetitive wishes about those objects, and can be represented as: *P wishes that x*, where *x* is one of four formally definable classes of consummatory acts, defined by the intersection of two dimensions, valence (Attraction–Repulsion) and activity (To–From). Table 6.1 shows the four generic emotional appetites, each with its generic wish and generic consummation.

ME emotions do not have objects, function as beliefs, and can be represented as: *P believes that y*, where *y* is information about the status of satisfaction or nonsatisfaction of appetitive and other significant wishes. The satisfaction of wishes results in the experience of *pleasure*, while nonsatisfaction results in the experience of *unpleasure*. Four generic classes are defined by the intersection of the two dimensions, valence (Positive–Negative) and activity (Active–Passive). Table 6.2 shows the tour generic ME emotions, each with its generic belief, unique experience, goal, and typical name.

From here on for the purpose of understanding and explaining two change events, I will largely disregard the Activity dimension and focus on the remaining four emotion categories. These will be referred to as follows: POS IT (for ATTRACTION TO/FROM IT), NEG IT (for REPULSION TO/FROM IT), POS ME (for POSITIVE ACTIVE/PASSIVE ME) and NEG ME (for NEGATIVE ACTIVE/PASSIVE ME). When any significant wish, including those implicit in the IT emotions, is activated, a computation to assess the possibility of fulfillment is automatically carried out and the outcome of this computation determines the resulting ME emotion. The ME emotions play a crucial role in conveying information about the state of fulfillment of all significant wishes, including those inherent in the IT emotions. The POS ME and NEG ME emotions function differently in this regard, a difference long recognized in a behavioral context as positive and negative reinforcement.

The causal effect of the POS ME emotions is that of facilitation in the sense of helping to stabilize the memory of the experience of satisfaction, promoting both its reactivation under suitable conditions and fantasies about the objects involved.[9] Conversely, the causal effect of NEG ME emotions is that of inhibition in the sense of a signal to invoke some kind of

TABLE 6.1.   The four generic emotional appetites (IT emotions), each with its generic wish, generic consummatory goal, and prototypic label

Generic wish	Goal: to perform consummatory act	Emotion
ATTRACTION TO IT	Take care of it	Love
ATTRACTION FROM IT	Explore it	Surprise
REPULSION TO IT	Get rid of it	Anger
REPULSION FROM IT	Escape from it	Fear

TABLE 6.2.   The four generic affects (ME emotions), each with its generic belief, unique experience, goal, and prototypic label

Generic belief	Experience (goal)	Emotion
POSITIVE PASSIVE ME		Contentment
Wishes have been satisfied	⎡ Pleasure ⎤	
POSITIVE ACTIVE ME	⎢ (repeat) ⎥	Elation
Wishes going well		
NEGATIVE PASSIVE ME		Depression
Wishes can't be satisfied	⎡ Unpleasure ⎤	
NEGATIVE ACTIVE ME	⎣ (get rid of) ⎦	Anxiety
Wishes not going well		

defense against: (1) the wish itself, that is, the activation of the memory of the experience of satisfaction, (2) the consummation of the wish, and/or (3) the NEG ME emotion itself. Depending on many factors a defense may or may not be invoked. Such defenses, if invoked, vary greatly in their effectiveness, particularly against the NEG ME emotion itself, often leading to auxiliary means, such as alcohol and other drugs, to get rid of the aversive quality of the NEG ME emotion. Different clinical syndromes can be identified that illustrate each of these defensive dispositions (see Dahl, 1978, pp. 396–397).

I have adapted a homely little scenario, created by Trabasso (1982), to illustrate a commonsense application of the theory. In Table 6.3, column 1 tells a story about John, column 2 lists some of John's emotions that one might plausibly infer from each event in the story, and column 3 translates these emotion names into the formal terms of the theory, including John's corresponding wishes and beliefs. The relationship between columns 1 and 2 is based on commonsense knowledge and that between columns 2 and 3 is based on (1) the empirically established relationships between emotion words and the classification dimensions and (2) the definitions of the present theory.

The Therapeutic Change Hypothesis (TCH)

Based upon the above theory of emotions, it is now possible to state a reasonably clear and clinically testable hypothesis (TCH):

> Therapeutic change is a causal result of specific changes in ME emotions that function as beliefs about the status of fulfillment of IT emotions and other appetitive and significant wishes. Moreover, such wishes and beliefs play a causal role in (1) the development of adaptive and maladaptive psychic structures and (2) in changing those structures later in life, most usually when a person undertakes some kind of psychotherapy.

TABLE 6.3. A story about John and Mary and Fred (adapted from Trabasso, 1982)

Narrative	John's emotions and affects	John's wishes and beliefs
John sees Mary, an attractive classmate, at a party.	Interested, curious	ATTRACTION TO/FROM IT Wish: *to get acquainted with Mary*
John feels attracted to Mary.	Fascinated, friendly, affectionate	ATTRACTION TO/FROM IT Wish: *to consummate his several appetites*
John imagines what he and Mary will do; he walks toward her.	Eager, enthusiastic, adventurous, bold, optimistic	POSITIVE ACTIVE ME Belief: *his wishes will be satisfied*
Mary suddenly turns to Fred, John's friend.	Anxious, distressed, upset, worried	NEGATIVE ACTIVE ME Belief: *his wishes may not be satisfied*
Fred joins hands with Mary and they leave together.	Dejected, depressed, discouraged, lonely	NEGATIVE PASSIVE ME Belief: *his wishes can't be satisfied*
John imagines that Fred has a serious accident.	Angry, jealous, envious	REPULSION TO IT Wish: *to get rid of Fred*

Note. Column 1 tells a simple story about John. Column 2 lists labels of some of John's emotions and affects that one might plausibly infer from each event in the story. Column 3 translates these emotion names into the formal terms of the theory, including John's corresponding wishes and beliefs.

Let me illustrate with two hypothetical examples. Suppose a child repeatedly experiences anxiety in interactions with his/her parents when he/she at first needs and later wants to be the object of the parents' appetites of love and affection. This sequence of wish followed by anxiety, through repetition, gradually becomes established as part of structures that Teller and I have called Frames (Dahl, 1988; Dahl & Teller, in press; Davies, 1988; Teller, 1988; Teller & Dahl, 1981, 1986). In this sequence, the child's anxiety functions as a belief that his/her wishes for love and affection are not going well, that they are not likely to be fulfilled. Once such a structure gets established, and especially if it generalizes to other significant wishes, the child's, and later the adult's, dispositions will, to a significant degree, be caused by the experience of anxiety and its many NEG ME variants.

The function of the anxiety can be translated into the proposition: *I probably will not get what I want.* This in turn leads to defensive behaviors and dispositions designed to reduce the anxiety. Regardless of whether or not the defenses succeed in getting rid of the anxiety, there are causal consequences in the form of inhibitions of whole classes of wishes, or repeated and failed attempts to satisfy them, symptoms, a pessimistic outlook, and inevitably, difficulties with other people.

Conversely, repeated experiences of fulfillment and satisfaction of significant wishes in interaction with caregivers becomes part of an event sequence that functions as a belief in the proposition: *I probably will get what I want*, a belief manifested in the whole range of POS ME emotions. It is easy to imagine the adventurous, bold, creative, free, and optimistic personality that would result from these entirely different interactions. It is easy because we already know from commonsense and clinical knowledge that both of the above hypothetical examples abound.

A person need not be aware (and perhaps most often is not) of the cognitive translation of the emotional state or disposition or temperament. He/she may not be able to put into words the correct functional equivalent of the experience of anxiety, and he/she may automatically invoke defenses against the experience of the anxiety. One's behavior, while completely understandable as caused by the belief that things probably won't work out, may be quite baffling to oneself. The task of changing can be seen as the task of changing the representation of the belief that is causally relevant, namely the anxiety. One can imagine a number of different routes toward altering the belief represented as a NEG ME emotion.

For example, Weiss (1986a,b), in a major revision of standard psycho-analytic theory, replaced a model of "automatic functioning" with one of "higher mental functioning," in which a patient suffering from chronic anxiety, for example, has an unconscious plan for getting well, a plan for altering his "pathogenic beliefs" about people. Weiss then postulated that a patient in treatment repeatedly tests the therapist to find out if the thera-pist's responses fit with the patient's own plan to discover what it is "safe" to say and do with the therapist. Although Weiss does not clearly specify and classify "pathogenic beliefs," the theory of emotions and the TCH offered here do in fact specify the class of these beliefs as the NEG ME emotions. According to the TCH, NEG ME emotions just are the key pathogenic beliefs that provoke inhibitions, defenses and symptoms and that must change if significant change is to occur. If the patient has successfully defended against conscious recognition of the NEG ME emotion itself, then that *re-*cognition is a necessary first step in the change process.

Standard psychoanalytic theory has it that such beliefs can be and often are altered by "emotional insight," by which is meant insight into the cognitive message, that is, the belief *things probably won't work out*, with concomitant change in the emotion, namely a diminution in the auto-matic experience of anxiety. Without the accompanying change in anx-iety the insight would remain "intellectual" and, it is widely held, would be ineffective since the cause (anxiety) would remain intact and influence behavior accordingly.

Other therapeutic techniques, such as behavioral desensitization, might reduce the anxiety (and hence the belief things probably won't work out) by systematic habituation of the response. Cognitive–behavioral techniques might attempt to change the cognitive belief that either preceded or accompanied the occurrence of anxiety, in effect reducing its rate of occurrence. Certainly all the therapies that emphasize the importance of "experiencing" are entirely consistent with this theory. Even without formal therapy there are a significant number of people who find in religious conversion a kind of transcendent joy (with its attendant belief things will work out, my wishes will be satisfied!) so pervasive that the causal consequences for behavior can be dramatic and long lasting. Chemotherapies that significantly diminish NEG ME emotions such as depression and/or anxiety can, for many patients, produce the same causal consequences as psychological therapies. Even negative therapeutic reactions, with increased anxiety and/or depression (and their attendant defenses), are accounted for by the hypothesis, since change may and does occur in either direction.

In this light, resistance to change consists not only in the defenses that are invoked, but in the beliefs, generically labeled anxiety and depression, that profoundly affect our expectations, and therefore the wishes we are willing to entertain and the tasks that we are willing to tackle and commit ourselves to. The use of "therefore" here is deliberate in order to emphasize the controlling feedback function of the ME emotions, that is, their role in selecting which wishes and actions are facilitated and which are inhibited.

The fact that the TCH is silent on exactly how to achieve changes in the NEG ME emotions suggests that there are many different routes to this accomplishment, an assumption that also underlies the title of this book, *Emotion, Psychotherapy, and Change.* The TCH offers us a theoretical basis for understanding this diversity. Finally, an unstated implication of the emotion theory from which the TCH is derived is that a certain minimum satisfaction and fulfillment of basic appetites, including IT emotions, is essential to a healthy life.

The Task–Goal–Technique (TGT) Congruence Hypothesis

If therapeutic change is as simple as the TCH implies, why then has psychotherapy research seemed such a formidable and difficult enterprise? Why have more than a quarter century of outcome studies mainly taught us that most treatments work some of the time and none works all of the time (Smith, Glass, & Miller, 1980)? Why have the advocates of different therapies and theories been at such pains and largely failed in the attempt to demonstrate the superiority of their own favorite techniques over others? In short, why does both everything and nothing succeed? This question strongly suggests that we need a very general outcome hypothesis, one that will explain why what works for one patient will not necessarily work for another and vice versa. For this I propose the *Task–Goal–Technique Congruence* hypothesis, which claims:

> In psychotherapy, other things being equal, the degree of positive or negative change is a function of the degree of Task–Goal–Technique Congruence.

These terms refer to: (1) the Task the patient is given in the beginning of the treatment, (2) what the patient does with this Task, (3) the patient's own Goal(s) for the treatment, (4) the relationship between the Task and the Goal, (5) the interaction of the Task and Goal with the therapist's Technique (e.g., in the case of psychoanalysis, the analyst's "analytic attitude"), and (6) the congruence, compatibility, or fit among these.

THE EXAMINATION OF TWO CHANGE EVENTS

With the TCH and the TGT Congruence hypothesis in mind, in the remainder of this report I shall examine two manifest change events that occurred in the course of a 6-year (1,114-hour) tape-recorded psychoanalysis. Unlike Rice and Greenberg's (1984) and Greenberg and Safran's (1987) single-case strategy, which involves the detailed investigation of a well-defined class of change events, I shall examine just two such events, their surrounding contexts, and their consequences. Moreover I will focus on the role of emotions, the Task of the treatment, the patient's Goal, and finally, the therapist's Technique.

The change events share three manifest properties: (1) They are statements by the patient that are significantly different from anything that preceded them; (2) they are steps toward the patient's Goal; and (3) they index the patient's involvement in the Task of the treatment. I shall analyze these events and their implications from several perspectives. There are key passages from verbatim transcripts that document each event and the background for it. The accompanying commentary focuses on the patient's Task and Goal and on the role of emotions in understanding the interaction of the Task and the Goal.

Two independent sets of evidence will be presented to establish the *fact* of the changes implied by the clinical description. The first of these is based on a study by Jones and Windholz (1990) and the second on reliable assessments of the patient's expression of emotions during treatment. Finally, we shall reconsider the TGT Congruence hypothesis in the light of the change events and suggest an answer to the question: What caused the changes?

Background for the First Change Event

The patient was a constricted, inhibited, obsessional married woman in her late 20s who sought analysis at the urging of her husband because she was unhappy with herself, her life in general, and her sex life in particular. The analysis began in Hour 1 as follows. (In all the verbatim text that follows, the analyst's speech is enclosed within slashes and the transcriber's comments are enclosed within parentheses in italics. Boldface is used to highlight words and phrases—especially those identifying emotions and affects—that appear to be particularly relevant to understanding the change events. Pauses are of 15 seconds to 1 minute and unqualified silences are 1–2 minutes in length. The symbol ¬ in brackets means "not.")

/ On the couch? /
Just lie right down?
/ Sure. /
I feel very funny. (*5-minute silence*) I'm finding it very hard to focus.
/ Your thoughts, you mean? /
Uhum.
/ That's not required. (*pause*) **The main requirement**, as I think I mentioned when you were here, **is that you say whatever you're thinking out loud.** /
I suppose the main thing that I'm thinking is, uh, I think of this more in terms of saying things that bother me and you know, working out why—you know, especially things that happen to be on my mind at the moment. And I had a very nice day today, (*nervous chuckle*) so I can't think of anything to say, (*nervous chuckle*) which is sort of an example of a negative way I look at things, I suppose. (*2-minute silence*) It does make me think, though, the fact that in most situations when I feel a little bit uneasy I always think I talk too much and say too much and don't listen or think first. And then now I can't. I feel very funny about talking at all. (*silence*)
/ Well, **it's hard to have so much freedom** isn't it? /
Hmm. Well, the other thing that happens is so many things fleetingly go through your mind. And, and now just, you have to select something of what's passing through and, and you keep thinking, that's not really important or, I guess a lot of things I feel sort of funny about saying. (*silence*) It does make me think of something though that I began to think, realize more clearly than ever before, just this fall. Uhm, that very often when somebody's just bringing up a subject in which I'm involved, I found myself very quickly becoming defensive and you know, almost saying, "I didn't do it" kind of thing and uhm, you know, immediately making excuses for something—that situation

that doesn't (*nervous chuckle*) even exist. (*silence*) So that made me wonder why I took things that way. (*2-minute silence*) I suppose another thing that's making it hard is, uh, I keep thinking there's a certain kind of thing to talk about here and I know I'm limiting myself very much when I think that way. (*pause*)

/ Well, it's a little trick you play on yourself to make it possible to not say what you think. /

Here the analyst focused on the patient's defenses against doing what he has explicitly asked her to do, namely to say everything out loud. And his putting it as, "a little trick you play on yourself" can easily be construed as implying that she could also stop playing the trick. Again she returned to her concern about talking:

(*silence*) I also keep thinking, well, I have to say it the right way, think about, in other words it has to come into my mind and then **I have to think about it awhile** (*nervous chuckle*) **so I say it the right,** you know, say it different ways in my mind **so finally I say it the right way,** (*nervous chuckle*) which I never do in real situations. (*nervous chuckle*) **I usually say things too quickly.** (*silence*) . . .

Soon she began to describe some of the sources of her concern about talking. She described how **"very tense and upset"** she felt whenever she was with her family. All her life they "never" listened to her and she was **never allowed to disagree** with them **or criticize** them:

. . . And whenever there's a, any sizable group and there's a discussion, it seems to me, and I again could be imagining this, that, uhm, neither of my parents particularly wants to hear anything that I have to say, which always gets **very upsetting** to me. And usually I end up, up, **feeling like having a tantrum.** I don't have one (*nervous chuckle*) but I end up just **feeling I can't control myself.** So I always have to leave.

/ At the thought that they don't want to really listen, you mean? /

Yes, . . . they won't pick it up or pay attention to it . . . and in my family it's a very competitive thing to get into a conversation . . . I just feel I **can't handle it** and . . . they just don't want to hear me . . . that they don't want to listen to me . . . I guess they just can't stand to have their own family saying things that are disagreeing . . . And **they're very aggressive** . . . even with friends of the family they're **extremely aggressive** . . . They, they aren't able to . . . see that perhaps other people don't agree. They just feel that what they think is right and there just can't be any way, any other way of thinking. And I just, I just

feel this is so unjust . . . I'm **afraid** they won't agree with me and that they'll **attack** me. Because they really just **attack** somebody who disagrees and **I never feel, I guess, strong enough** to stand up under that. (*silence*) . . .

Finally, near the end of the session, she told the following story about lighting up a cigar at a party:

> . . . And anyway, when I took this cigar, of course there were several comments. And I really, at the time I probably in a way knew it would make a sensation and **I was going to enjoy it.** But on the other hand, contradicting that, I don't like it when I do get the attention, because then **I never feel I can handle it** or know what to say or anything. But anyway, this was a very fleeting thing because I didn't make anything of it. There was a girl there who became **very jealous** of the fact that I had gotten this attention. And she was a type of girl that has to have it all the time and was dancing and doing things by herself so that everybody would look at her. And she was very good, and I, and I sincerely felt **I was enjoying it.** But later, but every time she had a chance she would **make a very sharp or nasty comment** to me, some of which passed over me, because at the time it just didn't occur to me that she would have been **jealous** of those 2 seconds that people hadn't been paying attention to her. Then I was kind of aware there was a certain **antagonism** and maybe I felt some for her, I don't know, because at the time I thought I was sincerely enjoying her act and thinking, **"Wouldn't it be nice if I could be that free?"**

Thus the analyst began the first session by restating to the patient the "basic rule," as analysts call it, to free associate. In other words he stipulated the patient's *Task* in the analysis. The patient, after documenting at length that no one in her family listened to her or allowed her to disagree with them, described her effort to outshine and take attention away from a young rival and confessed her own **wish to be that free.** In terms of the emotion theory that I have outlined we can now systematically represent her Wishes and Beliefs.

Wishes: To feel **free** [POS ME] to, among other things, **disagree** and criticize [NEG IT consummatory acts], to express a variety of NEG IT emotions, particularly **antagonism** and **jealousy** (as the other girl was "free" to do), and to attempt to satisfy the appetitive wishes implicit in these particular emotions by lighting up and smoking a cigar in a situation where she knew it would create a "sensation" and she would **enjoy** [POS ME] it.

Beliefs: That she is **not allowed to disagree** [NEG IT consummation] or make her own mistakes or assert herself, that she **will be rejected** [NEG IT] if she does.[10] This is chronically **upsetting** [NEG ME] and produces **tension** [NEG ME], which means that she believes she probably cannot fulfill her own NEG IT wishes, that is, carry out their appropriate consummatory acts.

In Hour 3, about two thirds of the way through the session, the analyst again mentioned the basic rule after she asked:

Is it better to force yourself to say something that you feel sort of not ready to say?

/ Well, **what was the rule I told you? Or what did I say was your job?** /

(*nervous chuckle*) I've been putting a lot out of my mind. (*pause*)

/ One thing I have noticed. I'm not sure what to make of it. Uhm, uhm, I'm not sure whether you're aware of it. I don't think you've referred to anybody by their name up to now. /

No. I have been aware of it every once in a while.

/ Is there a special reason for that? /

Well, I think it's the only time I become aware of the fact that there is a tape recorder and—

/ Ah. /

But that's not it entirely. I think it might be—probably too, I'm saying well, **some things I'm probably saying for the first time ever,** and **some things,** I'm saying that I just, you know **I would hardly ever say to anybody and only maybe to my husband or somebody really close.** So, I almost feel as if I can't bring, you know, I have to keep a certain anonymy [*sic*].

In the course of testing their own theory of psychotherapy, a group of researchers at San Francisco's Mount Zion Hospital (Weiss, Sampson, & the Mount Zion Psychotherapy Research Group, 1986) formulated their conception of this same patient's unconscious Plan for getting well. Caston (1986, p. 261) studied interventions that were judged according to their Plan Compatibility and reported that the above intervention (in bold face), in which the analyst restated the rule and mentioned her "job," got a score of 0.5 on a 7-point scale (0–6), meaning that judges regarded it as strongly opposed to the patient's unconscious plan for successful treatment. In other words, in their judgments, it strongly confirmed her pathogenic beliefs about other people's (including of course the analyst's) expectations of her and therefore was antitherapeutic. As we shall see, the story is more interesting than this judgment implies. It is just possible that the opposite was in fact the case.

A Puzzle

In Hour 38 (a Monday session), just before the first change event, the patient reported a dream about the analyst, a dream that poses a significant clinical puzzle whose solution will help us to explain the occurrence of both the first and the second change events. So let's see what role the patient assigned to the analyst:

> . . . And something else that's coming to my mind now, although it didn't at all yesterday—and yet on Saturday it was very much in my mind when we were going up to the North Shore—is, is **a dream I had**. And it was, well, I could remember enough of it so—I was practically awake when I had it. It was right before I got up on Saturday. And the details of it are sort of vague now. But somehow it was a gathering of people that had something to do with this dance. And, I don't know, we were sitting around talking and you were there. And I can just remember in the dream feeling a progressive **need to withdraw** more and more and, I don't know, just a greater **feeling of discomfort**. And then, at one point you sort of indicated to me that you knew what I was doing and that I'd better stop doing it. And I think I woke up then, but I had the feeling that I could stop doing it. And just somehow thinking about that during the day was **very comforting** to me and I **didn't get nearly as nervous** as I thought I would before the dance. (*clears throat*) But then **it bothered me that I was kind of using fantasy to escape in**. And it just did seem like an **escape** to me . . .

After some associations to a movie about a young girl who was a true free spirit who charmed everyone, whom everyone adored and whom the patient envied, the analyst returned her attention to the dream.

> / You said that, uhm, in the dream I said to you, in effect, "You know what you're doing and stop it." Right? What was it? /
>
> I—what you said?
>
> / Yeah, I mean, what was it that, ah was being referred to? Do you recall? /
>
> I think I was actually sort of, uhm, gradually **hunching up** more and more and **putting my face in my hands** and just kind of **hiding my face**.
>
> / Ah, that's what I was referring to. /
>
> Sort of gradually, yeah. But beyond that, what feelings I was feeling that was making me do that. But it **wasn't a harsh** kind of a thing. I don't know, it was almost a **feeling of being understood** and somebody who expected something else from me and yet **because they understood** what, what I was doing, **cared** and could be **gentle**

about it. I don't know, it was, it was, uhm, just a **very comforting feeling** that I got from thinking of it . . . But even while I was feeling that, I was also **feeling upset** that I had a dream that you were in, because somehow, I think even before I started analysis, I was **afraid of fantasizing about you** and making you something you weren't **and having you take an importance with me** that was just fantasy. (*silence*)

Now we have the ingredients of what common sense tells us is a paradox. On the one hand, she felt a certain feeling of freedom, but on the other hand, she dreamed that the analyst gave her orders to stop hunching up and hiding her face. I call this a paradox because not only does common sense tell us that people do not normally like to be told to stop what they are doing, but also obeying such an order, on the face of it, would seem to be the opposite of satisfying the freedom she had wistfully longed for at the end of the first analytic hour.

Another detail is relevant, namely her fear of "fantasizing" about the analyst, of his taking on "an importance" that was "just fantasy." What does this mean? Why should she have been reluctant for the analyst to become important to her and feel upset that he appeared in her dream? So the puzzle is twofold. First, she was afraid that the analyst would become too important to her (and presumably that she might find herself dreaming about him). And second, she dreamed that he found her withdrawing and hiding at a party and told her to stop doing it, which, paradoxically, she found comforting and a sign of his gentle caring about her.

By now it is obvious that in the dream, and her associations to it, the patient has expressed a range of emotions.[11] So another way to state the puzzle is: In the face of an unspecified danger she felt **afraid**, wanted to consummate this by **escaping** and, when told to stop **hiding** she felt **comforted** and **cared for** until she woke up and felt **upset** that she had used fantasy to **escape**. The main wishes and beliefs involved are:

> *Wishes:* **Afraid** [NEG IT] of fantasizing about the analyst and wanted to **escape** [NEG IT consummation], presumably, the dangers associated with expressing her lifelong NEG IT wishes.

> *Beliefs:* **Comforted** [POS ME] when the analyst ordered her to stop hiding her aggressive wishes, but **upset** [NEG ME] that he was becoming important in her fantasies.

The First Change Event

In this context, the first change event occurred near the end of Hour 38. She continued her associations to the dream:

. . . But I think also **your being in the dream represented some-thing more than, than just you.** I mean, it was sort of a feeling that I have about being here—and I don't always have it—but that, **well, I am feeling more and more that what I am thinking I can say and that at least there's not any horrible thing happening to me for saying it or any rejection for saying it.** I don't know, **I can't really find words for this feeling but there is a certain feeling of freedom.** (*pause*) At least, there wa—, there is when I'm not here. **Sometimes when I'm here I can't believe that there is because I just feel so tense or disturbed** because the thoughts that I'm, I keep having are disturbing ones but—(*pause*)

This newfound, if fragile, feeling of freedom in saying what she was thinking stood in marked contrast to her usual state of: **"I'm not free to think . . . I'm not free within myself . . . I'm just not feeling free."** Here, for the first time since the wish, **"Wouldn't it be nice if I could be that free?"** was expressed near the end of Hour 1, the patient's belief that she was not free has changed to a new belief, however temporary, that **"there is a certain feeling of freedom"** associated with **"not any horrible thing happening to me for saying it or any rejection for saying it."** Let us review her wishes and beliefs at the end of the first change event:

Wishes: Unchanged since Hour 1, namely to feel **free** [POS ME] to **disagree, criticize** and **have a tantrum** [NEG IT consummation] and feel **antagonism** and **jealousy** [NEG IT] and **afraid** [NEG IT]. And presumably, to **enjoy** [POS ME] lighting up a cigar and being the center of others' fascination [POS IT] with her.

Beliefs: In Hour 1 her *belief* was that she was **not free** [$\neg$ POS ME] ("I couldn't handle it"; "can't control myself") [NEG ME] to fulfill any of her negative appetites [NEG IT]. However, by Hour 38 she was able to express a **feeling of freedom** [POS ME] to say what she was thinking, a feeling that she attributed to the **absence of any horrible thing** [$\neg$ NEG IT] or any rejection [$\neg$ NEG IT] happening, in other words, to the absence of feeling attacked or frightened. Nonetheless her old beliefs, represented in feeling **tense** [NEG ME] and **disturbed** [NEG IT/ME], promptly returned.

How shall we understand this immediate retraction of the feeling of freedom? Of course it can be understood as a classic example of defensive undoing, substituting a negative state for the positive one. But what would be the motive for such a defense? A classic psychoanalytic answer might be that the "freedom" indirectly signaled a danger that some unacceptable unconscious wishes might be permitted into consciousness, hence the need for the immediate re-emergence of NEG ME emotion and reinforcing defenses. Whatever the merits of that view, it seems equally likely that this switch was a regression to an earlier more persistent and stable state, a switch from a ME emotion whose message is "my *wishes are going well* and I *probably will get what I want*" to her predisposition (at least as an adult) for emotions whose messages are "my *wishes are not going well* and I *probably won't get what I want.*" After all, the NEG ME emotions have been her nearly constant companions and the newfound feeling of freedom is just that, new and fragile and easily replaced by the old companions.[12]

The Solution to the Puzzle

The solution to the puzzle posed by her seemingly contradictory emotions will become clear if we focus on two things: the *Task* that the patient was given in the analysis and her *Goal* (central Wish) in the treatment. Both were explicitly described in the first analytic session, which followed an earlier initial interview in which the analyst and patient had agreed on the terms of the analysis. In that interview the patient consented to having the analysis tape-recorded for research purposes and was told that her task would be to say out loud what she was thinking. Then, as we have seen, the analyst described her task again in Hours 1 and 3. We now have the information necessary to solve the clinical puzzle posed by the apparent contradiction between the content of her dream in which the analyst told her to stop what she was doing, and the comforting, gentle, caring feeling that followed this order.

The solution lies in understanding that the Task, to say out loud whatever she was thinking, though at first perceived by the patient as very difficult, fit precisely into her own central wish (Goal) to become free. The first freedom, of course, given the Task, was to say whatever was on her mind. Much of the content of the first session revolved around her perceived lack of freedom in her own family. The analyst, noting her difficulty in talking said: "Well, it's hard to have so much freedom isn't it?"[13]

In particular, during Hour 1 she had focused at length on the struggle she felt to be heard in her own family, to be free to disagree with her parents and siblings, and of her deep resentment that they did not seem to pay attention to her or take her opinions seriously. From this perspective, smoking the cigar can be seen as a variation on the freedom to speak, in this case in competition with another woman at a party, rather than with the members of her own family as she grew up. So a basic question on her mind from the very beginning was, "Am I worth listening to?" The analyst's giving the basic rule to free-associate implicitly answered this with a resounding, "Yes, not only are you worth it, but I insist on listening to you." Then, during the weekend before Hour 38 she constructed a dream[14] in which the analyst, while ostensibly ordering her to stop what she was doing, in effect was telling her to *stop hiding* and *speak up!* Her seemingly paradoxical positive reaction to his order is no puzzle at all when seen in this light. Moreover, her feeling that the analyst's "being in the dream represented something more than just him" was right on the mark. He represented her own wishes to stop hiding, to speak up, to disagree, to smoke a cigar, in short, her wish to be free to assert herself and her own wishes and have them taken seriously. By Hour 38 she has clearly been persuaded that nothing "horrible" or "any rejection" would result.[15] In other words, her emotional beliefs have changed, and this is reflected in her statement of a new belief, namely a feeling of freedom.

At this point we already have a number of clues that suggest possible answers to an obvious question: Freedom to do what? At a minimum, from her manifest statements in the first hour, we can already predict that the patient should feel free to say what she thinks, to disagree, to criticize, to compete, and to feel jealous and envious.[16] The second change event will confirm this prediction in large measure.

Background for the Second Change Event

The second change event occurred during a period of the analysis that can be characterized as the height of the "transference neurosis," a term psychoanalysts use for a period in which a patient's central conflicts are re-enacted in the relationship with the analyst.[17] Loewald (1980, p. 309) described this aspect of a psychoanalysis as follows:

> Transference neurosis is not so much an entity to be found in the patient, but an operational concept. We may regard it as denoting the retransformation of a psychic illness which originated in pathogenic interactions with the important persons in the child's environment, into an interactional process with a new person, the analyst, in which the pathological infantile interactions and their intrapsychic consequences may become transparent and accessible to change by virtue of the analyst's objectivity and of the emergence of novel interaction possibilities.

This event occurred in Hour 727, an hour before a summer vacation at the end of the fourth year of the analysis. The patient's own words capture the central quality of the struggle in which she was then engaged with the analyst. It was quite literally a battle to defeat him and his efforts to analyze her aggressive wishes and behavior—to resist changing by keeping what she had described as a "balance" between her own hostile wishes, those of her husband for her to change, and her beliefs about the possible disadvantages of not changing. It was manifestly a recapitulation of a recurrent battle with her parents during her childhood. In Hour 716, she described the victory she was beginning to savor—the fulfillment of her lifelong angry [NEG IT] wishes—when she said:

Yeah, but then I'm remembering, uhm, well, I suppose even with my father I had this, uhm, but sometimes I'll interpret things here or I'll think of **what if you said that was all, you weren't going to continue or that clearly I wasn't going to get anywhere so you were going to stop** or I, I mean I've even specifically, I can't recall now, but interpreted your remarks sometimes to be **your sort of saying you're not going to be stuck with me.** And I don't know. (*sighs*) And, and I know with my father, too, there must have been times. **But it, I** suppose the main feeling, though, still is that **basically I feel fairly secure that, that you're stuck with me.**

Then the analyst, referring to their very first interview before the analysis began, continued:

/ Well, you know, you were very concerned about that at the very beginning, the very first time we ever talked here. That was one of your main questions, you know, you, eh, what would happen if something about the research or the recording or anything like that? Would I continue to see you without it? In other words, would I make a real, you know, firm commitment? That was on your mind even then. /

(*pause*) Well, I was also just thinking about that. I mean basically **things are a bit less secure,** I mean in, in the way I see it, with Dave. But even there, I, I suppose I've seen this already, but I'm just seeing it (*sighs*) again, perhaps a little more clearly, how **I've used coming here for hi—** against **him in that that's how I've kept myself fairly secure** and, and **able to continue fighting him by saying, "Well, I'm coming here, so give me more time."** And, and also I suppose, **playing on his basic feeling of not really wanting to get divorced.** But I was also just thinking of, of, uhm, when I even think about it, **in feeling you're stuck with me, I still feel** (*laughs*) that you are. Because I, I mean I was thinking about whenever I think of not coming anymore, it's always thinking **I would decide, not you would.** (*pause, sniffles*)

As a young girl she had often provoked her mother to kick her out of the house, and at one point she believed that the members of her family no longer wanted her around because they found her behavior so disagreeable. Now, in the transference relationship with the analyst, she has finally gotten her revenge. His professional obligations to her meant that indeed **he was "stuck" with her,** that is, in her view, **trapped**[18] [NEG IT]. In fact, in the initial evaluation interview, he had told her that if in his judgment the recording was interfering with the analysis he would discontinue it but continue treating her. Her laughter [POS ME] specifically expressed her satisfaction in fulfilling these very old NEG IT wishes. Now it was the analyst who was stuck (trapped), not she.

The Second Change Event

The second change event occurred in Hour 727, the next to the last session before a summer vacation at the end of the fourth year of the analysis:

> The next thing I was thinking is, uhm—(*pause, sigh*) well, I, I think the way I was thinking it is not quite what it really is but, uhm, I, I think I was thinking of the fact that **here I am, not even at the point I'd reached yesterday. I'd forgotten some of the things and can't put it together again.** And then I thought, it's almost like **I want to ask you, "Doesn't this drive you crazy, that, sort of, I go forward a bit and then go back more?"** Uhm, and I suppose at first I was thinking that—(*Analyst **laughs** first and then she **laughs** too.*)
> / Is that as transparent to you as it is to me? /
> Yeah, well, **I wanted to drive you crazy.** (***laughs***)
> / Of course! /
> But first I was thinking, oh, I wanted you to say, "Oh no!" sort of, "I understand," or something.

Again, her joining in with the analyst's laughter, coupled with her own laughter [POS ME] while acknowledging NEG IT wishes ("I wanted to drive you crazy"), signaled with POS ME emotions the fulfillment of her wishes. Of course, her latent anxiety also was reflected in her immediate undoing ("I wanted you to say, 'Oh, no!'"), but only after this dramatic realization and expression of her beginning acknowledgment of and satisfaction in her fighting and resistance.

The answer to the question posed by the first change event, "Freedom to do what?" is provided by the second change event. Part of her freedom was, just as we anticipated, to disagree, to criticize, to be antagonistic, to fight, in short, to be as aggressive and demanding and as uncaring for the consequences as she had described her own parents in Hour 1! The analysis of the dream that preceded the first change event led us to postulate that the patient's Task in the analysis, to say everything (and anything) out loud, perfectly matched her own Goal to be free and, far from being an onerous order that she had to obey, was implicit permission to end up saying, "Doesn't this drive you crazy?" But the other part of her freedom was to enjoy saying it, to enjoy feeling that the analyst was stuck with her and could not abandon her, as she had repeatedly feared that her parents could do. This is exactly what the emotion theory stipulates: The pleasure (POS ME emotion) functions as a belief that the wishes (in this case negative appetitive) have been fulfilled.

Three questions remain to be answered. First, is there any independent evidence that a transference neurosis in which the second change event was embedded did in fact occur? Second, is there any independent evidence for the fact of the kinds of changes in emotions implied by the analysis of the two change events? Third, is there any evidence that might suggest a possible cause for the patient's ability to achieve her wish to be free and to express her powerful negative appetitive wishes? Evidence relevant to these questions is presented in the next two sections.

Other Empirical Evidence for Change

The Development and Resolution of the Transference Neurosis

Although it is very difficult to be precise about the beginning and end of a transference neurosis (and thus certify its existence), an independent investigation of this case helps us estimate the boundaries. In a study designed to describe systematically the course of this psychoanalysis, Jones and Windholz (1990) selected as data seven blocks of ten sessions each, beginning with hours 1–10 and ending with hours 936–945. Their measures were 100 Psychotherapy Process variables that had been carefully selected in previous studies to describe fundamental characteristics of both the therapist's and the patient's behavior as well as their interactions. Their method was to have judges read through each of the 70 randomly ordered verbatim transcripts and then do Q-sorts of the variables on each session. Among the many results they reported for this case were patterns of statistically highly significant changes in certain variables over the course of the analysis. Of particular interest here are the changes they reported between two blocks covering the early third to the early fourth year of the analysis and between two blocks covering the early fifth to the beginning sixth year. They concluded that the patterns of increases and decreases that they found were important evidence for a "transference neurosis."

Here is a partial listing[19] of statistically significant variable changes from Hours 429–438 to 596–605, covering the period of the developing transference neurosis:

Variables that increased from the earlier to the later block:
Patient resists examining thoughts, reactions or motivations related to
    problems.
Patient has difficulty beginning the hour.
Patient is distant from her feelings.
Silences occur during the hour.
Patient experiences discomforting or troublesome painful affect.

Variables that decreased:
Patient is introspective and readily explores thoughts and feelings.
Patient brings up significant issues and material.
Patient talks of being close to or needing someone.

The following selected significant variable changes occurred between the blocks of Hours 765-774 and 936-945, the period of the beginning resolution of the transference neurosis:

Variables that increased during the resolution:
Patient's dreams and fantasies are discussed.
Patient seeks greater intimacy and closeness with analyst.
There is an erotic quality to the therapy relationship.
Love and romance are discussed.
The analytic relationship is discussed.

Variables that decreased:
Patient is self-accusatory and expresses shame or guilt.
Patient experiences painful affect.
Patient has difficulty understanding the analyst's comments.
Patient verbalizes negative feeling toward analyst.
Patient rejects the analyst's comments and observations.
Patient is anxious and tense.

Taken together, these changes appear to be evidence for the clinical changes that preceded and followed the second change event. The judgment of Jones and Windholz—that they constitute substantial evidence for the development and resolution of a transference neurosis—is entirely consistent with my position.

Changes in the Distribution of Emotion Categories

The sessions chosen to study the expression of emotions were picked independently of the analysis of the change events. They included a sample of three each of early, middle, and end hours that had already been selected for a study of the Frame structures that Teller and I had discovered in the same case (Teller & Dahl, 1981, 1986). The early hours chosen were 5, 8, and 38. Hour 5 has been extensively and intensively studied for other reasons (Bucci, 1988; Dahl, 1988; Dahl & Teller, in press; Hoffman & Gill, 1988; Luborsky & Crits-Christoph, 1988; Teller, 1988) and has been published as "The Specimen Hour" (Anonymous, 1988). Hours 8 and 38 were picked because they contained dream reports for use in an entirely different study and thus were handy. The middle hours, 726, 727, and 728, were chosen because, as indicated above, they occurred in the middle of the transference neurosis, just before the analyst's summer vacation at the end of the fourth year. The end hours, 1112, 1113, and 1114, were simply the last 3 hours of the psychoanalysis and thus of intrinsic interest.

For the present study, I wanted to determine what differences, if any, there were in the distribution of the patient's expression of different emotions during these three phases of the treatment. Transcripts of these nine sessions were examined for the occurrence of manifest expressions of emotions as specified by the theory summarized above, including emotion labels, references to consummatory behaviors (e.g., fighting as a consummation of anger) and typical motor expressions identified in the transcriber's comments (e.g., nervous chuckles, laughing, and crying).

The procedure was as follows: One experienced judge identified manifest expressions (labels, consummatory behaviors, enactments) of each of the 12 categories (8 main + 4 intermediate) of emotions in each of the nine transcripts. Typical expressions, included here under the main four categories, were:

POS IT: approval, close, friendly, intimate, support, surprised

NEG IT: angry, annoyed, argue, criticism, disapprove, fight, find fault, subdue, bothered, afraid, horrified, shocked

POS ME: fine, good, quiet, free, happy, laughing, enthusiastic, strong, successful

NEG ME: inadequate, inferior, sad, stupid, awful, guilty, uncomfortable, anxious, distressed, disturbed, tense, upset

Then two judges (one experienced and one inexperienced) independently classified each expression into one of just the four major categories—POS IT, POS ME, NEG IT, and NEG ME emotions—with a reliability of .76 (kappa) for a subsample of 292 expressions.[20]

Figure 6.2 is a graph of the mean frequency of each emotion category per 1,000 patient words and Table 6.4 shows the main results of a $2 \times 3 \times 2$ factorial analysis of variance (ANOVA) of the data.[21] There is an overall difference ($p < .01$) in total emotions over time with significant linear ($p < .05$) and quadratic ($p < .025$) trends and with the lowest total expression in the middle hours. There is also an overall difference ($p < .001$) in the NEG/POS ratio of 2/1, confirming what clinicians already know, that patients do not usually enter treatment to talk about how good things are.

More interesting are the two significant interactions. The IT/ME by TIME interaction ($p < .001$) is evident in the graph. Although NEG IT and ME emotions are both high in the early sessions, the NEG ME emotions drop significantly during the middle sessions and then rise to their earlier level at the end ($p < .001$), while the NEG IT emotions increase in the middle hours ($p < .025$) and then significantly drop at the end ($p < .001$). The POS ME emotions, which drop in the middle, rise again at the end ($p < .06$), while the POS IT emotions are not significantly different in the three phases.

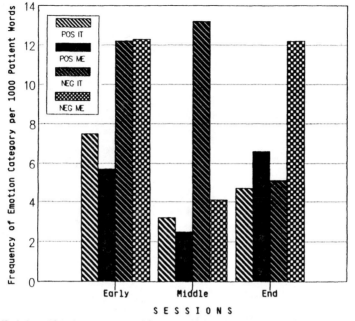

FIGURE 6.2. The distribution of four major emotion categories—POS IT and ME and NEG IT and ME—over time. $N = 3$ each of early, middle, and end sessions from the psychoanalysis. The measures are of the frequency of expression of each category per 1,000 patient words.

It should also be noted that the breakdown of the NEG IT category into REPULSION TO IT and REPULSION FROM IT shows the Anger/Fear ratio jumping from 2/1 in the early hours to 9/1 during the middle hours and back to 5/2 at the end, which makes clear that it is the patient's REPULSION TO IT (anger and fighting) that accounts for the increase in NEG IT emotions during the middle hours and confirms the conclusions derived from the second change event analysis. In fact the data at this point appear to support the conclusions reached on the basis of both change events. The patient's predominant early emotions are both NEG IT and NEG ME, while the main emotions during the middle transference neurosis hours are NEG IT.

What then are we to make of the other striking finding that appears to go against the TCH, namely, the large and significant rise in the NEG ME emotions at the end of the treatment? The answer to this apparent anomaly lies in the simple fact that high level of NEG ME emotions at the end reveals the patient's major preoccupation with *sadness* and with feelings of *wanting to cry* over the imminent prospect of termination. These emotions reflect her belief that she will no longer be able to satisfy her wishes

TABLE 6.4. The results of a $2 \times 3 \times 2$ factorial design analysis of variance of two emotion dimensions, Valence (POS/NEG) and Orientation (IT/ME), over three TIME periods (early, middle, and end)

Source	SS	df	MS	F	p
A (POS/NEG)	208.8	1	208.8	31.6	<.001
B (TIME)	82.3	2	41.2	6.2	<.01
C (IT/ME)	1.8	1	1.8	0.3	ns
A × B (POS/NEG × TIME)	15.1	2	7.6	1.2	ns
A × C (POS/NEG × IT/ME)	0.5	1	0.5	0.1	ns
B × C (TIME × IT/ME)	135.4	2	67.7	10.3	<.001
A × B × C (POS/NEG × TIME × IT/ME)	75.3	2	37.7	5.7	<.01
Within hours (ERROR)	157.8	24	6.6		
Total	677.0	35			

Note. The scores for each session were expressed as a rate: the number of emotion expressions per category per 1,000 patient words spoken in a session. $N = 3$ sessions per time period.

about the analyst, that she has to separate and give up the relationship with him. Although her emotional response conveys a belief that certain wishes cannot be satisfied, there is clearly a significant clinical difference between a depression in which major wishes are believed unsatisfiable and sadness at giving up a satisfying relationship.[22]

The congruence between the patient's Task to say everything out loud and her stated Goal to be free seems clear enough already. The question now is: What is the connection, if any, between this congruence and the therapist's technical stance, that is, the "analytic attitude"? Jones and Windholz's study sheds light on this question. Among their 100 variables were a number of analyst characteristics that did not significantly increase or decrease across the entire set of seven blocks of hours. Here is their list of the most and least characteristic:

Variables most descriptive:
Analyst is neutral.
Analyst accurately perceives therapeutic process.
Analyst conveys a sense of nonjudgmental acceptance (vs. disapproval, lack of acceptance).
Analyst is confident or self-assured (vs. uncertain or defensive).
Analyst emphasizes patient feelings in order to help her experience them more deeply.

Variables least descriptive:
Analyst acts to strengthen defenses.
Analyst is directly reassuring.
Analyst adopts a supportive stance.

Analyst's own emotional conflicts intrude into relationship.
Analyst gives advice and guidance (vs. defers even when pressed).

Taken together this set of characteristic analyst behaviors captures much of the "analytic attitude." This attitude of neutrality and abstinence is taught to every candidate; maintaining it was a central goal for the psychoanalyst who conducted this analysis. Above all, he wanted to demonstrate that it was possible to engage in a characteristic psychoanalytic process while tape-recording. Not too long ago, Schlesinger (1974), speaking for a great many practicing psychoanalysts, seriously wondered if this was possible. Here we have evidence that it is.

Task–Goal–Technique Congruence

If we can accept for the moment that the above measures truly represented the essence of the analyst's treatment "technique," then it seems quite clear that in this case there was a nearly perfect fit between the analyst's Technique and the patient's Task and Goal. This attitude, to the extent that it was characteristic of the analyst's behavior, would have provided a climate of maximum freedom and minimal interference with the patient's expression of powerful negative appetitive wishes and permitted her finally to satisfy them in the transference relationship with pleasure. Only then could she be expected to give them up and go on to other goals in her life. Of course it is clear that this one case does not prove the hypothesis, but it does suggest the importance of further testing of the TGT Congruence hypothesis.

In a commentary titled "Give Choice a Chance in Psychotherapy Research" (Dahl, 1983a), I proposed an experimental design for outcome studies where, after initial assignment to either an experimental or control group, experimental patients would be offered a choice of both type of treatment and therapist, whereas the control patients would be randomly assigned to treatments and therapists. The TGT Congruence hypothesis suggests that it is time to extend the notion of giving choice a chance to single-case designs. In each case, measures of TGT Congruence would be used as predictors of the outcome measures derived from the TCH, namely, the POS ME and NEG ME emotions related to the patient's significant somatic and emotional appetitive wishes.

CONCLUSION

Since so much of this examination of two change events has involved "listening" to the patient's struggles in the treatment, it seems only fitting to end with a passage in which the patient spontaneously described her own perception of the analyst's attitude toward her. In Hour 1112, while summing up the roles she had played with the men in her life (e.g., her father, husband, and colleagues at work), the patient said, "I would alternate between being, you know, sort of the cute little girl, or being a real bitch." A bit later the analyst asked:

> / Do you think you have been only, uh, a cute little girl, or a bitch, here? /
>
> (*sigh*) No, but uhm, (*pause*) well, I was going to say, but this is different. And, I suppose in some ways it's not. Because then I start to feel **very sad** thinking it's different, and it's not something that—uhm, you know, **it's something I'm losing**. And then I think, well, why should I, because **really what I've been here is just myself**. And sometimes I've been both those things. But I guess, you know, I've been able to be other things, too. And uhm, but still, it is different. I don't know w—, quite what makes it different. Whether it's that, in a way, **your not reacting, somehow, you know, in any kind of a personal way, your personal feelings, or just what**. But somehow, it just seems like it's different. (*pause*)
>
> I don't know, (*sigh*) now I'm coming to something that I, i __, seems like it's **very conflicting**. Because I'm thinking, well, it's also, maybe **it's what I meant by your not reacting personally, or according to your own feelings. Uhm, but I was thinking, well I can trust you, or count on you, you know. If I say that I'm having fantasies about you sexually, you will not take me up on it and think that's an invitation to go ahead and have an affair with me or something. Which I've always had, you know. I might have those fantasies, but I didn't want it to happen.**

Recall for a moment a question raised but left unanswered at the end of the first change event: Why should the patient have been "afraid of fantasizing" about the analyst and at the same time bothered by his taking on "an importance" that was "just fantasy"? Now she has given us an answer. At the time of Hour 38 she was not yet able to "count on" or "trust" the analyst not to take her fantasies as "an invitation to go ahead." She wanted her wishes fulfilled and not fulfilled at the same time. In the end, in the case of her sexual appetites, she settled for fulfillment in fantasy rather than reality, and in the case of her emotional appetites of anger, fulfillment in the transference relationship. These outcomes are what the analytic attitude was designed to permit.

Near the end of the session she continued:

> I don't know, I was thinking again of that initial feeling today when I felt like **crying**, uhm, and then, you know, my thinking about **crying** the last day. A_ and uhm, there's something about it that I

don't want to do, and uhm, I think it's because i_ it's sort of, if I'm feeling like **crying**, i_ it's, you know, out of trying to say, "**Don't leave me**," or uhm, last night, I guess right before the end, I was saying, "**Don't forget me**." And, and uh, maybe that's why in particular I felt like **crying** last night, I don't know. Uhm, but it's a, it's, I don't know, it just seems to come out of **feeling dependent** somehow. Uhm— (*silence, sigh, 3-minute silence*)

Well, I guess what I was just mainly thinking is, thinking that I think I want to **feel independent**. And then, I don't, I w—, just may be that this doesn't even exist, but I was thinking, well probably in a lot of different animal families at some point the parent animals uhm, push the young ones when they're ready, you know, sort of out of the nest. And uh, (*sigh*) the, you know, I was sort of imagining the kind of feeling they might initially have. But then, they would be able to be **independent**. And I don't even know if there's some uhm, factual information that I have read about that, or whether I'm just thinking it might be. And then I was thinking about a book on wolves that I've read, and they are not that way, unlike what a lot of people had thought. But uhm, (*sigh*) I don't know, I guess I was then just sort of thinking, well, I **feel ready**, even if I'm **feeling reluctant**.

/ Well, it seems like a good note to stop on today. /

And a good place to end our investigation as well.

ACKNOWLEDGMENT

I wish to thank Virginia Teller for her many helpful comments during both the reformulation of my theory and the investigation of the change events.

NOTES

1. See Dahl (1977, 1978, 1979) and Dahl and Stengel (1978) for the previous versions as well as background and support for the major claims. For a fuller account of the revised theory see Dahl (in preparation).

2. These terms from our common sense were first given a more formal status in Heider's (1958) "commonsense" or "naïve" psychology and later in intentional system theories, for example, Dennett (1978, 1987, 1988), Searle (1983), and many others.

3. Among those who have proposed n-dimensional schemes, only de Rivera among emotion researchers, along with Descartes (see Stone, 1980) and Freud, has stressed the importance of the Subject–Object (IT–ME) dimension. No theoretical

(as distinguished from commonsense) rationale for this distinction is provided by any other major theory except perhaps that of Pribram and Melges (1969). The terms "orientation," "valence," and "activity" provide abstract terms intended to capture the essential properties of the dimensions.

4. Of the 371 words, 65% were decided at $p < .05$ on all three dimensions; for 153 words the splits were significant at $p < .001$ on all three dimensions (a joint chance probability of less than 1 in 1 billion). An appendix to Dahl and Stengel (1978) lists all the words and the splits on each dimension.

5. Brenner claimed (1974) that each emotional experience is unique and consists of pleasure or unpleasure, plus a related idea, a view that is not consistent with these data.

6. Such as behavioral expressions (Darwin, 1872), instincts (McDougall, 1923), facial expressions (Ekman, 1973; Izard, 1971, 1977; Tomkins, 1970), and others (Davitz, 1969; Plutchik, 1962).

7. This definition is adapted from Freud's (1900/1953) famous seventh chapter of *The Interpretation of Dreams* (cf. Dahl, 1965, 1978, 1979, 1983b), in which he proposed two very different models of motivation: one based on wishes, a very modern-looking cognitive model, and the other on instinctual energy. It was the instinctual energy model that survived as the standard for psychoanalysis and has given rise to the current "crisis" of theory. How different psychological history might have been had the cognitive model survived instead! I have been trying to resurrect it since 1965.

8. Koob and Bloom (1988, p. 720), as a result of their studies of "cellular and molecular mechanisms of drug dependence," have in a sense reinvented the wheel (*wish* in this case) in their attempt to account for the intense craving experienced by opiate and cocaine addicts undergoing withdrawal. They wrote, "If craving is defined as a memory for the pleasant aspects of the drug, then . . . various external and internal signals can act as discriminative stimuli for eliciting the memory of drug experiences and these memories may serve as motivational factors in drug recidivism."

9. Frijda (1986, p. 38) claims that "joyful behavior has no function in the sense that angry or fearful behavior has. It has no purpose, it is just there." So here we have clearly contradictory hypotheses.

10. These are examples of her parents' NEG IT appetites directed toward the patient; her NEG ME responses of being upset and tense represent her belief that she probably could not consummate her counter-NEG IT-appetitive wishes of anger and/or fear toward them.

11. Before the dream she was **afraid** of fantasizing about the analyst, of his becoming too important to her. Then she dreamed of feeling **discomfort** at a party where the analyst observed that she was **withdrawing, hunching up, hiding**; he told her to stop what she was doing; she felt **not nervous** and that he was **not harsh**,

cared, was gentle, and comforting. After the dream she was upset and it bothered her that she had used fantasy to escape.

12. Although I have labeled this feeling of freedom a "change" event, it should be clear that I make no claim about the permanence of the patient's new feeling; the immediate data clearly establish its temporary, even momentary, nature. But, as we shall see, the freedom was nonetheless a harbinger of the future.

13. Although this was the analyst's only use of the word "freedom" in the first 38 hours, one can speculate on a question that Grünbaum (1984, 1986) might raise: Did his use of the term inadvertently function as a suggestion and shape all the patient's subsequent associations that led up to this change event? Alternatively, did it presciently code the latent wishes and beliefs in her initial silences and concern about talking "too quickly" without stopping to "think first" when she felt uneasy? This study cannot definitively decide between these alternatives. Nonetheless I believe that the line of reasoning and arguments that offer a solution to the clinical puzzle also implicitly support the second over the first of these hypotheses.

14. That dreams are constructed is a premise that I simply take for granted.

15. Persuaded by what? The analyst's conduct of the analysis? Outside events? This of course is the key causal question, the one that researchers need to continue to address. How can we establish in single-case designs firm causal links between what the therapist does and changes in the patient?

16. Weiss, Gassner, and Bush (1986, p. 161) focused on her "wishes to be strong, independent, loving, and uninhibited."

17. Although it is difficult to be precise about the beginning and end of a transference neurosis, an independent study of this case by Jones and Windholz (1990), reported below, helped establish the boundaries.

18. When a word of interest occurred that was not among those classified by Dahl and Stengel's (1978) judges, I have searched Figure 3 and the Appendix in that publication for likely synonyms.

19. I have included only those variables that reflect either some defensive operation or the expression of an emotion as specified by the theory.

20. POS IT and NEG IT are shorthand for ATTRACTION and REPULSION TO/FROM IT. In two earlier studies the emotion categories were used to assess the expression of emotions in psychoanalytic and psychotherapy transcripts. The average reliability attained by Silberschatz's (1978) two trained judges, $r_2 = .82$, was comprised of coefficient alphas computed separately for the eight main categories, with a low of .63 for fear [REP FROM IT] and a high of .94 for anxiety [ACT NEG ME]. Seidman's (1988) coefficient alphas for two trained judges ranged from a low of .62 for guilt [NEG ME] to a high of .86 for love [ATT TO IT] and .94 for lack of emotion.

21. The statistical analysis was based on a model by Edwards (1964, pp. 201-205, 240-247), which assumes independence of the error components in the sampled

units (hours in this study). The independence of successive observations was established by three intercorrelation matrices of the four dimensions: (1) a first-order correlation, $n = 9, \bar{r} = .05$; (2) a +1 lagged autocorrelation, $n = 8, \bar{r} = .05$; and (3) a -1 lag, $n = 8, \bar{r} = -.02$. Only 1 of the 18 correlations reached the .05 significance level.

22. My theory does not offer a principled explanation of the difference between sadness and depression. Although both reflect beliefs that important wishes are unsatisfiable, it seems likely that their clinical differences are the result of differences in defenses that are evoked. To experience sadness and to know what wishes cannot be satisfied is clearly quite different from being depressed and not knowing what wishes are at stake and judged unfulfilled. Nonetheless, the obvious clinical distinction between depression and sadness calls for further study.

REFERENCES

Anonymous. (1988). The specimen hour. In H. Dahl, H. Kächele, & H. Thomä (Eds.), *Psychoanalytic process research strategies* (pp. 15-28). New York: Springer-Verlag.

Brenner, C. (1974). On the nature and development of affects: A unified theory. *Psychoanalytic Quarterly, 43*, 532-556.

Bucci, W. (1988). Converging evidence for emotional structures: Theory and method. In H. Dahl, H. Kächele, & H. Thomä (Eds.), *Psychoanalytic process research strategies* (pp. 29-49). New York: Springer-Verlag.

Caston, J. (1986). The reliability of the diagnosis of the patient's unconscious plan. In J. Weiss, H. Sampson, & the Mount Zion Psychotherapy Research Group, *The psychoanalytic process: Theory, clinical observations, and empirical research* (pp. 241-255). New York: Guilford.

Dahl, H. (1965). Observations on a "natural experiment": Helen Keller. *Journal of the American Psychoanalytic Association, 13*, 533-550.

Dahl, H. (1977). Considerations for a theory of emotions. Introduction to: J. de Rivera, *A structural theory of emotion (Psychological Issues*, Monograph 40, pp. 1-8). New York: International Universities Press.

Dahl, H. (1978). A new psychoanalytic model of motivation: Emotions as appetites and messages. *Psychoanalysis and Contemporary Thought, 1*, 375-408.

Dahl, H. (1979). The appetite hypothesis of emotions: a new psychoanalytic model of motivation. In C. E. Izard (Ed.), *Emotions in personality and psychopathology* (pp. 201-225). New York: Plenum.

Dahl, H. (1983a). Give choice a chance in psychotherapy research. *Behavioral and Brain Sciences, 6*, 287.

Dahl, H. (1983b). On the definition and measurement of wishes. In J. Masling (Ed.), *Empirical studies of psychoanalytical theories* (pp. 39-67). Hillsdale, NJ: Analytic Press.

Dahl, H. (1988). Frames of mind. In H. Dahl, H. Kächele, & H. Thomä (Eds.), *Psychoanalytic process research strategies* (pp. 51-66). New York: Springer-Verlag.

Dahl, H. (in preparation). *A cognitive motivational theory of emotions for psychotherapy research.*

Dahl, H., & Stengel, B. (1978). A classification of emotion words: A modification and partial test of de Rivera's decision theory of emotions. *Psychoanalysis and Contemporary Thought, 1,* 269-312.

Dahl, H., & Teller, V. (in press). Characteristics and identification of frames. In N. Miller, L. Luborsky, J. Barber, & J. Docherty (Eds.), *A handbook for dynamic psychotherapy research and practice—a how to do it guide.* New York: Basic Books.

Darwin, C. (1872). *The expression of the emotions in man and animals.* London: John Murray.

Davies, J. (1988). *The development of emotional and interpersonal structures in three-year-old children.* Doctoral dissertation, Derner Institute for Advanced Psychological Studies, Adelphi University.

Davitz, J. (1969). *The language of emotion.* New York: Academic Press.

Dennett, D. (1978). *Brainstorms: Philosophical essays on mind and psychology* (pp. 3-22). Cambridge, MA: MIT Press.

Dennett, D. (1987). *The intentional stance.* Cambridge, MA: MIT Press.

Dennett, D. (1988). Précis of the intentional stance. *Brain and Behavioral Sciences, 11,* 495-546.

de Rivera, J. (1962). A decision theory of emotions. *Dissertation Abstracts International.* (University Microfilm No. 62-2356)

Deutsch, J. A., & Deutsch, D. (1966). *Physiological psychology.* Homewood, IL: Dorsey Press.

Edwards, A. (1964). *Experimental design in psychological research.* New York: Holt, Rinehart & Winston.

Ekman, P. (Ed.). (1973). *Darwin and facial expression: A century of research in review.* New York: Academic Press.

Freud, S. (1953). The interpretation of dreams. In *Standard Edition* (Vols. 4 & 5). London: Hogarth Press. (Original work published 1900)

Freud, S. (1957). Instincts and their vicissitudes. In *Standard Edition* (Vol. 14, pp. 117-140). London: Hogarth Press. (Original work published 1915)

Frijda, N. (1986). *The emotions: Studies in emotion and social interaction.* Cambridge, England: Cambridge University Press.

Greenberg, L. S., & Safran, J. D. (1987). *Emotion in psychotherapy: Affect, cognition, and the process of change.* New York: Guilford.

Grünbaum, A. (1984). *The foundations of psychoanalysis: A philosophical critique.* Berkeley: University of California Press.

Grünbaum, A. (1986). Précis of the foundations of psychoanalysis: A philosophical critique (with commentary). *Behavioral and Brain Sciences, 9,* 217-284.

Heider, F. (1958). *The psychology of interpersonal relations.* New York: Wiley.

Hoffman, I., & Gill, M. (1988). A scheme for coding the patient's experience of the relationship with the therapist (PERT): Some applications, extensions, and comparisons. In H. Dahl, H. Kächele, & H. Thomä (Eds.), *Psychoanalytic process research strategies* (pp. 67-98). New York: Springer-Verlag.

Izard, C. (1971). *The face of emotion.* New York: Appleton-Century-Crofts.

Izard, C. (1977). *Human emotions.* New York: Plenum.

Jones, E., & Windholz, M. (1990). The psychoanalytic case study: Toward a method for systematic inquiry. *Journal of the American Psychoanalytic Association, 38,* 985–1009.

Koob, G., & Bloom, F. (1988). Cellular and molecular mechanisms of drug dependence. *Science, 242,* 715–723.

Loewald, H. (1980). The transference neurosis: Comments on the concept and the phenomenon. In *Papers on psychoanalysis* (pp. 302–314). New Haven, CT: Yale University Press.

Lorenz, K. (1965). *Evolution and modification of behavior.* Chicago: University of Chicago Press.

Luborsky, L., & Crits-Christoph, P. (1988). The assessment of transference by the CCRT method. In H. Dahl, H. Kächele, & H. Thomä (Eds.), *Psychoanalytic process research strategies* (pp. 99–108). New York: Springer-Verlag.

McDougall, W. (1923). *Outline of psychology.* New York: Scribners.

Nachman, P., Stern, D., & Best, C. (1986). Affective reactions to stimuli and infants' preferences for novelty and familiarity. *Journal of the American Academy of Child Psychiatry, 25,* 801–804.

Plutchik, R. (1962). *The emotions: Facts, theories and a new model.* New York: Random House.

Pribram, K., & Melges, F. (1969). Psychophysiological basis of emotion. In P. Vinken & G. Bruyn (Eds.), *Handbook of clinical neurology* (pp. 316–342). Amsterdam: North-Holland.

Rice, L. N., & Greenberg, L. S. (Eds.). (1984). *Patterns of change: Intensive analysis of psychotherapy process.* New York: Guilford.

Schlesinger, H. (1974). Problems of doing research on the therapeutic process in psychoanalysis. *Journal of the American Psychoanalytic Association, 22,* 3–13.

Schwartz, R., & Trabasso, T. (1984). Children's understanding of emotions. In C. Izard, J. Kagan, & R. Zajonc (Eds.), *Emotions, cognition and behavior* (pp. 409–437). Cambridge, England: Cambridge University Press.

Searle, J. (1983). *Intentionality: An essay in the philosophy of mind.* New York: Cambridge University Press.

Seidman, D. (1988). *Quantifying the relationship patterns of neurotic and borderline patients in the initial interview.* Doctoral dissertation, Teachers College, Columbia University.

Silberschatz, G. (1978). Effects of the analyst's neutrality on the patient's feelings and behavior in the psychoanalytic situation. *Dissertation Abstracts International, 39,* 3007-B. (University Microfilm No. 78:24277)

Smith, M., Glass, G., & Miller, T. (1980). *The benefits of psychotherapy.* Baltimore: Johns Hopkins University Press.

Sroufe, L., & Waters, E. (1976). The ontogenesis of smiling and laughter: A perspective on the organization of development in infancy. *Psychological Review, 83,* 173–189.

Stone, M. (1980). Modern concepts of emotion as prefigured in Descartes' "Passions of the Soul." *Journal of the American Academy of Psychoanalysis, 8,* 473–495.

Teller, V. (1988). Artificial intelligence as a basic science for psychoanalytic research. In H. Dahl, H. Kächele, & H. Thomä (Eds.), *Psychoanalytic process research strategies* (pp. 163–177). New York: Springer-Verlag.

Teller, V., & Dahl, H. (1981). The framework for a model of psychoanalytic inference. *Proceedings of the Seventh International Joint Conference on Artificial Intelligence, 1*, 394–400.

Teller, V., & Dahl, H. (1986). The microstructure of free association. *Journal of the American Psychoanalytic Association, 34*, 763–798.

Tomkins, S. (1970). Affect as the primary motivational system. In M. Arnold (Ed.), *Feelings and emotions: The Loyola symposium* (pp. 101–110). New York: Academic Press.

Trabasso, T. (1982). The importance of context in understanding discourse. In R. Hogarth (Ed.), *Question framing and response contingency: New directions for methodology of social and behavioral sciences* (pp. 77–89). San Francisco: Jossey-Bass.

Tzeng, O., Hoosain, R., & Osgood, C. (1987). Cross-cultural componential analysis on affect attribution of emotion terms. *Journal of Psycholinguistic Research, 16*, 443–465.

Weiss, J. (1986a). Two psychoanalytic hypotheses. In J. Weiss, H. Sampson, & the Mount Zion Psychotherapy Research Group, *The psychoanalytic process: Theory, clinical observations, and empirical research* (pp. 22–42). New York: Guilford.

Weiss, J. (1986b). Unconscious pathogenic beliefs. In J. Weiss, H. Sampson, & the Mount Zion Psychotherapy Research Group, *The psychoanalytic process: Theory, clinical observations, and empirical research* (pp. 68–83). New York: Guilford.

Weiss, J., Gassner, S., & Bush, M. (1986). Mrs. C. In J. Weiss, H. Sampson, & the Mount Zion Psychotherapy Research Group, *The psychoanalytic process: Theory, clinical observations, and empirical research* (pp. 155–162). New York: Guilford.

Weiss, J., Sampson, H., & the Mount Zion Psychotherapy Research Group. (1986). *The psychoanalytic process: Theory, clinical observations, and empirical research.* New York: Guilford.

Wolff, P. (1966). *The causes, controls and organization of behavior in the neonate. (Psychological Issues,* Monograph 17). New York: International Universities Press.

Section C

Experiential Approaches

Experiential approaches to therapy have traditionally placed greater emphasis on the experiencing and expression of emotions than either the cognitive behavioral or psychoanalytic approaches. In the client-centered tradition, theorists such as Carl Rogers and Eugene Gendlin have emphasized the role of bodily felt experiencing as an important form of knowledge and the maintenance of an ongoing openness to such experiencing as the essence of psychological well-being. Fritz Perls viewed emotion as a biologically adaptive orientation system that continually guides adaptive action. He saw people's attempts to control and/or eliminate their emotions as a primary source of dysfunction potentially associated with the pathology of self-control and self-manipulation.

Two important emphases in the experiential tradition have been on the healing aspects of: (1) accessing and exploring tacit information contained in bodily felt experience and, (2) accessing and expressing emotional experience that has been interrupted. The chapters in this section do an excellent job of teasing out the similarities and differences between these processes and in clarifying the mechanisms underlying both of them.

Engle, Beutler, and Daldrup focus on the use of the empty chair intervention from Gestalt therapy to facilitate the expression of angry feelings that have been interrupted. They attempt to model the processes involved in this change event and to analyze the relevant mechanisms in theoretical terms.

Rice and Greenberg examine two different affective change processes. The first one emphasizes the healing effect of expressing painful, disavowed emotions in the presence of an accepting and validating therapist. The second emphasizes the process of accessing and symbolizing tacit information that is carried in emotional experience.

The final chapter by McGuire attempts to further clarify similarities and differences between emotional change processes that are cathartic in nature versus those that are more oriented toward the symbolization of meaning implicit in bodily felt experience. She explores the change process involved in Eugene Gendlin's focusing procedure and examines the similarities and differences between this and change processes that are more cathartic in nature. McGuire's chapter is then followed by a commentary from Eugene Gendlin in Part III of this volume.

7

Focused Expressive Psychotherapy: Treating Blocked Emotions

DAVID ENGLE
University of Arizona

LARRY E. BEUTLER
University of California at Santa Barbara

ROGER J. DALDRUP
University of Arizona

INTRODUCTION

Focused Expressive Psychotherapy (FEP) is an experiential method for resolving blocked affect. It provides a methodology for finishing the tasks, the abortion of which results in feelings that are restricted and problematic, so that patient's feelings become incorporated into the gestalt of their experience. This therapeutic approach works with the full range of inhibited emotions (grief, sadness, joy, fear, anger), with particular emphasis on the range of emotion that surrounds the aborted expression of anger. The approach is based on the principles of Gestalt therapy as delineated by Perls, Hefferline, and Goodman (1951) and developed by others (Polster & Polster, 1973; Zinker, 1977). However, many of the concepts and techniques are related to other theories, but have been drawn together into a psychotherapy specifically tailored to those persons who have constricted emotions.

FEP'S THEORY OF EMOTION

Since FEP is based upon Gestalt therapy concepts, emotions are placed in the context of a holistic approach to personhood. Emotions are only a part of the changing system of behavioral, cognitive, affective, and sensory experiences that are in interaction with a constantly changing environment.

Gestalt theory does not provide a comprehensive theory of emotion. Mermin, however (1974), has extracted from the work of Perls et al. (1951), what he believes to be the salient principles defining and governing emotion. According to Mermin, emotion is a composite of differentiating sensations (heat in the face, clenched fist), "excitement" (heightened metabolic activity and increased energy), and awareness of the relationship between the organism and the environment of field. The function of emotion in human beings is to return balance to the perceptions of the organism. Perls et al. (1951) consider emotions to be the organism's direct evaluative experience of the organism's environmental field. That is, in Gestalt therapy emotion is regarded as a component of cognition (Greenberg & Safran, 1987). Experience is not mediated by thoughts and verbal judgments, but is immediate and incorporates thoughts and judgments. It is unclear whether this idea is in conformity with the recent concepts of Zajonc (1981, 1984) that "preferences need no inferences." Emotion is also viewed, by the Gestalt authors, as the crucial regulator of action, because it creates the basis for awareness of what is important for the organism and mobilizes energy for action.

Emotion does not reflect physiological change alone, but identifies physiological changes in an environmental context which, Mermin (1974) believes, introduces a cognitive component to the process. Perls took the view that emotions need to be discharged, but was careful to state that mere catharsis is not sufficient for lasting relief of emotional distress. Senselessly discharged emotions will not bring satisfaction. Beneficial discharge must occur in the context of contact with an appropriate object in the environment. Therefore, although FEP is generally based upon Gestalt principles, it must look to other theorists for a comprehensive view of emotion.

Current Work on Models of Emotion

Clinicians are growing in their recognition of a need for models to explain adequately both the nature of emotion and the role it plays in psychotherapy. Discussion and debate by theoreticians have moved toward such an end; witness the discussion about the relationship between cognition and emotion (Lazarus, 1982; Lazarus, Averill, & Opton, 1970; Zajonc, 1980, 1981, 1984). A number of other psychotherapy theorists have also begun to discuss the role of affective factors in personal dysfunction and therapeutic change (Davison, in Goldfried, 1980; Goldfried, 1982; Lang, 1970; Mahoney, 1980; Rachman, 1980).

Greenberg and Safran (1984) have reacted to the ongoing discussion by attempting to delineate different mechanisms by which change in emotional processing can bring about therapeutic change. They propose that affect is important in creating change, and must not be looked up simply as a *dependent variable* in the equation of human functioning. They strongly advocate the view that there is a complex interdependence of thinking, feeling, and action systems, and therapeutically useful models will reflect this interdependence. Greenberg and Safran are more in agreement with Lazarus, Coyne, and Folkman (1982) in proposing that thoughts, emotions and motive (to which they add behavior and physiology) are "fused" in nature.

The viewpoint of Greenberg and Safran is consistent with that proposed by Kaplan and Kaplan (1985). These authors argue that Gestalt therapy is essentially nonlinear; whatever is happening at a given moment is a unitary or holistic relationship involving whatever aspects of the system are currently active. Activity is integral as it occurs. Although language used to described such a process represents it as a linear process, this misrepresents the degree to which every aspect of a person's functioning is simultaneously an aspect of the whole. The Kaplans believe a person is involved in a moment-to-moment process of creating configurations. The person is a continually changing unitary configuration in an ongoing relationship to an ever-changing environment.

FEP accepts the model of emotion articulated by Leventhal (1979). In Leventhal's model, there are three distinct mechanisms operating in the process of emotional experience: (1) a facial–motor mechanism, (2) a schematic or emotion memory, and (3) a conceptual system that stores rules and beliefs about emotional experience. They are arranged in a hierarchical order and operate in an integrated fashion. In the end, emotional experience is not the product of a conscious inferential process, but rather a preattentive, synthetic process through which emotion is constructed from component elements. While Greenberg and Safran (1984) do not see Leventhal's model as all-conclusive, they believe it to be a useful background theory for the discussion of emotion in the context of psychotherapy.

As to the question of whether perception is theory-driven or data-driven, that is, whether perceptual processing takes place from the top down (guided by concepts, expectations or schemata) or from the bottom up (guided by stimuli), Greenberg and Safran (1984) articulate our own philosophy that it is more useful to think of emotional processing as proceeding from bottom up and top down with equal ease. Information from the conceptual, schematic, and perceptual–motor level may be thought of as constantly feeding into the emotional process simultaneously rather than being linearly or unidirectionally related. Viewed from this perspective, "it is not entirely accurate to conceptualize affect and cognition as operating as two independent systems in human experience, one of which precedes and causes an occurrence in the other. In a sense, there is no affect without cognition and no cognition without affect" (Greenberg & Safran, 1984, p. 569). Any approach that focuses upon either cognition or affect, to the exclusion of the other, ignores the integral nature of affect and cognition; in fact, separation of "feeling" and "thinking" may actually be a sign of dysfunction.

FEP attempts first to access schematic memory by directing attention to potential sources of the development of those memories (i.e., interactions with parents, spouses, children, or siblings). Therapy then is designed to heighten the intensity and expression of emotion associated with the memories so that new schematic structures can be realized.

Emotions Are Neutral

In contrast to some theories, such as the rational–emotive therapy of Ellis or the cognitive therapy of Beck (Kuiper & MacDonald, 1983), FEP contends that emotions are neither positive nor negative, good nor bad; they simply exist. Consequently value can only be placed upon what is done with emotions, not upon the class or set of emotions being experienced.

People possess the capacity to experience a full range of opposite emotions, directed toward a variety of objects in the environment. Plutchik (1980) believes emotions can be thought of as polarities of experience in which different emotions represent opposite ends of a continuum, from love to hate, sadness to joy, fear to excitement. FEP assumes that while these polar feelings are actually experienced by everyone, they may not be acknowledged or allowed awareness within some channels of experience. For example, emotions may be experienced at the sensory but not at the cognitive level. Because of social fears (fantasies and predictions) and past histories (schematic memories) people may become unwilling to access the bipolar representation of these experiences. FEP encourages the abandonment of value judgments that inhibit the experience of both poles of each emotion.

Gestalt Formation and Completion

The formation and completion of the gestalt cycle as outlined by Zinker (1977) follows the path of (1) sensation, (2) awareness, (3) mobilization of energy, (4) contact, and (5) withdrawal. When acting freely, a person moves naturally through this cycle, satisfying the needs of the organism in the context of the environment. However, one can interrupt the cycle at any place in the process; a person may have clenched fists and a tightly set jaw (physical sensations), and not allow awareness of these sensations, while another person may be aware of mobilized physical energy, but will not allow that energy to contact the proper object in the environment. "If I express my anger toward him, he may reject me." These interruptions of the expression of emotion are aided by rationalization, intellectualized judgments, and denial. On the other hand, mobilization of the intellectual, physical, and emotional forces can move a person from a state of conflict to a completed gestalt, signified by a state of rest within the organism.

The cycle, which proceeds from sensation to awareness, mobilization, contact, and withdrawal, is governed by the principle of homeostasis. This principle is assumed to apply to emotional systems as easily as it does to biological systems. If there is a natural uninterrupted flow to the cycle, then the need of the organism is aroused and driven to a state of completion. This natural tendency toward completion, if interrupted by injunctions forbidding the expression of certain emotions, for example, leaves one in a state of imbalance where the emotional expression is excluded while the awareness experience still exists. These excluded experiences strain toward integration, intruding into one's current gestalt. Prolonged endurance of such imbalance may cause both physical and psychological stress, necessitating a restructuring of early schematic memories.

Restructuring Schematic Memories

Strategies for recognizing, expressing, or denying emotions are learned in childhood because the child introjects the prescriptions of others, usually parents. Children are dependent upon the environment and have little choice other than to follow the parental (environment) messages. Children make inherent attempts to reconcile the discrepancies among what is told to them about their experience ("Don't be angry.") and what is actually experienced ("I feel angry."). Often those parental messages are sanctions about the expression of feelings. It's difficult for children to throw off introjects because they sense, often correctly, that adults will not approve of them if they do. Therefore, children seek out compromise solutions that are designed to ensure that safety is not threatened. They can choose, at a preattentive state, to deny the event, deny feelings about the event, or convert one affective state for another (e.g., convert hurt and anger to guilt and shame; "I must be bad because my father left").

These childhood experiences create a world view, which is composed of cognitive/affective schemata. A schema is a representation of a specific emotional experience that has taken place in the past, along with key perceptual features that have elicited a particular response to eliciting stimuli (Leventhal, 1979). Schematic processing links these eliciting stimuli to emotional experiences through a type of emotional funneling. Since multiple stimuli are processed through very similar cognitive schemata, the result may be fixed, automatic emotional responses. In order to restructure these fixed schemata, FEP encourages the acknowledgment of intense experience and the broadening of the emotional, physical, and intellectual components of the schematic memory. Theoretically, emotional experiencing takes place at an automatic, *preattentive* level, the components of that experience (stimulus events, reactions, expressive-motor, and conceptual meaning) are synthesized outside focal awareness. When the therapist stimulates the unfinished emotional experience by drawing attention to sensory, muscular and perceptual-motor behaviors, physical changes are produced that bring emotional states alive. Once the emotional state is experienced in full intensity by the patient, the interrupted action tendency can be allowed to complete itself, thereby allowing cathartic relief. At the same time, the intense emotional experience unpacks the preattentive expressive-motor, memorial, stimulus, and conceptual components. The patient then uses current processing capacities to reinspect and reprocess these components, now at an attentive level, into new experientially derived schemata. The re-enactment or reprocessing that takes place both within and following therapy sessions leads to a restructuring of emotional schematic memories, and thereby, to a selective broadening in the internal representation of a whole class of memories (Daldrup, Beutler, Engle, & Greenberg, 1988; Greenberg & Safran, 1987; Kaplan & Kaplan, 1985).

The Particular Problem of Anger

In keeping with a holistic posture, FEP attends to any of a full range of emotions which may be blocked or inhibited (fear, sadness, grief, joy), but particular attention is given to anger because it is especially problematic. Many authors believe that anger affects the sexes differently (Kaplan, Brooks, McComb, Shapiro, & Sodano, 1983; Miller, 1983). They propose that women tend to grow up in a subordinate role in society and develop feelings of weakness, unworthiness, and a sense that they have no right to be angry, while males are given messages to fear not being aggressive enough (Lerner, 1977).

Others dissent from the view that anger affects the sexes differently (Averill, 1983). While sex difference may occur in prevalence rates, practitioners of FEP find that the nature and type of problems of constricted anger affects both males and females similarly. FEP generally concentrates on freeing up overly controlled emotional awareness and expression of anger.

Primary versus Reactive Emotions

FEP subscribes to the view (Greenberg & Safran, 1987) that not all expression of emotion is therapeutically productive. Greenberg and Safran propose a threefold division of emotion, based on clinical assessment, of primary, secondary (reactive), and instrumental emotion. Only *primary* emotions lead to therapeutic effects, while *secondary, reactive* emotions or *instrumental* emotions do not facilitate change. Primary emotions are defined by Greenberg and Safran as those experienced in the moment without any secondary gain. They are "authentic," relatively unenduring (because they are adaptive responses to specific situations), and incorporate body responses and images ("My pain is so deep"). Most often, primary emotions are experienced as anger, sadness or fear, and the patient takes personal ownership or agency of the emotion ("I resent him" . . . "I am so angry I could kill"). Such emotions are usually not in full awareness when someone enters therapy but are underlying or denied, while still seeking to complete the sequence of resolution described earlier.

Secondary, reactive emotions, referred to in FEP as "defensive" emotions, are learned, dysfunctional responses that interrupt the therapeutic process of resolution. The patient exhibits or reports troubling emotional reactions and enlists the therapist's aid in getting free of them. However, if emotions are reactive, that is, the end product in a chain of reactions, the therapist must acknowledge the emotion and then search for the underlying, precipitating factors. Only with training and clinical experience can the therapist differentiate between primary and secondary emotions. Greenberg and Safran caution that to accept and work with these defensive emotions is a therapeutic error, since such emotions act to strengthen the patient's defensive stance. For example, anger can be a reactive emotional response as well as a primary one, and thus used to hide underlying fear, which ultimately must be resolved so that the patient can give up the protective anger.

Finally, instrumental emotions, driven by secondary gain, attempt to blame, change or punish others, in contrast to primary emotions, which are released solely for the purpose of achieving a state of release, that is, to finish unfinished business. Instrumental emotional response are well learned and used by the patient to achieve a sense of security, especially by controlling or manipulating others into getting what one wants. Greenberg and Safran offer a simple test for the presence of either instrumental or defensive emotions. Patients in a state of primary emotion will be less able to respond to therapist interruption (e.g., a request for information) than those in either defensive or instrumental emotions. The goal, when working with primary emotions, is to express the emotion until some sense of closure is achieved, while the goal with defensive emotions is to come to access the underlying precipitating factors and the primary emotions that accompany them. The goal with instrumental emotion is to increase the patient's awareness of the function served by the emotion, rather than increased awareness or arousal of the affect itself. Therefore, it is critical that therapists attend not only to the patient's affect, but also to the form that affective state takes, because it dictates which intervention strategies will be effective. Failure to distinguish among primary, defensive, and instrumental emotions has contributed to the confusion in the debates on the role of emotions in therapeutic change (Greenberg & Safran, 1987).

The Role of Emotional Release in Psychotherapy

Literature examining the benefit of discharge of emotions during psychotherapy is not unified in its results. However, this literature does give essential support to the value of emotional discharge. Nichols and Zax (1977) found that 7 of 11 analogue studies that they surveyed demonstrated emotional discharge to be beneficial. Bohart (1977) and Bohart and Haskell (1978) found that expression of emotion along with cognitive processing produced the most significant psychotherapy outcome.

In a comprehensive review of psychotherapy research over the past 35 years, Orlinsky and Howard (1986) found evidence to support the value of expressive therapy experiences. In a rare long-term study of feeling–expressive therapy, Pierce, Nichols, and DuBrin (1983) found that those who do not express feelings do not change, while also finding that those who show the most catharsis do not necessarily show the most change. The significant criteria for change appeared to be the expression of previously avoided conflict-laden or unconscious feelings, accompanied by a cognitive understanding of the work, and a clear increase above the baseline amount of expressiveness.

In a comprehensive study of psychotherapy procedures representative of experiential and analytical perspectives, Beutler and Mitchell (1981) concluded that experientially oriented therapy was more powerful than analytically oriented therapy for treating both depressed and impulsive patients. The authors cautioned that their feelings must be interpreted within the limitations set by setting, source of funding, and the quasi-random method of assigning patients.

A few studies of expressive psychotherapy have found beneficial changes in physiological measures such as electroencephalogram, blood pressure, and rectal temperature (Karle, Corriere, & Hart, 1973; Woldenberg et al.,1976), and in beta-endorphin levels (Beutler et al., 1987).

Psychosomatic literature generally supports the finding that inhibition of emotion in general, and the containment of anger specifically, may be related to the development of chronic diseases (Achterberg-Lawlis, 1982; Greer & Morris, 1981; Levey, Herberman, Maluish, Schlein, & Lippman, 1985; Spergel, Erlich, & Glass, 1978). The biological mechanisms by which this happens are not yet clear but are under investigation (Pennebaker, Kiecolt, & Glaser, 1988; Shavit, Lewis, Terman, Gale, &

Liebeskind, 1984). It is recommended by some authors that the treatment of such disorders ought to include the expression of emotion as part of the treatment regimen (Beutler, Engle, Oro-Beutler, Daldrup, & Meredith, 1986; Greenberg & Safran, 1987).

WHO IS APPROPRIATE FOR FEP TREATMENT?

FEP may be most beneficial for individuals who have problems because of excessive emotional constriction as manifested in restricted emotional expression and focus. At present, caution is advised about the use of FEP with those whose expression of anger is undercontrolled. Patients can be taught, through FEP, to identify the appropriate environmental provocation of their anger, and to express that anger in controlled, safe ways. Undercontrolled patients often have not made such an identification (lack focus) and indiscriminately express their anger at indirect targets (innocent people) or in inappropriate ways (physical abuse). Such patients may benefit from assistance in identifying the focus of their anger and in learning safe modes of anger expression. One study has demonstrated that FEP has a significant positive effect on prisoners' self-rating of change in a penal setting (Schramski, Feldman, Harvey, & Holiman, 1986). However, it has also been demonstrated that as poorly controlled patients come to feel better during experiential psychotherapy, their acting out behavior may increase (Calvert, Beutler, & Crago, 1988). Therefore, because of the present lack of convincing evidence, caution must be exercised with undercontrolled or poorly integrated patients.

Because the emphasis of FEP is upon the failure to resolve interpersonal anger, we believe that FEP also will be most appropriately applied to those who can identify significant others with whom they have aborted interpersonal relationships or with whom they have failed to complete interpersonal experience because of intimidation, fear, hurt, anger, and so on (Daldrup et al., 1988).

THE FIVE-STEP PROCESS OF FEP

The affective change events targeted by FEP are those changes experienced by the patient during resolution of "unfinished business." In order to avoid painful feelings or because of fear of unwanted emotion, people will block their own natural drives toward action. Such a block leads to "unfinished business," that is, incomplete experience and unchanneled excitement. Unfinished business is a state where tension is aroused but not released, excitement mounts but is not discharged, and the flow of need into behavior is interrupted (Greenberg & Safran, 1987). A marker of

unfinished business is established when the individual manifests four behaviors: (1) a *current lively experience* of emotion (anger, sadness, hurt,
or grief), (2) the experience of this emotion is related to a *significant
person*, such as a parent or spouse, (3) the experience and expression of
the alive feeling is *currently interrupted or constricted*, and (4) the
experience of the feeling and its interruption is *presently problematic* for
the person, as indicated by direct acknowledgment or indirect nonverbal
cues. The appearance of these four behavior indices marks the presence of
an affective disturbance amenable to FEP intervention.

Step One: Identification of Focus and Task

The literature is in agreement (Gendlin, 1969, 1981; Mahrer, 1983;
Strupp & Binder, 1985) that the presence of a strong focus in psychotherapy is beneficial to outcome. In FEP, the therapist makes a direct and
straightforward attempt to elicit a response to those areas in a person's life
where there is unfinished business. Although there may be a range of
unfinished situations in a person's life, those found to be most salient for
therapeutic work seem to be unfinished relationships with four groups of
significant others: parents (or parental figures), intimate love relationships
(spouses or lovers), one's children, and one's siblings. This narrowing of
focus helps to heighten the experience of the unfinished issues and clarifies
the nature of the work to be done. This focus is attained in the following
excerpt:

> T1: As I listen to you describe your relationship to your alcoholic
> mother, it seems clear that even though you have not lived with her for
> years, you are still angry with her.
> P1: Yeah, but I don't know what to do. She still calls me from Califor-
> nia and I always end up in a mess at the end of those calls. . . . I tell myself
> that I won't get upset, but it always happens.
> T2: So you are aware of old emotions getting stirred up when you talk
> with her, is that so?
> P2: Right. . . . I feel a bit of it while we are talking.
> T3: What I'd suggest is that you focus on your unfinished issues with her
> right in this session. I believe there are ways to finish old, unfinished business.
> We can start by switching from talking about her, to talking to her.

This invitation to change from "talking about" a person to "talking to"
a person is important in activating the whole of the schematic memory.
Once activated, earlier life experiences with emotions can be re-expe-
rienced and schematic memories attached to those experiences can be
restructured.

Step Two: Commitment to the Work

The second step in the FEP model is to obtain a commitment to enter into an experimental or imagined engagement with a significant other. The therapist is discouraged from proceeding to step three (the working experiment) if the person is clearly unwilling, or if the tone of the commitment is more reluctant than ready. Obtaining a commitment to the process of conflict resolution is rather brief if the patient gives a definite "yes" to a straightforward invitation. But this step can be quite involved if conflict splits or introjections about the expression of emotions are dominant in the patient's presentation. When such issues surface, they must be resolved before attempting additional steps in the process.

> T1: You sound and look as if you are really angry with your ex-wife. Would you like the opportunity of being free of that anger?
> P1: It sure isn't doing me any good. I have felt angry for several weeks, but I can't shake it. I guess I don't know how.
> T2: I believe I can suggest some ways to do it. It would involve asking that you make your ex-wife present in this chair across from you, so that you can express your anger here and now. Are you willing to do that?
> P2: Yes, anything is worth a try. . . . I'm tired of feeling the way I do.
> T3: Just take a moment to make her present to you, and as you do that, notice all that you can about how your body reacts to her presence [inviting notice of benchmarks].

At this point the therapist helps the patient to establish the current psychophysiological experience or "benchmarks." These signs or symbols, typically physical/sensory in nature ("I have a pain in my gut"; "My breath is shallow and I find it hard to swallow"), are elicited from the patient. Benchmarks are mentally filed by the therapist, to be used as assessment points during the next step of the process and at the conclusion of the session.

Step Three: Working through Unfinished Business

Often this work phase utilizes a large part of the session. It is during this phase that the patient experiments with the experience and expression of anger that has previously been prohibited. The therapist's role at this point is to assist the patient effectively to heighten the experience and expression of emotion, so that there is a mobilization of the energy that drives the person toward expression, contact, and release. Some discussion of appropriate interventions will follow later in this chapter. A more thorough discussion can be found in Daldrup et al. (1988).

The working relationship upon which the process of this and the previous steps in treatment are built must be a collaborative one (Orlinsky & Howard, 1986) in which there is a contractual agreement on the nature of therapeutic roles between the patient and the therapist. The contractual agreement must be monitored by the therapist, because one experiment can sometimes evoke work at a deeper level, requiring a new contractual agreement, as when work on anger at one person (e.g., boss or spouse) arouses more poignant work with another person (e.g., parent). An ongoing assessment is achieved by checking continually on the benchmarks and concomitant level of emotional intensity: "As you tell your father those things, tell him also how the black knot in your stomach is doing."

The predominant experiment used in this phase of the work is the classical Gestalt dialogue exercise. This out-loud dialogue is helpful for both the patient and the therapist. The therapist can observe all the verbal and nonverbal behavior characterizing the exchange, while the patient can experiment with the expression of material which is too risk-laden for an actual confrontation.

As the work progresses, the task is to access the schematic memory with its full emotional intensity so that both the prior and present life experience come to bear on the unfinished material, allowing both emotional release and cognitive restructuring of the event. Such work is completed when the benchmarks have changed from unpleasant to acceptable experiences and when the patient professes changes in both emotional arousal and stance toward the significant other. More will be said about this in step four (evaluation).

In the following dialogue, the therapist and patient began working with a conflict or split until it was clear that one side of the split had the same voice and content as the patient's grandmother. At that point they mutually decided to bring grandmother into the empty chair and to address the patient's unfinished business with her. The benchmarks have already been established.

T1: What I'm gonna invite you to do right now is to say to Grandma what you didn't dare say as a kid.

P1 (*to grandmother in empty chair*): You are so mean. I hate you. I do love you, but I hate you. You embarrass me, you dirty old woman. You remind me of death. I don't want to live with you [she has just regressed in age]. You scare me. (*Face looks young and her voice sounds hurt and fearful. She also experiences conflict between love and hate.*)

T2: Try out, "I'm angry at you for scaring me." [Introduces an attempt to help her give up the hurt and find her strength.]

P2: No, I feel scared. [Attempt was premature, and the patient directs the therapist to what is true.]

T3: OK. Feel the fear and express that to Grandma.

P3: I hate being here with you. You constantly talk about dying and death, death, that's it, every day, every day.

T4: "I resent you talking about death every day." [attempt to move her from blaming language to language of ownership]

P4: I resent you talking about death every day. Every day! You talk about how my mother died, and my father died and this one died. You constantly talk about dying yourself. [She has slipped back to "you" language, which means that the expression can be instrumental, rather than primary anger, but then switches to "I" language.] I don't want to talk about dying. I'm a little girl. I want to live! I want to be a child, not somebody just waiting to die. (*Voice is fearful again.*)

T5: How are you doing right now? [an invitation to the patient to monitor her present experience]

P5: I'm all right, just nauseous [new benchmark], like, you know, I just feel all this awful fear.

T6: Do you want to get past this fear?

P6: Yes. [This checks the commitment before introducing an intervention that will grade up the intensity of the experiment.]

T7: I'm gonna ask you to experiment with getting really angry with your grandmother, to give back to her all the anger that you didn't dare express as a kid.

P7: OK.

T8: Tell Grandma what goes on with you when I suggest that to you.

P8: It makes me . . . I want to hit you. I did hit you. Sometimes I pushed you.

T9: Right now, right this moment, what are you experiencing? [bringing awareness to present experience]

P9: I feel like I might hit you . . . but then you will start screaming. [This prediction can block movement toward expressive action.]

T10 [intervening with the prediction]: Well, here tonight is your opportunity to take care of you and not have to pay those awful consequences. You can make her sit here and simply take it from you without retaliating.

P10 (*strikes with bataca*): It feels so strange to hit you. [For a while, with the encouragement of the therapist, the patient works in a deliberate, practicing manner, seeking out the anger beneath the defensive stance of fear. As she experiments with the anger, the usual fearful voice and manner continue to return. Each time the therapist asks her to notice the tone and strength of her voice, and with renewed awareness she strengthens her voice. Slowly the "as if" anger gives way to spontaneous anger.]

T11: Tell her how you are doing right now. [progress check]

P11: I'm getting angry and I feel (*strike*) better when I tell you how I feel. I resent you for taking me (*strike*) and keeping me instead of letting me live with Aunt Edith. And I resent (*strike*) you for never letting me have a pet. I always wanted a (*strike*) dog, something to love . . . and you never let me . . . you always said (*strike*): "Here's the money" and then you took it back.

T12: "And I resent you for that . . ."

P12: Oh . . . I *resented* that. (*strike*) You never let me have anything of my own. I resent you! (*Voice strong, angry, and spontaneous—memories are coming quickly.*)

T13: Just feel it, feel it in your jaw. [Therapist sees her jaw is tight and her teeth are set.] Stay with the anger until you give it back over here and out of your body.

P13: I resent the times that you called me a tramp. (*strike*) I was never a tramp! You always said, "You'll become (*strike*) pregnant." I never did things like that. But you always said that I was no good, a slut.

T14: "And I resent you for that . . ." [looking for the anger attached to the statement]

P14: I resent you for that . . . And I resent you for not trusting me, for not letting me be a young person. I resent you for dragging me to cemeteries to see dead graves. . . . I *resent* that (*repeated heavy blows with the bataca*). . . . I *hated* that. I resent that you always took me to cemeteries and made me think about dead people. (*repeated heavy blows*) That's all you talked about, was dying, dying, dying. I resented you for making me call when I was gone for 20 minutes. I resented you for not trusting me, for worrying constantly about me. I *hated* you when you worried about me.

T15: Tell her how you are doing. [checking on benchmarks and progress]

P15: I just . . . I feel . . . I feel stronger now. I feel stronger. I'm in control, not you.

T16: How do you know that in your body? What do you feel is different? [checking to see if benchmarks are shifting]

P16: I feel like I don't have such a scared feeling in here. (*pointing to chest and stomach*) I'm not shaking like I was. I feel more awake.

T17: Uh-huh. Your voice sounds different.

P17: When I'm awake I feel more adult.

T18: Hmm.

P18: I feel more adult-like.

T19: OK. Sounds like an important thing to notice.

P19: I feel more relaxed. I don't feel anger or resentment right now. [signs that it is appropriate to move toward closure]

T20: Look at your grandmother. Tell her what you just did for you and then say good-bye.

Note: "You" language is indicative of the patient's desire to blame, change, or punish the significant other. This is referred to as instrumental expression of emotion. The word "you" places the focus on the behavior of the other, not on the unresolved emotion of the patient and the expression of affect is used as a manipulative strategy. "I" language, on the other hand, returns the focus to the present unresolved reactions of the patient.

Step Four: Assessment of the Work

At the fourth step of the process, the therapist and patient evaluate the work just completed. The principal assessment is obtained by asking the patient to bring full attention to him/herself and to report all self-awareness. Benchmarks established at the beginning of the work phase are re-examined to determine if these have shifted in any way; unchanged benchmarks may indicate the absence of real therapeutic change. The assessment includes the sensory, the affective and the cognitive domains; that is, the therapist will ask the patient to report on present physical sensations (benchmarks), level of emotional arousal, and new insights or cognitions resulting from the experiments just concluded. This assessment phase also acts as a reinforcement for the future self-monitoring.

Step Five: Homework and Planning for the Future

Therapy is not considered to be an isolated, once-a-week event, but an ongoing effort to effect change. Thus, once the session has been completed, the therapist assists the patient in planning how to utilize the new insights and perspectives in the future outside the session. Sometimes this requires rehearsal to prepare the patient for implementation of newly reorganized approaches to coping with life. For example, the therapist and patient may work out a homework task that will either enhance the work of the session, keep the patient aware of incomplete work, or celebrate a breakthrough achieved in therapy.

PATIENT PERFORMANCE IN FEP

Since FEP attends specifically to the identification and resolution of unfinished business, as indexed by changes in sensory markers, it is important to identify the competencies or performance steps through which the patient will go in order to reach a satisfactory conclusion of his/her work. Researchers have proposed a variety of methodologies for the analysis of the process of psychotherapy (Greenberg & Pinsof, 1986; Rice & Greenberg, 1984).

Greenberg (1984) advocates the use of a task analysis process, which he believes is highly congruent with Gestalt therapy. In general, the task-analysis process identifies a recurring event or marker in psychotherapy and then discerns the performance steps necessary for successful resolution. The first step in the task-analysis process is to develop an ideal model of the changes or steps experienced by the patient in a successful resolution of a common therapeutic issue. Such a model can be developed by combining theoretical constructs of FEP with clinical experience supported by transcripts of sessions identified as "successful." Such an ideal rational model can lead to development of an understanding of probable resolution strategies, which the client uses in an attempt to resolve painful issues, in this case unfinished interpersonal conflict.

Once a theoretical model for resolution of unfinished business has been constructed, the next step is empirical verification of that model. Actual tape transcripts of FEP sessions are compared with the theoretical model. The transcripts of the tapes are divided into transitional segments and the segments are aligned with the model, determining to what extent the model is representative of actual performance. Where there are discrepancies, the theoretical model is amended and other transcripts of successful resolution sessions are again divided into transitional segments and compared with the theoretical model.

At this point, the FEP theoretical model for resolution of unfinished business has been compared with several transcripts of sessions identified as successful resolution sessions and one identified as an unsuccessful resolution session to identify erroneous patient strategies that interfere with therapeutic change. These comparisons have led to a revised working model.

The next stage of work in the development of this task analysis will be actual empirical verification of the model. The transitions identified as discrete stages in the process of therapeutic resolution will have to be supported by the application of appropriate therapy process measures. Although this work is still in progress, the present working model has helped to develop plausible hypotheses about some of the patient's significant change events that must occur for successful resolution of unfinished business.

The FEP working model presented here is in agreement with the theoretical model for resolving unfinished business proposed by Greenberg and Safran (1986). However, our working model has both technical and theoretical differences from the preliminary empirical model of those authors, as will be discussed later. Shown here are both the Greenberg and Safran theoretical model (Figure 7.1) and the present FEP working model (Figure 7.2).

Comparison of Models

As illustrated in Figure 7.1, a theoretical comparison of the theoretical model presented here and the model of Greenberg and Safran suggests

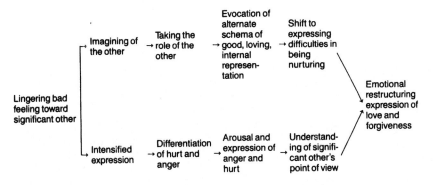

FIGURE 7.1. Preliminary empirical model of finishing incomplete experience. From *Emotion in Psychotherapy* by L. S. Greenberg and J. D. Safran, 1987, New York: Guilford. Copyright 1987 by The Guilford Press. Reprinted by permission.

several areas of essential agreement. In FEP the presence of unfinished business is established by a sensory or behavioral marker. FEP evokes the schematic memories by identifying a focal significant other (internalized object) and by establishing experimental dialogue with the significant other in the empty chair. During this experimental phase the therapist and patient work with facial-motor mechanisms, emotional memories and with the conceptual system of rules and beliefs (schematic components). Finally, resolution in the FEP model is evidenced by changed posture toward the significant other and toward the self, changes in psychophysiological experience when evoking the memory of the significant other, and by the absence of angry affect (restructured schema).

In spite of their similarities, FEP also is distinguished from the model of Greenberg and Safran on several theoretical and technical points. For example, in resolving unfinished business with a significant other, the latter authors propose that the patient identify with the projection of the significant other by taking on that role in the experimental phase of the session. They ask the patient, in the role of the significant other, to explain the thoughts, feelings, and behavior of the significant other to the patient. Taking on the alternate role is thought to increase cognitive understanding and empathy of the patient, thereby facilitating a shift in posture toward the significant other. Our model, on the other hand, proposes that resolution of unfinished interpersonal conflict usually occurs without having to see the world from the other person's eyes. Certainly both models are working with the projected significant other, but we believe that it is not necessary to role-play the projected significant other in order to achieve resolution. In evaluating this difference of procedures, it is apparent that Greenberg and Safran stress a more conscious movement between affect and cognition during the therapy experiment than we do in FEP. We take

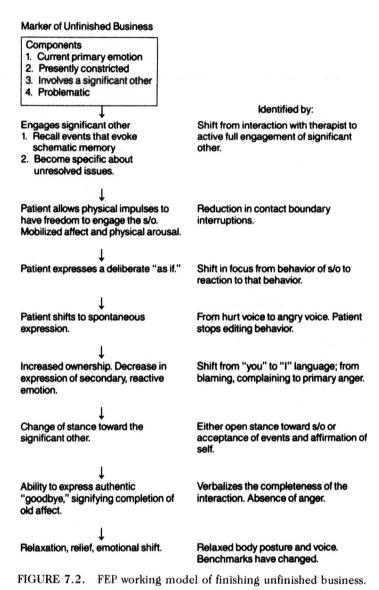

FIGURE 7.2.   FEP working model of finishing unfinished business.

an approach that places trust in the assumption that cognitive restructuring will occur spontaneously, once the toxic, unexpressed anger and resentment have been expressed.

Another difference between these two models resides in how the issue of boundaries between the patient and the significant other are approached. Whereas Greenberg and Safran seem to desire a reduction or softening of boundaries, with the patient working to forgive the significant other as a goal, we do not believe that always desirable or beneficial to encourage a softening of boundaries. For example, those who have been physically or sexually abused by the significant other may not be benefited or motivated to forgive, only to be rid of anger, resentment, and hurt, which inhibit productive living. Therefore, we emphasize the completion of all unfinished, unproductive affect rather than rapprochement. These differences may then lead to variance in the techniques and interventions selected by the two approaches even though both look toward the use of affective material to bring about the restructuring of schematic memories.

Heightened Physiological and Emotional Involvement

Using the working model described in the foregoing, we can follow some of the change events as they occur during the session. First, once an indentification of the four components of a marker of unfinished business has been verified by both the patient and therapist, the therapist can suggest that the patient engage the significant other through the experiment of imagined dialogue. The first request is to make the significant person present. For example, the patient is asked to change from talking to the therapist about father to engage in a direct verbal confrontation with father in the empty chair.

T1: Make your father present in the empty chair and attend to what you experience.
P1: Oh. . . . Just seeing him there makes me want to run. My body feels very tight. It's uncanny . . . I feel like I'm a little kid again.
T2: These are feelings that are difficult to experience, but today, I'm encouraging you to stay with your feelings and experience them as long as you can. Tell him what is going on right now!
P2: I feel like I always do when I talk with you.

When the experiment is established and the patient is no longer talking about an event, but is facing the significant person in that event, an importance change occurs. The patient shifts into a heightened state of emotional arousal simply by engaging in an experimental contact with the significant other, rather than talking about that person. This contact with the significant other through experiment brings vague and ill-defined issues into sharp focus. A general statement ("I hate my father") now is fleshed out with the vivid re-experiencing of critical events which, although now often outside conscious awareness, have driven the sense of hatred.

The most essential therapist intervention at this stage is the introduction of the experiment, which must be done in a way that enhances the opportunity to access the full range of cognitive, physiological, and emotional components. The therapist follows the basic Gestalt guidelines (Harman, 1974; Levitsky & Perls, 1970; Polster, 1985; Zinker, 1977), which promote the development of experiment as facilitative strategy.

Physiological Mobilization toward Action

A second change event appears to occur when the patient continues in an intense, contactful dialogue with the significant other. The continuing dialogue elicits a mobilization of physiological energy, the appearance of which is sometimes more obvious to the therapist than to the patient.

T1: I'm aware that you have restricted your breathing and that your left hand continues to make a fist, as you talk to your son. Tell him what you experience in your body as you talk to him.

P1: Sometimes . . . sometimes, I just want to kill you. I get so damned angry that you are ruining your life. I want to pound some sense into you.

T2: Are you aware of wanting to pound right now?

P2: Yeah, my whole body is full of anger at him. He's my son and I love him, but boy. . . . I am angry.

T3: You don't have to leave here with that anger, you can pick up this foam bat and see what it is like for you to release the anger that you feel right now.

Mobilization of angry impulses allows the patient to both feel and understand the opposing forces that are occurring and that often have occurred in the body before; there is a part of the patient pushing toward release and a part defending against release of emotions. Through the experiential and experimental framework of the session, the patient becomes aware of how unresolved issues are associated with a sensory experience that drives the organism toward expression and completion. "I was never aware of holding my breath before, but now I realize that every time I feel angry, I hold my breath instead."

Appropriate and useful interventions at this stage include an array of therapist questions and statements that help the patient to become aware of heightening emotion, on one hand, and of containing the expression of that emotion on the other. The therapist is careful at this point to help the patient attend simultaneously to two tracks; one is the content track, where patient speak of issues, beliefs, specific events, and so on, and the other is the process track, where the patient learns to attend to the moment-to-moment experience of the self in the context of the unfolding story. "As you say that to your mother, pay attention to what you are doing with your breath—fist—eyes. Then tell your mother what you are experiencing." "Are you aware that after each thing you say to your father that you smile as if trying to soften what you say?" These interventions are relatively straightforward, but often bring the patient to awareness of important but neglected self data, especially about the physiological results of emotional constraint.

Physical Expression

Another important transition takes place if the patient can be encouraged to experiment with overt expression of the inhibited emotion, whether it be anger or some other feeling. When initially engaging in expressing the inner-felt and physically present emotion, the patient goes through a period of *deliberately acting "as if."* They report, when first allowing some release of their experience, feeling strange, embarrassed, or hesitant, and their overt behavior is controlled and restricted, both in voice and physical movement. There is often a tendency to retreat to more familiar and safer behaviors. Initial expressions of anger sometimes seem to surprise the patient, as if he/she cannot believe the intensity of what was just said or expressed physically. If the patients can be encouraged, at this critical stage of the process, to avoid retreating to safer ground and to continue to "act as if" angry, resentful, or hurt, often they begin to experience a spontaneous expression of intense feeling.

The nature of the patient–therapist interaction then changes; the therapist no longer has to be in a "coaching mode," instructing the patient to try sentences or to repeat behaviors that express affect ("hit the cushion again . . . say that again . . . say it with more force," etc.). The patient now moves directly and spontaneously into the expression of the previously constricted emotion and acknowledges and allows the impulses to enter awareness as they occur physically. Breathing, physical expression, verbal language and voice quality all merge into a congruent, spontaneous expression.

P: Boy . . . does this feel good to be giving you back all this crap. . . . I resent you for lying to me about your affair . . . (*voice strong and body expresses anger physically*) I resent you for leaving me all those nights with the kids . . . (*more physical expression*) I resent you for making me believe your work was keeping you away. . . . Oh . . . and I really resent you for not being home on Sarah's birthday. . . . That really pisses me off.

In this example, we can see that the patient no longer needs the coaching of the therapist to express angry feelings. The patient has taken charge of herself and of the therapy session. The therapist can become part of the supportive background for the moment, only occasionally emerging to remind the patient to check on the physical benchmarks, or to reinforce new cognitive understandings as the patient moves through the work; that is, as the patient comes to understand that changes are happening as emotions are being expressed. The therapist re-enters the process more actively when/ if the patient becomes conflicted, finishes with the expressed emotion, or runs out of time for that session. The change from a deliberate "as if" expression to an expression of spontaneous and felt emotions demonstrates the emergence of new strength and self-understanding, and usually is accompanied by vocal changes (e.g., from a hurt to an angry voice).

     P: I didn't believe that I could do that. I have been so scared to let me be angry at you. I just gave most of it back to you and I feel good. And you know what? . . . no guilt . . . I didn't allow you to make me feel guilty about getting angry at you. I know that if more anger comes up, I can take care of me.

     Therapist interventions at this point in the process have a distinctly different flavor from those at earlier stages. A clear agreement about task has been established, along with a commitment to enter a working experiment. The therapist's stance changes from one of eliciting thoughts, feelings, and behaviors to one of directing the action. The therapist now directs the patient to experiment with behaviors that encourage the patient both to stay at the heightened level of emotional arousal and to express that emotional arousal in the context of the experiment. The directive, encouraging stance of the therapist is especially important when the patient is trying on expressive behaviors that previously have been constricted and prevented. Once the patient shifts to a more spontaneous flow of expression, the therapist again can assume a less active role.

Language Change

It is somewhat unclear whether increased ownership of and decreased blame for emotions are developed concomitantly with the development of spontaneous emotional expression. In either case, a language shift does appear to be a characteristic change event in the FEP process. With a shift from blame to ownership, instrumental emotional expression and language, designed to blame, change, or punish a significant other, gives way to primary emotional expression and language.

Stance toward Significant Other

A change in the patient's stance toward the targeted significant other is one genuine indicator that the patient is achieving resolution of the unfinished business. Unfinished interpersonal conflict in a patient generally will manifest itself in an antagonistic posture toward the significant other. As the emotion (anger, resentment, hurt) is expressed toward the targeted person, there is noticeable shift away from the initial posture. The patient may shift spontaneously from the expression of anger/resentment to the expression of appreciations, affection, acceptance. While a shift to a loving, open stance is not likely to happen if the object of the anger expression is an object of general contempt or objective hurt, like, for example, a rapist, the patient may still shift his/her therapeutic posture to one that is an acceptance of the event and an affirmation of the self. Body posture is more relaxed and open, and the angry, hurt, or fearful tone of voice has given way to one that conveys completion.

The change event just described may be confirmed as such by observing the way in which the patient concludes the session, that is, when the therapist instructs the patient to tell the significant other what was just accomplished and then actually to say good-bye. If the unfinished business is resolved in the session, the good-bye can be expected to be clear and straightforward. If only part of the work is done or if the patient has been expressing reactive, secondary emotions rather that primary emotions, the patient's hesitancy may reveal that the letting go that is symbolized in the statement of a good-bye is an issue of conflict.

The therapist needs to be alert to the close of a piece of experimental work to see if closure has actually been achieved. The therapeutic task is to challenge the patient whenever there is evidence that the material comprising the conflict with the significant other is not being addressed directly or feelings have not been fully expressed. The need for more work is evidenced by benchmarks that remain unchanged or are exacerbated after work is finished.

State of Relaxation and Rest

The final change event is achieved when the patient experiences a state of relaxation or relief. When this occurs, nonverbal cues and self-reports confirm that such a change has taken place.

P: I feel tired, like I just did a good workout, but I feel good. It is a nice tired. I'd like to just go to my hammock and be there. My body is mine again. . . . I don't feel all the pain in my gut. . . . you know, I feel very good right now.

At this transition point, the therapist will need to balance the benefits of eliciting information about what cognitive restructuring has occurred against the benefits of reinforcing the newly discovered state of balance and relaxation. Too much therapist–patient talk and information gathering could dissipate these new experiences. Verification procedures are needed to clarify the change events experienced by patients as they move through the FEP process of resolving unfinished business.

RESEARCH ISSUES

Efforts at both process and outcome research for FEP have been underway for several years. Initial efforts concentrated on patients with different pain conditions. A study of patients with rheumatoid arthritis (Beutler et al. 1987) studied the effects of FEP on beta-endorphin levels, and significantly reduced depression levels of the patients. Rheumatology dimensions and pain levels did not change.

A subsequent study of depressed psychogenic pain patients concentrated on standardizing the training of FEP and on the development of valid and reliable measures of therapist compliance and competence. In this latter study, FEP was found to reduce depression, but not to a significantly greater degree than an educational contrast condition. The consistent finding that FEP is effective in reducing depression but does not directly affect pain, lends support to the proposal that pain and depression, while sharing some common mechanism, are essentially distinct phenomena (Beutler et al., 1986). This latter study of depressed psychogenic pain patients also revealed that decreases in pain were most closely associated with family/marital stability (Beutler et al., 1988). That is, when the pain patient and the spouse had a congruent view of the relationship, FEP had a beneficial effect, while those couples exhibiting an incongruent view of the relationship did not improve. The implication for research is that family-oriented rather than individual treatment may be a productive treatment modality for patients with chronic pain.

A recently concluded study developed more refined indicators for predicting differential effects of FEP, cognitive therapy, and a self-help program among patients having unipolar depression. This study provided both a test of FEP efficacy and extended understanding of how patient predispositions and characteristics influence specific treatment programs (Beutler, Mohr, Grawe, Engle, & MacDonald, in press; Beutler, Engle, et al., in press).

CONCLUSION

In this chapter we have described Focused Expressive Psychotherapy (FEP), a therapeutic intervention found useful in working with patients who have blocked affect, especially that associated with unfinished interpersonal issues. FEP is based on Gestalt therapy principles and is supported by a nonlinear theory of emotion described by Leventhal. We have referred to the growing body of literature that describes the importance to positive outcome of emotional expression. The chapter outlines the five-step FEP process: (1) identification of a focus, (2) achievement of commitment, (3) development of experimental dialogue, (4) assessment of completed work, (5) assignment of homework tasks. We compared our working model of the patient's change process with that of Greenberg and Safran and we detailed some of the change steps consistently found in patients who successfully resolve unfinished business. We believe this form of psychotherapy fits comfortably within the widening interest in the role of emotional expression in psychotherapy. FEP continues to show promising results in the alleviation of depression and in the resolution of unfinished interpersonal conflict.

ACKNOWLEDGMENT

Preparation of this chapter was supported by a National Institute of Mental Health Grant MH 33859-03A1.

REFERENCES

Achterberg-Lawlis, J. (1982). The psychological dimension of arthritis. *Journal of Consulting and Clinical Psychology, 50,* 984–992.
Averill, J. R. (1983). Studies on anger and aggression: Implications for theories of emotion. *American Psychologist, 38,* 1145–1160.
Beutler, L. E., Daldrup, R. J., Engle, D., Guest, P., Corbishley, A., & Meredith, K. (1988). Family dynamics and emotional expression among patients with chronic pain and depression. *Pain, 32,* 65–72.
Beutler, L. E., Daldrup, R. J., Engle, D., Oro-Beutler, M., Meredith, K., & Boyer, J. (1987). Effects of therapeutically induced affect arousal on depressive symptoms, pain and beta-endorphins among rheumatoid arthritis patients. *Pain, 29,* 325–334.
Beutler, L. E., Engle, D., Mohr, D. C., Daldrup, R. J., Bergan, J., Meredith, K., & Merry, W. (in press). Predictors of differential response to cognitive, experiential and self-directed psychotherapeutic procedures. *Journal of Consulting and Clinical Psychology.*
Beutler, L. E., Engle, D., Oro-Beutler, M. E., Daldrup, R., & Meredith, K. (1986). Inability to express intense affect: A common link between depression and pain? *Journal of Consulting and Clinical Psychology, 54,* 752–759.
Beutler, L. E., Mohr, D. C., Grawe, K., Engle, D., & MacDonald, R. (in press). Looking for differential treatment effects: Cross-cultural predictors and differential psychotherapy efficacy. *Journal of Psychotherapy Integration.*
Bohart, A. C. (1977). Role playing and interpersonal conflict reduction. *Journal of Counseling Psychology, 24*(1), 125–24.
Bohart, A. C., & Haskell, R. (1978, April). *Ineffectiveness of a cathartic procedure for anger reduction.* Paper presented at the 58th annual convention of the Western Psychological Association, San Francisco.

Calvert, S. C., Beutler, L. E., & Crago, M. (1988). Psychotherapy outcome as a function of therapist–patient matching on selected variables. *Journal of Social and Clinical Psychology, 6,* 104–117.

Daldrup, R. J., Beutler, L. E., Engle, D., & Greenberg, L. S. (1988). *Focused expressive psychotherapy: Freeing the overcontrolled patient.* New York: Guilford.

Gendlin, E. T. (1969). Focusing. *Psychotherapy: Theory, Research, and Practice, 6,* 4–15.

Gendlin, E. T. (1981). *Focusing.* New York: Bantam Books.

Goldfried, M. R. (Ed.). (1980). Psychotherapy process [Special issue]. *Cognitive Therapy and Research, 4,* 269–306.

Goldfried, M. R. (1982). *Converging themes in psychotherapy.* New York: Springer.

Greenberg, L. S., & Pinsof, W. (Eds.). (1986). *The psychotherapeutic process: A research handbook.* New York: Guilford.

Greenberg, L. S. (1984). A task analysis of intrapersonal conflict resolution. In L. N. Rice & L. S. Greenberg (Eds.), *Patterns of change: Intensive analysis of psychotherapy process.* (pp. 67–123). New York: Guilford.

Greenberg, L. S., & Safran, J. D. (1984). Integrating affect and cognition: A perspective on the process of therapeutic change. *Cognitive Therapy and Research, 8,* 559–578.

Greenberg, L. S., & Safran, J. (1987). *Emotion in psychotherapy: Affect, cognition, and the process of change.* New York: Guilford.

Greer, S., & Morris, T. (1981, August). *Psychological response to breast cancer: Eight year follow-up.* Paper presented at the American Psychological Association meeting, Los Angeles.

Harman, R. L. (1974). Techniques of Gestalt therapy. *Professional Psychology, 5,* 257–263.

Kaplan, A. G., Brooks, B., McComb, A. L., Shapiro, E. R., & Sodano, A. (1983). Women and anger in psychotherapy. *Women in Therapy, 2,* 29–40.

Kaplan, M. L., & Kaplan, N. R. (1985). The linearity issue and Gestalt therapy's theory of experiential organization. *Psychotherapy: Theory, Research, and Practice, 22*(1), 5–15.

Karle, W., Corriere, R., & Hart, J. (1973). Psychophysiological changes in abreactive therapy: I. Primal Therapy. *Psychotherapy: Theory, Research, and Practice, 10*(2), 117–122.

Kuiper, N. A., & MacDonald, M. R. (1983). Reasons, emotion and cognitive therapy. *Clinical Psychology Review, 3,* 297–316.

Lang, P. (1979). A bio-information theory of emotional imagery. *Psychophysiology, 16,* 495–512.

Lazarus, R., Coyne, J., & Folkman, S. (1982). Cognition, emotion and motivation: The doctoring of Humpty-Dumpty. In R. W. J. Neufeld (Ed.), *Psychological stress and psychopathology* (pp. 218–239). New York: McGraw-Hill.

Lazarus, R. S. (1982). Thoughts on the relations between emotion and cognition. *American Psychologist, 37,* 1019–1024.

Lazarus, R. S., Averill, J. R., & Opton, E. M., Jr. (1970). Toward a cognitive theory of emotions. In M. Arnold (Ed.), *Feelings and emotions* (pp. 207–232). New York: Academic Press.

Lerner, H. (1977). The taboos against female anger. *Menninger Perspective*, 8(4), 5-11.

Leventhal, H. (1979). A perceptual motor processing model of emotion. In P. Pliner, K. R. Blankstein, & I. M. Spigel (Eds.), *Advances in the study of communication and affect: Vol. 5. Perception of emotions in self and others*. New York: Plenum.

Levitsky, A., & Perls, F. S. (1970). Rules and games of Gestalt therapy. In J. Fagen & I. L. Shepherd (Eds.), *Life techniques in Gestalt therapy* (pp. 93-107). New York: Harper & Row.

Levy, S. M., Herberman, R. B., Maluish, A. M., Schlein, B., & Lippman, M. (1985). Prognostic risk assessment in primary breast cancer by behavioral and immunological parameters. *Health Psychology*, 4(2), 99-113.

Mahoney, M. (1980). Psychotherapy and the structure of personal revolutions. In M. Mahoney (Ed.), *Psychotherapy process: Current issues and future directions* (pp. 157-180). New York: Plenum.

Mahrer, A. R. (1983). *Experiential psychotherapy: Basic practices*. New York: Brunner/Mazel.

Mermin, D. (1974). Gestalt theory of emotion. *The Counseling Psychologist*, 4(4), 15-20.

Miller, J. B. (1983). *The construction of anger in women and men*. A work in progress, The Stone Center, Wellesley College, Wellesley MA.

Nichols, M. P., & Zax, M. (1977). *Catharsis in psychotherapy*. New York: Gardner Press.

Orlinksy, D., & Howard, K. (1986). Relation of process to outcome in psychotherapy. In S. L. Garfield & A. E. Bergin (Eds.), *Handbook of psychotherapy and behavior change* (3rd ed., pp. 311-384). New York: Wiley.

Pennebaker, J. W., Kiecolt, J. K., & Glaser, R. (1988). Disclosures of trauma in immune function: Health implications for psychotherapy. *Journal of Consulting and Clinical Psychology*, 56, 239-245.

Perls, F., Hefferline, R. E., & Goodman, P. (1951). *Gestalt therapy*. New York: Julian Press.

Pierce, R. A., Nichols, M. P., & DuBrin, J. R. (1983). *Emotional expression in psychotherapy*. New York: Gardner Press.

Plutchik, R. (1980). *Emotion: A psychoevolutionary synthesis*. New York: Harper & Row.

Polster, E. (1985). Imprisoned in the present. *Gestalt Journal*, 8(1), 5-22.

Polster, E., & Polster, M. (1973). *Gestalt therapy integrated*. New York: Brunner/Mazel.

Rachman, S. (1980). Emotional processing. *Behaviour Research and Therapy*, 18, 51-60.

Rice, L. N., & Greenberg, L. S. (Eds.). (1984). *Patterns of change: Intensive analysis of psychotherapy process*. New York: Guilford.

Schramski, T. G., Feldman, C. A., Harvey, D. R., & Holiman, M. (1984). A comparative evaluation of group treatments in an adult correctional facility. *Journal of Group Psychotherapy, Psychodrama and Sociometry*, 36(4), 133-147.

Shavit, Y., Lewis, J. W., Terman, G. W., Gale, R. P., & Liebeskind, J. D. (1984).

Opioid peptides mediate the suppression effect of stress on natural killer cell cytotoxicity. *Science, 223,* 188-190.

Spergel, P., Erlich, G. E., & Glass, D. (1978). The rheumatoid arthritic personality: A psychodynamic myth. *Psychosomatics, 19,* 79-86.

Strupp, H., & Binder, J. L. (1985). *Psychotherapy in a new key: A guide to Time-Limited Dynamic Psychotherapy.* New York: Basic Books.

Woldenberg, L., Karle, W., Gold, S., Corriere, R., Hart, J., & Hooper, M. (1976). Psychophysical changes in feeling therapy. *Psychological Reports, 39,* 1059-1062.

Zajonc, R. B. (1980). Feeling and thinking: Preferences need no inferences. *American Psychologist, 35,* 151-175.

Zajonc, R. B. (1981). A one-factor mind about mind and emotion. *American Psychologist, 36,* 102-103.

Zajonc, R. B. (1984). On the primacy of affect. *American Psychologist, 39,* 117-123.

Zinker, J. (1977). *Creative process in Gestalt therapy.* New York: Random House.

8

Two Affective Change Events in Client-Centered Therapy

LAURA N. RICE
LESLIE S. GREENBERG
York University

Affect has a central role in both the theory and practice of client-centered therapy. A cornerstone of Rogers's view of optimal human functioning, as well as optimal client process in psychotherapy, is the ability to experience fully in awareness one's own emotionally toned reactions to inner and outer events (Rogers, 1963; Seeman, 1984). Before describing and illustrating the two different kinds of affective change events, we will discuss some of our basic assumptions concerning the role of emotion in human functioning and in psychotherapeutic change.

BASIC ASSUMPTIONS ABOUT THE ROLE OF EMOTION IN HUMAN FUNCTIONING AND PSYCHOTHERAPEUTIC CHANGE

The first and most basic assumption in a client-centered view of human functioning is that human beings are fundamentally motivated toward growth and wholeness, toward developing their full potential. This involves not only meeting "deficiency needs" but also moving toward growth, autonomy, and creativity (Maslow, 1954). People are motivated to engage in creative new experiences even when these experiences may actually increase tension (Butler & Rice, 1963; Rogers, 1959). A further assumption is that the growth principle can function optimally only when people can attend to their own affectively toned organismic experience. In other words, emotion cannot serve its biologically adaptive function in the complex human environment if emotionally toned experience is not attended to with accuracy and immediacy.

The second assumption concerning human functioning is that people have what Rogers has called the "gift of awareness" (Rogers & Skinner, 1962). That is, they have the basic capacity to turn attention inward and become aware of a level of immediate, emotionally toned experience that reflects the presence of emotions, needs, reactions, and perceptions, in the immediate present. This kind of inner tracking of feelings provides a window on the state of the organism at that moment. Rogers's (1959) definition of "experiencing a feeling" captures the focus of this inner tracking.

> It denotes an emotionally tinged experience, together with its personal meaning. Thus it includes the emotion but also the cognitive content of the meaning of that emotion in its experiential context. It thus refers to the unity of emotion and cognition as they are experienced inseparably in the moment. (p. 198)

This perspective on the unity of emotion and cognition experienced inseparably in the moment implies some internal processing mechanisms that integrate many different levels of information (Greenberg & Safran, 1987). Thus awareness of feelings provides meanings that capture experience better than just words or reason alone. Rogers's (1959) claim that the person is wiser than his/her intellect alone, thus refers to the inner integrative process that combines information from a variety of sources and provides us with this information as a type of feedback. If we are open to this experiential feedback (i.e., able to symbolize it in awareness), we are more congruent and more likely to act adaptively in the world.

Another interesting point about the client-centered view of emotion in human functioning has been made by Gendlin (1962). He emphasizes the intentionality involved in emotion. He stresses the point that we are always "angry at" or "afraid of" and that it is the meaning of the feeling in context that is of greater significance than the emotion of anger or fear itself.

The above two basic principles of human functioning have immediate implications for the role of emotion in psychotherapeutic change, and for the role of client and therapist in the therapeutic process. The first assumption is that the growth principle applies to all people during the different stages of their lives, but that growth can be impeded or blocked for many people by the ways in which they have learned to process their experiences in relation to self and environment. If these blocks and impediments can be overcome, the growth principle can be counted on to function effectively. Thus crucial client tasks in therapy involve becoming able to process emotionally toned experiences in more effective ways. It is neither necessary nor desirable for the therapist to make assumptions about what would be satisfying or ideal goals for the client. If the dysfunctional modes of processing are changed, then one can rely on the basic growth motivation. The goal is to change processing in order to open the person to more internal and external information, rather than to predict an ideal product of processing.

A second assumption important for the conduct of therapy is that the client is the expert on his/her own inner experience, and that this inner experience is trustworthy. Under favorable conditions, anything that is potentially available to human awareness can be symbolized accurately in awareness without the need for external observation and interpretation. We are not saying that this "inner track" is necessarily an accurate statement of "reality" in an external, consensual sense, but that it offers the most accurate data on the state of the organism at this moment. This view of the client as an expert on his/her experience is consistent with the view of emotion as the product of a complex integrative feedback system that provides information to organisms about their reactions to situations (Leventhal, 1979; Greenberg & Safran, 1987). Thus emotion provides us with information that helps us orient in the world so that we can survive and grow. This is the information function of emotion.

Most client-centered therapists have stressed the importance of focusing on the level of feelings rather than on "sheer emotion" (Gendlin, 1979). Feelings are a cognitive–affective functional unit, a higher-level integration of emotion and meaning. Although there are times when a client-centered therapist would reflect "pure" emotions such as being "sad" or "afraid," usually they would also try to facilitate the client in getting a differentiated sense of the sadness, such as "feeling over the hill," or of the fear as feeling "small and exposed." In other words, the assumption is that the information function of emotion can usually be best accessed through more idiosyncratic feelings.

Thus the therapist is usually tuned to the client's internal frame of reference, reflecting the feelings that seem to be live and poignant for the person at that moment. This fosters in the person an intense inward deployment of attentional energy, directed toward exploration, discovery, and reprocessing of new inner experience. Thus feelings are viewed as trustworthy, subjective, and available to the client only from the inside.

The third perspective on the role of emotion in therapy is not one stated by Rogers, nor did he subscribe to it as a way of functioning in therapy. Nevertheless it is, in our opinion, highly consistent with the previous two assumptions. Our assumption is that, in working with affectively toned experience, it is important for the therapist to respond differentially to different classes of "affect markers" (Rice & Greenberg, 1984). Although "process diagnosis" involves the therapist's adopting an explicit selective focus, it is certainly consistent with the client-centered procedure of not formulating a treatment plan in advance concerning the content areas in which the client needs to change. What we are advocating here is that the therapist can become aware of process markers indicating that at this moment the client needs to access his/her own inner track in a particular way, and that the person is currently ready for this particular allocation of attention. The judgment of need does not concern a particular content or a theory of psychopathology, but rather an apparent present processing style or underlying processing deficit involving emotionally toned experience that is amenable to intervention. Furthermore the particular kind of intervention that is likely to be most effective for the client is different at different times. Thus different affective markers signal to the therapist the importance of particular modes of responding.

The two different kinds of affective change events to be described in this chapter involve different kinds of affect markers. In both kinds of event, the therapist is responding to feelings, but the style of responding is quite different, leading to different kinds of change, and following different paths.

SELECTIVE RESPONDING TO FEELINGS

Rather than focusing on a single kind of affective change event in client-centered therapy, it seems more illuminating to focus on two quite different kinds of events. Not only does this promise to be theoretically interesting, but also it is important for therapists to learn to distinguish between them in order to be maximally facilitative. There seem to be at least two basic process dimensions involved in successful client-centered change events. Most client-centered sessions contain elements of both, but we think it is profitable to consider the kinds of change events that each dimension makes possible. These two dimensions can be characterized as "interpersonal experience" and "experiential search." In the present chapter we will describe one kind of affective change event from each of these dimensions.

Responding to feelings has always been considered primary in client-centered therapy, and trainees are taught to listen for them and to focus on them in their reflections. The basic assumption has been that feelings are closer to an organismic level than are most other kinds of content. Thus if people could be helped to focus on what their organisms were telling them, then the actualizing tendency could function more effectively. Experienced therapists are probably often aware of differences in the different kinds of client feeling states at such moments, and do respond differentially, but this is seldom explicated. Therapists receive little explicit training in recognizing and reflecting different kinds of feeling states, nor has there been an attempt to explicate ways in which different

kinds of therapist focus on affective experience could be maximally facilitative of different kinds of client change. With a few exceptions (cf. Anderson, 1974; Gendlin, 1984; Gurney, 1984; Rice, 1983; Wexler, 1974),
client-centered therapists have avoided the use of particular kinds of interventions that are deliberately selected for a particular person at a particular moment. In his most complete exposition of his theoretical position,
Rogers (1959) mentioned in a footnote that clients who engage in certain
kinds of therapy process might conceivably need different kinds of interventions but he considered it "neither necessary nor helpful to manipulate
the relationship in specific ways for specific kinds of clients" (p. 214). This
reluctance was based on a fear that such selective responding would
interfere with the genuineness of the relationship. Our position is that
focusing on different kinds of client tasks need not interfere with the
genuineness of the relationship, provided that the kinds of interventions
chosen do not violate the primary relationship conditions and are consistent with the basic assumption that the client is the expert on his/her own
experience.

The two change events that we describe and illustrate are the interpersonal affirmation event and the evocative unfolding of problematic reactions.

CHANGE EVENT I—THE CLIENT'S SENSE OF AFFIRMATION: EMPATHIC PRIZING AT A VULNERABILITY MARKER

The Change Process That Occurs

Experienced emotion reflects the current state of the organism. If some
emotional experiencing has to be inhibited when one is relating to other
people, there is a kind of fragmenting of the person's sense of self. Some
aspect of one's own experience is interrupted because of a fear of where it
might lead. Having this experience is regarded by the person as unacceptable or abnormal. Often clients feel cut off from other people by such
seemingly abnormal feelings. There is often the fear that if these emotions
are expressed, they themselves will be overwhelmed by them or that the
therapist will find them unacceptable or even be frightened by them. Thus
such feelings are avoided or played down.

To be able to express an intense present experience, such as fear of
the future or despair about one's life, can have an extremely powerful
effect if it is recognized and reflected in a way that clearly indicates that
the therapist senses the feeling in its full intensity, is not made anxious by
it, and is clearly valuing the client without reservation. This effect is more
than simply catharsis. For the client there is a sense of making contact with
a feared aspect of experience and of being totally accepted as a person,

even though one feels extreme, different, or even strange. Because the intensity of the feeling, which has previously made it seem beyond the bounds of normal or acceptable feelings, is being fully recognized, this full acceptance can have substantial impact on the client. There is a sense of being an acceptable human being, expressing a shared human experience, which breaks the sense of isolation. For example, when one shares a sense of the total desperation involved in one's inability to connect with anyone, or the vulnerability one feels at a loss, or the rage and overwhelming desire for revenge when violated or shamed, these feelings can be seen, not as totally unacceptable inhuman emotions, but rather as understandable humanly acceptable feelings. These feelings, once shared and accepted, no longer disrupt the client's sense of coherence. There is a sense of being a whole person again, not a fragmented person with an "unspeakable" part.

For some clients there is the fear that if the emotion is fully experienced it will be bottomless or engulfing. Entering into it and experiencing the kind of affirming therapist responses we are referring to allows them to have the courage to experience it fully and not be overwhelmed by it. It is as if going to the very bottom and letting it be fully felt enables the person to start up again. Rather than being more frightened by these feelings, clients experience a sense of release, even a sense of being energized. One no longer needs to use one's energy and attention to keep from being overwhelmed by the feelings, and can function as a whole person again.

But what does it mean to "hit rock bottom" and emerge with the energy to start up again? Our assumption is that the full experiencing and expression of the emotion has been inhibited by the anxiety associated with it. The supportive, affirming stance of the therapist enables the person to overcome this anxiety and experience the dreaded feelings and thoughts. The struggle against the feelings ceases, and the resources of energy become available to strengthen the person. In addition there is the incontrovertible evidence that after the emotion has been experienced, the person has not disintegrated or dissolved, and neither has the therapist. Clearly the therapist does not view the experience as "bad" or frightening, and is not negatively evaluating the client or being pushed away by it. Thus through the affirming, prizing, nonjudgmental attitudes of the therapist the person feels able to allow the feeling and feel whole again.

This experience of affirmation of one's being is powerful in itself, but for many clients it can lead to a further productive process. For instance it can lead to an experiential search. At this stage, one not only has the energy to explore, but also feels stronger and can now afford to take the risks involved in exploring oneself. Affirmation can also lead to an emerging change in one's view of self, with a spontaneous focus on more positive, creative aspects of self. These aspects can be seen as real, not just as feeble attempts to cope with or disguise the negatives. For some clients there is the sense of being motivated to do something, or to stop doing something such as pretending. Some people begin to reveal to the therapist a cherished but hidden part of themselves that had previously been felt as too vulnerable to destructive criticism.

Although these further explorations can be important and productive, we consider that the most fundamental effect of this kind of change event is the affirming quality and the resulting sense of wholeness. The client at this moment feels, "This is me! I'm acceptable! I can respect myself."

Therapist Interventions

In discussing the therapist interventions that would facilitate this kind of affective change event it is important to note some directions that are likely to be hindering rather than facilitative. At this kind of client marker one would not push for inner exploration and try to help the client explore the edges of his/her experience. One would stay solidly with the experience as expressed. One would not focus on the situational determinants, nor would one focus on possible alternatives or solutions. In other words, one should not be trying to do anything with it at this point.

The primary interpersonal relationship conditions must be clearly and genuinely present. The therapist is clearly prizing the client as a worthwhile and truly respected person, thus enabling the client to respect him/herself. The therapist is empathically resonating to the emotional experience and is genuinely not frightened or disturbed by the feeling. Much of this special message cannot be put into words, but will come out in the voice, the look, and the manner, not only as caring, but with a solid sense of strength, being a separate person who is sharing the feeling but is not enmeshed in it or overwhelmed by it.

Process Markers for This Change Event

What are the markers that signal readiness for this kind of therapist responding? For what kinds of clients is it important? For some clients, especially those diagnosed as "borderline," such moments are not uncommon, especially in the earlier phases of therapy, and it is crucial to respond to them. For other clients they may occur rarely, but when they do occur, they can lead to important turning points. Rather than identifying kinds of clients, however, we find it more useful to identify momentary process "markers" that indicate that the client is intensely vulnerable at this time.

There are several aspects that, together, define these "vulnerability markers": (1) The feeling is usually not connected with a specific situational experience, but is a more pervasive one that colors a variety of experiences. (2) There is a sense of a reluctance to express the feeling, but also a quality of newness, of its being directly expressed for the first time. (3) The third quality is hard to describe in words, but comes through in voice, posture, sighing, and facial expression. It has a quality of being "at the end of the road," a sense of finally recognizing how bad it feels.

Some examples of the vulnerability markers are given below.

> "I guess maybe I feel like a—a—damaged person. I'll never be like other people, so why try." (*voice trembling*)
> "I feel finished—like I have no more energy left. The struggle is too much." (*voice flat*)
> "I just don't have any real friends. People come and go but I'm just not connected—ever." (*hopelessness in voice*)

Transcript of an Interpersonal Affirmation Event

The following excerpt is from the eighth session with a 34-year-old woman. Her husband died 3 years ago and her only brother died 6 months before that. She had had approximately 6 months of therapy with a different therapist a few months after these events and she continued to function adequately, retaining her job as a librarian. She came to the present therapist complaining of intense avoidant anxiety and depression.

The transcript begins about 35 minutes into the session. She has been talking about her attempts to avoid things that remind her of her husband and brother.

C1: Just now I was thinking about someone at the library mentioning a woman who took her own life. She just couldn't take it any more. I can understand that—the pressure. It's not that I'm thinking of doing it, but I could understand it's the pressure that eventually can get to you. I just thought—there is so much going on—the pressure—it doesn't quit. Then I think, "I just have to keep going."

T1: So there's pressure—day after day. But you just have to keep going.

C2: I'm dealing with it on the outside. But inside I don't feel very strong. It's like I don't have anything left. It's like I'm pulling from something but I don't feel like there's much there.

T2: Uh huh. So it's like pulling from an empty well. And there just isn't anything left right now.

C3 (*cries*): Yeah, the well is empty. It's been too long, just too long. The last 3 years I've been struggling with this.

T3: Yeah. It's been a long, long struggle.

C4: Like I don't want to go on.

T4: If they are gone, it's like I don't want to carry on any more.

C5 (*crying*): Yeah, I just can't seem to carry on without both of them.

I just feel like I'm not whole. When I feel like this I need to go back to running things through them. If they're not here then I don't have them to run things through—then there isn't me here. Only a quarter of me is here without them.

T5: So without them here to check things out with it's like a large part of you is missing. You're just not whole.

C6: Yeah, I just can't seem to carry on without them. I just feel like I'm not whole.

T6: Yeah. It's not so much I need them to support me in the world. More, inside of me I just don't feel like I can hold together, and just feeling kind of desperate about it.

C7: I have to be able to tell myself I'll be OK.

T7: It gets so scary, you need to be able to reassure yourself.

C8: Sometimes I'm not sure. I feel I might go stark raving mad.

T8: Um huh—

C9: Sometimes it feels dark. I feel confused. I lose myself. And I guess it's a feeling of going through the motions, just doing things—and I'm aware of my own fragility. It's like I'm on my own.

T9: So you're saying "ultimately I'm on my own. And I don't know if I can make it on my own."

C10: I have been so buffered for so long. I don't know if I know how to be in the world. I mean we did things, I did things on my own—but somehow it was always "we." You know I've been getting through on my weakness not on my strengths.

T10: Mhm. Somehow the "I" doesn't feel very strong—ready to move on.

C11: Like when I could have taken that new job and gone out West. I'm so aware of what I clamp off—all that excitement—the possibilities of what I could do. I get depressed knowing how much I'm missing, about all the things I'm missing.

T11: Yes, and you really want to be able to live and enjoy things.

C12: Yeah, I do . . . It's been important for me to be able to talk like this—because it's me.

T12: Yeah, if you don't you feel cut off and isolated.

C13: Yeah, like all bottled up inside and not able to be myself with anybody. This is really important for me to be able to say what's really going on inside.

Commentary

There seem to be at least two recognizable shift points in this kind of change event. The first is a point at which the therapist's responses accurately reflect the full quality of the person's feelings, clearly sensing what it is like for the person. This is not an attempt to intensify the feeling nor to play it down, but simply an attempt to recognize it with full empathy and respect. This seems to happen here at T2. The client feels understood and supported, and thus able to begin to experience the feeling fully. She cries and begins to go down into the feeling.

The second kind of shift point is the point at which the client begins a small shift upward that seems to signal that the person has reached the bottom and is beginning to come up again. For the present client this seems to happen only slightly, right at the end of the session at C11, when she begins to express impatience, a sense of wanting to get on with her life. The therapist clearly recognizes this in T11. For some clients this might signal the start of a new self-exploration. For this person, however, the most important awareness at this time is her relief at having been able to express to the therapist the full extent of her pain and desperation. The real sense of coming up again doesn't seem to happen until the next day. At the beginning of the next session, the therapist asks how she feels. She says that the hopeless feelings were still there for the rest of the day, but that gradually they faded away, and she felt much better. "Just being able to connect with you was very helpful. It helped me somehow to ride the wave and come out on the other side."

CHANGE EVENT II—EXPERIENTIAL SEARCH: SYSTEMATIC EVOCATIVE UNFOLDING AT A PROBLEMATIC REACTION MARKER

The Change Process That Occurs

The second kind of emotional change event leads to therapeutic change by means of a client process we call "experiential search," a process that is quite different from that of interpersonal affirmation. Although prizing and therapist congruence are still essential background conditions, the emphasis is on helping clients to get in touch with the edges of their own affectively toned experience, and thus to discover and synthesize crucial elements of experience. As mentioned earlier, one of the basic client-centered assumptions is that a person's differentiated awareness of his/her affectively toned inner experience provides the most accurate data on the state of the organism at that moment. The assumption underlying the process of experiential search is that when clients are describing troubling incidents in their lives, there is potentially available to them a store of affective-cognitive information that was not fully processed in awareness at the time of the incident. Therefore, if the incident can be vividly re-evoked under conditions of safety, empathic understanding, and systematic experiential focus, it can be reprocessed more slowly and completely. Through this process of experiential search clients can arrive at new meanings that are more accurate representations and organizations of their own experiences of self in the world. In other words, this new information forces reorganization of the inadequate or distorted self-schemata through which their experience was formerly processed, thus leading to fuller and more accurate processing of inner and outer events (Rice, 1974). This in turn provides a base from which people are able to make more satisfying choices leading to personal growth.

Most good exploration carried out in the client-centered mode depends to some extent on this information function of emotion, but the process can take different forms, and can lead to varying degrees of positive change. The kind of change event that will be described here involves an attempt by the therapist to engage clients in a systematic process of experiential search at times when clients are describing incidents in which they have found themselves reacting to a particular situation in ways that they regard as exaggerated, unexpected, maladaptive, or otherwise problematic.

Clients often spontaneously describe such incidents with a sense of surprise, as if they had violated some expectation of themselves. Such problematic reactions may have involved some clear behavioral component, or they may have been primarily internal reactions. For instance, one client described an incident in which he replied to a seemingly friendly comment with an antagonistic response, while another client described a situation in which he suddenly felt small and insignificant. The implications of such incidents are often ignored by therapists, who view them as merely the recounting of stories. The significance of these stories lies in the fact that the clients are aware of some discrepancy between their view of an appropriate or self-consistent reaction and their own actual reaction, and are thus motivated to explore and understand it.

The avenue that we have found most productive at such "markers" is to embark on a systematic evocative unfolding of a particular incident that involved such a problematic reaction (Rice, 1983, 1984; Rice & Saperia, 1984). There are a number of different stages in this evocative unfolding process, each with a different focus and with emotions serving somewhat different functions in each. The first four stages involve the deliberate accessing of the relevant emotion schemata. According to Leventhal (1979, 1984) schematic emotional memory contains representations of the key features of stimulus situations, combined with expressive–motor and conceptual responses to the situations, all coded together in a tight associational structure. Schemata thus organize our experience, integrating different particulars, such as expressive–motor actions with perceptions of the situation, images, and memories, to create a complex integrated emotional experience. When new situations are encountered, if they evoke a particular schematic structure through the similarity of the salient pattern of its features, the whole structure is activated and determines the person's response.

When working with people to unfold problematic reactions to situations, one evokes the relevant schema by eliciting one or more components of its structure, such as the situational stimuli, subjective feelings, or expressive or autonomic responses.

Each of the five stages involves its own goal, and each stage could be used separately. In fact, a client-centered therapist would recognize some of these stages as processes that seem to take place when a therapy is going well. In the present change task they are instigated in sequence, with the completion of each stage leading to the beginning of the next. Each stage builds on and is made possible by the previous one. The whole unfolding process will usually require most of an hour. Each stage is discussed below, together with a description of the "goal" of each stage, and a brief description of the way in which the therapist is trying to facilitate the process.

Stage 1: Staying with the Primary Reaction

The first important task of the therapist is to maintain the focus on the reaction that is felt by the client to be problematic, rather than letting his/her energy get diverted into a focus on the reaction to the reaction. This reaction to the reaction is a secondary response and is similar to what Greenberg and Safran (1987) have referred to as a "secondary emotional reaction," such as frustration, depression, or anxiety. In a problematic reaction these secondary reactions are often feelings of shame or self-disgust. The reaction felt by the client to be problematic should be dealt with as the primary reaction, even though the secondary reaction, such as despising onself for being so childish, may contain the clearest and most intense feeling at the moment. For instance the therapist might respond "even though it seems childish to you now, I guess the part that really puzzles you is your reaction then—just wanting to lash out." The feeling of wanting to lash out is the clear focus of this statement. It is this emotional output that is the synthesis of a complex set of internal processes in response to the situation. In responding this way, the therapist is making a discrimination rather than just "reflecting feelings." This kind of therapist response serves two functions: It prevents the client from "short-circuiting" the primary reaction and focusing primarily on the self-disgust. In addition it serves to confirm just which part of the reaction was felt by the client as puzzling. If the client confirms this, then the therapist suggests exploring that incident in detail. If the client expresses interest and willingness for such exploration, then the next stage is begun.

The goal of this stage is threefold: (1) to defuse the secondary emotional reaction if necessary, (2) to maintain the focus on the reaction that was actually felt to be puzzling, and (3) to establish a climate in which there is an explicit intention to embark on a shared journey of exploration.

Stage 2: Building and Re-Entering the Scene

At this point the client is asked to describe the situation just before the reaction occurred "so that we can get a feel for it." This would involve both the scene as perceived and the client's inner state just before the reaction was triggered. The client is encouraged to describe the incident as vividly as possible, thus re-evoking the sights and sounds and feelings experienced at the time. Thus the client "re-enters" the scene, re-experiencing freshly the moment when the reaction was triggered. This evocation provides immediate, emotionally toned experience that can be tracked by the client.

The goal of this stage is to make it possible for the client to retrieve the "episodic memories" (Bower, 1981; Tulving, 1972) that would not be available without the emotional re-experiencing. These memories are somewhat state-dependent. They are evoked when sufficient experiential cues at the sensory–motor level, both kinaesthetic and visual, are attended to. Stated in terms of Leventhal's (1984) perceptual–motor model of emotion, the client is thus able to access the relevant emotional schemata. As Greenberg and Safran (1987) have stated, "These structures provide a representation of specific emotional experiences that have taken place in the past, as well as the key perceptual features that have elicited these emotional experiences" (p. 150). Once this emotion schema has been evoked a host of new information is available to the client, information that was not remembered because it was not stored in conceptual memory. Thus this stage serves as priming for stages 3 and 4.

Stage 3: Recognizing Salience in the Eliciting Stimulus

Once the scene has come alive and the emotion schemata are evoked, clients are encouraged by means of open-ended reflections to identify the aspect of the stimulus situation that was salient for them at the time the reaction was triggered. We have found that at this point most clients are able to access the automatic perceptual–emotional appraisals made at the time and thus to recognize the aspect of the eliciting stimulus that had had emotional impact on them. This spontaneous recognition of what it was about the stimulus situation that effected them places this salient aspect and its experienced impact in focal awareness, and provides the material for the next stage.

Stage 4: Tracking the Idiosyncratic Personal Meaning of the Stimulus as Construed

Once the salient aspect of the stimulus situation is in focal awareness the therapist's job is to facilitate the client's retrieving and exploring the way in which the impact or potential impact of the eliciting stimulus was construed and experienced. When this exploration is successful, the client discovers the link between the stimulus impact as construed and the nature of the reaction that was triggered. This tracking involves a process of explicit awareness that was not possible at the time of the original incident. It is now possible because of the following three aspects of the therapeutic climate and the exploratory focus. In the first place, the processing that had previously been automatic is now slowed down and made a focus of attention. Secondly, there is intense inward deployment of the client's attentional energy. The third and crucial aspect is that the client's emotional arousal makes the emotion–schematic memory system accessible.

For some clients the most vivid awareness at this point is the affective quality of their own inner reaction to the salient aspect of the stimulus situation. Therefore, the therapist first tries to facilitate their exploration of the differentiated quality of the feeling, since this will contain the most accessible information at this moment. As mentioned above, we view the term "feeling" as involving a complex blending of emotion and cognition rather than the quality of "raw" emotion. Thus two clients might both refer to the experience of "anger," but when they were able to explore the differentiated feeling quality, one of them might become aware of having felt a kind of helpless anger, of being "put down" or "weakened," while the other client might become aware of a belligerent sense that "someone is infringing on my territory." Getting in touch with a differentiated feeling has an information function, telling the client something about the way in which the eliciting stimulus was construed. Tracking the quality of the feeling reaction enables clients to become aware of the meaning the stimulus had for them, their "experienced reality" at the moment when the reaction was triggered.

For other clients, although there is some emotional arousal, the most vivid awareness seems to be the quality of the eliciting stimulus, and therefore client and therapist focus directly on the nature of the client's subjective construal of its assumed impact. This is not done in an objective, analytic manner, but is explored as if it were happening right now. This is possible because the whole emotion schema, including the eliciting stimulus, has been re-accessed and can become the focus of attention. The salient features of the eliciting stimulus are linked in schematic memory with expressive–motor responses and autonomic responses. Thus when the eliciting stimulus situation is re-evoked and the client's attention is focused on it, all of these become available. Because of the link between stimulus features and expressive–motor responses, idiosyncratic stimulus construals such as the "look on his face" or the "empty hallway" always carry an implied affective quality, such as feeling put down or feeling alone.

Stage 4 is completed when the client discovers the nature of his/her subjective construal of the potential impact of the stimulus situation, and recognizes self as agent in this construal. We call this the "meaning bridge" because it involves the discovery and owning of the causal link between the nature of one's own construal and the nature of one's own puzzling problematic reaction.

Stage 5: Exploring One's Own Mode of Functioning— Broadening, Deepening, and Owning

The previous stage was completed when the client recognized that his/her problematic reaction was a direct response to his/her own idiosyncratic construal of the stimulus situation and of the feelings thus aroused. Once this idiosyncratic link has been recognized, clients usually spontaneously recognize that the way in which they were functioning in this situation was an instance of a more pervasive and general mode of functioning. The client has identified in a compelling way a personal style of functioning that was clearly operating and that is inconsistent with his/her own self-expectations. The person is now motivated to explore this personal style of functioning and its consequences as a means of making sense of his/her experience in the world.

Stage 5 is characterized by the client's instigating a broadening and deepening of the self-exploration. It is still clearly an experiential search process but it seems to be guided by some implicit questions. "What is this personal style? What is it for? How does it fit with the rest of my experience?" This intensive exploration seems to be motivated by much more than curiosity. There is a sense that some aspect of one's life is not going right, isn't really satisfying one's own needs. This self-guided search leads to an exploration of one's own needs and wants, values and basic beliefs, fears, and capabilities. Links are made between them, not primarily through intellectual analysis, but through checking inside. It is as if the needs and wants, fears, values, and beliefs about self are being "tasted" in relation to each other. This tasting process is a set of complex internal operations that is quite recognizable on the level of observable process. For instance, the client at a particular moment may feel some of the need or want, and then experiences a complex emotional response to the need. This response may contain some very positive feelings but also a sense of apprehension, of pulling back. Then the person focuses on this sense of apprehension and its personal meanings, and realizes that it no longer has much power in relation to the other feelings. In the context of this experiential search process the client is able to attend to these emotional reactions and their implication rather than automatically drawing his/her conceptually laden conclusions, thus generating important new data.

When this phase of the experiential search is successful, the client reaches a point that we consider to be the resolution of an affective problem. "Resolution" is defined as "new awareness of important aspects of one's own mode of functioning in a way that restructures the issue. Though still experientially involved, one now has a sense of what one wants to change and a sense of having the power to instigate the change."

Following this resolution point there is usually some further exploration and "emotional tasting" of one's own needs and wants, values and "shoulds," fears, and capabilities, but their relative emotional valences seem to have shifted. For instance our observations confirm an interesting distinction made by Hart (1983), between needs stated by a client as "problems" and those stated as a personal declaration of what one needs and wants. He regards this as one of the crucial shifts that takes place in a successful therapy.

Some evidence for this emergent sense of power and possibility was provided in a study by Wiseman (1986; Wiseman & Rice, 1989) in which Interpersonal Process Recall, using a Client Mood Scale (Elliott, 1986), was administered at various stages of the video playback of the sessions in which problematic reaction points were successfully resolved. The mood was essentially negative for all clients at the time of stage 2, when the scene was re-entered, and there was little upward shift at the time of the Meaning Bridge, even though there was an awareness of new discoveries at that point. At the point of "resolution," however, there was a strong positive shift in the mood of each of the clients.

This emotional change event concludes differently for each person. For some clients new options are immediately apparent and new plans are made and tried out during the week. For other clients the new view is recognized, but its full impact only makes itself felt during the next week or two. For others the new view seems to tap into an even broader issue. No immediate new options are seen, but the resolution provides a new vantage point from which to explore this broader issue.

THERAPIST INTERVENTIONS

Although this change event must take place in the context of a good interpersonal therapeutic relationship, most of the therapist interventions are quite different from those in the first kind of change event. The therapist is attempting to facilitate the client's engaging in an experiential search process rather than affirming the client's experience. Most of the therapist interventions are reflections or reflective questions, in which he/she is trying to grasp the idiosyncratic flavor of the client's inner experience as it is being expressed. Most reflections are said in a way that conveys the expectation that the client will check them with his/her own inner experience and correct them or carry them further.

Although the therapist is clearly "process-directive" in the sense of keeping the client focused on this particular experience, and has a "map" of the essential steps in the search process, the therapist is not "content-directive" in the sense of pursuing his/her own hypotheses concerning the content of the discoveries that the client needs to make. Our experience has been that the crucial links discovered are quite idiosyncratic, and that if the therapist attempts to suggest or steer the client towards some hypothesized connection, even if the hypothesis seems correct, the link would be oversimplified and its impact would be diluted.

Most of the therapist's empathic reflections leave the "open edge" on the aspect that seems to be alive (truly felt) for the client at the moment, but that has not yet been explored to the edges of the experience. Although client and therapist are both aware of entering purposively into a special kind of experiential search, the basic relationship conditions are maintained, and the emphasis is clearly on the client as the expert on his/her own experience.

It is important to note that the two major shift points, the Meaning Bridge and Resolution, are not therapist-initiated. They are moments at which the client's own experiential search process has led to an important shift in perspective.

The Process Marker for This Change Event

The marker that signals a readiness for this kind of experiential search must contain three elements as follows: (1) a particular incident, (2) a reaction involving feelings or behavior or both, and (3) an indicator that the client finds his/her own reaction problematic in some way.

The most important criterion for deciding to use evocative unfolding at such a point is that the client seems to be experiencing a real sense of discrepancy and puzzlement at this moment. Often such problematic incidents seem directly relevant to the themes that are being dealt with in therapy. At other times, however, the incident may seem unrelated or even trivial, and yet its unfolding may yield important and very relevant data. There are some negative indicators for trying to unfold a problematic reaction, especially the more habitual emotional reactions. When clients are obviously distressed and deeply disturbed by their own reactions, it may be much more helpful not to initiate exploration at this point. To be able to express what they feel and to be truly heard and valued and affirmed is much more important at such a time. Exploration can come later.

Some clients recount such incidents quite often, while others seldom do. We have found that for people who do not spontaneously bring in such incidents, we can describe and illustrate a problematic reaction point and suggest that they might find it interesting to notice one and bring it in to explore. Somewhat to our surprise, once they are alerted to such points, clients are often able to do this, and to unfold the problematic reaction point quite successfully. Our sense is that for clients who do not spontaneously question their own reactions this can lead not only to new awareness but also to a greater tendency to recognize and question such discrepancies between their own reactions and their self-expectations.

Transcript of the Unfolding of a Problematic Reaction

This transcript is from the fourth session of a brief, time-limited therapy. The client is a 21-year-old, female, university student. Her presenting issues involved lack of confidence in herself and her own decisions. She wanted to be able to decide to leave home, but did not want to leave with a sense of bitterness toward family members.

This transcript will be presented in two parts, with a commentary after each part. The first part begins with the marker for a problematic reaction point and concludes with the Meaning Bridge (stages 1-4). The second part continues through stage 5, ending with the point of Resolution.

C1: There was something that happened last week. I don't really understand it. It was kind of weird. I went to a sort of party. I do volunteer work with this kid and it was her family. And I went there on my own to this get-together and I just hated it. Like . . . I . . . It's probably just the way I was feeling . . . And then ah . . . I just wasn't into it. Like, I just wasn't into being there by myself kind of thing. I just . . .

T1: So, somehow um . . . what you feel puzzled about at this point is being there and feeling uncomfortable, or . . .

C2: It happens once in a while. I just sort of . . . It sort of overwhelms me. Like I really feel kind of . . . um . . . (*short pause*) Like a big weight is on me kind of. It's weird. It's a really weird thing. I'm not . . . It's not even really depression. It's (*short pause*) It's just like . . . I don't know. I can't explain it. Maybe it's because I was tired or something. But afterwards when I remember . . . like feeling this when I went home. Sort of really strange and I didn't understand it.

T2: So it's the feeling of being really heavy and bogged down that's strange for you?

C3: Yeah. It was weird. It's just sort of um . . . Well, probably I was overtired for one thing.

T3: I wonder if we could go back into that situation? (C: OK.) And um, sort of re-create it and see if we can get a sense of . . . of um . . . what was happening for you. You went over in the evening . . .

C4: It was after . . . OK my sister and brother were there for dinner. So I went after dinner—around seven.

T4: So you had a family kind of meal together? (C: Right.) And how had that gone? How were you feeling after it?

C5: Oh . . . Let's see. Not bad. I guess . . . It was okay sort of thing. There's a lot of . . . I guess I always had . . . There are a lot of feelings that I . . . with regards to my family in a lot of ways, and maybe it doesn't put me always . . . maybe it has something to do with, maybe the way I was feeling afterwards . . .

T5: So, you were feeling a little tense at dinner?

C6: Maybe. I'm not sure. I mean there are um . . . I think I sort of tend to sort of feel, or have always felt that it's been always hard to express my opinion.

T6: So around the dinner table at home—you're kind of feeling a little bit uneasy. You want to kind of participate and don't know how?

C7: In a way . . . It's . . . I don't know. It sounds kind of weird but it . . . I mean . . . that is nothing new . . . Um . . . in itself. I guess maybe that sort of—maybe put me into some kind of different mood. But then afterwards—that's when it . . .

T7: So, then we get to um . . . to the party.

C8: To that party, and I just wasn't feeling like being there.

T8: What was happening when you arrived?

C9: Well . . . People were talking and walking around . . . people talking a lot. I feel accepted. Like, their family definitely accepts me, and I don't know about the other people. But I guess I didn't really feel that comfortable. It wasn't really the party. I think it was just the mood I was in. I just wasn't . . . in the mood for it. I guess—that night. I just wasn't feeling like being there.

T9: Well, can we kind of go back into the situation and see when the mood kind of started—when you started feeling bogged down? When you arrived—I take it, you were feeling a bit edgy and insecure . . . But you didn't feel that sort of heavy weight?

C10: No . . . Not . . . Not at the beginning . . .

T10: You're sitting at the party and um . . . kind of . . . I don't know . . . feeling a little bit on the outside?

C11: Oh yeah . . .

T11: Because you're not a family member?

C12: Yeah. Sort of . . . And I just . . . Yeah. For some reason I was really detached, sort of.

T12: Just feeling very detached?

C13: Yeah.

T13: And kind of—what—the observer?

C14: Exactly . . . I just wasn't really participating and I just didn't feel like I was a part of it.

T14: So somehow you didn't really jell with them . . . And . . . and become part of them.

C15: Yeah . . . Whereas, I might have . . . I think it had something to do with being on my own too in a way. Um . . . Sort of tired of being there by myself . . .

T15: So there's something about going there by yourself?

C16: Yeah. (*short pause*) Like I . . . I don't know . . . It just kind of bothered me being, you know, going by myself kind of.

T16: Is there something about being alone there that is kind of disturbing?

C17: In a way . . . (*short pause*) It just sort of reminds me that I don't really have a boyfriend at the moment . . . and being at this party by myself . . .

T17: So, I'm not sure then um . . . kind of being alone at the party— was it that aloneness, that feeling kind of—almost . . .

C18: Kind of overwhelmed or . . . Um . . .

T18: Was that the heavy feeling?

C19: I'm trying to think of that . . . Um . . . It sort of happened. Like, it was maybe I'd been there just for awhile at the party . . . Um . . .

T19: And kind of feeling that maybe you're sticking out like a sore thumb because you're a lone girl there . . .

C20: I guess that was part of it

T20: So, you're sitting at the party and you're feeling alone and you're not really part of the scene and having a fine time. Just kind of sitting on the outskirts—watching everyone . . . And what's happening?

C21: I guess . . . just lots of people there . . . You know, there was music. The kids were dancing and things like that . . . It was just chaos.

T22: So, there's this chaos . . . the dancing, the talking and . . . you're kind of surrounded by this noise . . .

C23: Like just confusion . . .

T24: And you're just sort of stuck in the middle of this confusion, just watching it.

C25: Yeah, like I didn't know what to do . . . just looking . . .

T25: A kind of looking . . . Almost looking through a window and wondering how you can get in and kind of talk to these people . . . something is holding you back . . .

C26: Yeah. It was like that. It was like watching from a window actually. It was just sort of . . . I felt like I wasn't even there sort of thing.

T26: Like you didn't exist? That you're almost like a shadow that is looking through the window and there's this big party going on inside and . . .

C27: But I knew that people were noticing me, you know, that I wasn't really participating. But I just couldn't bring myself to for some reason . . . I just basically just wanted to sit there . . . I think.

T27: So you just wanted to sit in the corner, or . . .

C28: Yeah. I didn't want to be there. Or I didn't feel like being there.

Maybe that was my way of not wanting to . . . just acting like that or whatever . . .

T28: So in a way you felt coerced being there . . . you were there against your will.

C29: Sort of. Maybe it was my way of just, you know, like sort of a quiet rebellion or something, you know. So finally I just sort of slipped out . . . like . . .

T29: And is the heaviness . . . Are you starting to feel the heaviness?

C30: It's kind of . . . Like I wasn't feeling like that sort of weighted feeling until I started driving.

T30: So you left the party . . . got into the car . . . And you're feeling kind of "Oh, it was a miserable evening, I didn't want to be there,"and you're driving along and . . . I don't know. Was it being in the car alone that suddenly made you feel flat, or, I'm not sure . . .

C31: I think it was a combination of things, thinking about the evening—not wanting to be there and then—just felt like it was a waste in a way.

T31: Somehow you felt you had wasted your time?

C32: Yeah, for some reason. Like I often feel like that when I go over . . . because I don't think the family really . . . I'm supposed to be helping this kid and I try, but they don't do anything to help her. They don't cooperate. I mean . . . all my efforts sort of seem worthless . . . sometimes . . . they sort of think I'm a miracle worker, I guess. And I go over . . . and it's like I'm making all the effort and no one in the family is making any effort.

T32: So you've been putting out and . . . kind of they're not really trying to help themselves. Is there something about feeling that you're carrying the weight of this responsibility that . . . that sort of disturbs you?

C33: Yeah. I get tired of that. So now I get tired of going over. I sort of get that feeling that I'm responsible for her, you know. Or . . . It's weird . . . Yeah . . . I just don't feel like it . . .

T33: It's kind of you feel that you're responsible for the child . . . that you have to carry the weight entirely.

C34: Yeah. And maybe I'm sort of getting to the point where I don't want to do it any more, but I don't want to affect this kid in a negative way . . . like have her think that I really don't want to do this any more.

T34: So you don't want to reject the child, but you're getting really tired. (*short pause*) So you get into the car, and you're feeling very flat and kind of wasted. I'm not sure what the feeling is—that I'm not achieving anything here?

C35: Sort of. And maybe it's . . . I don't know if it's time for a change, or (*short pause*) I think it's maybe saying something. Maybe I really don't want to do it. Maybe . . . I think in a way . . . I sort of feel like that when I end up—that sort of feeling comes around when I end up doing something I really don't want to do, but I can't change it.

Commentary

In C1, near the beginning of the session, the client brings up an incident in which she reacted in a way that she didn't understand. Her reaction is an internal one of feeling a heavy weight on her, rather than a behavioral reaction. At T1 the therapist reflects in a tentative way the part of the reaction that the client felt to be puzzling; then the client corrects or elaborates on the description. At T2 the therapist checks again which part felt puzzling and strange. When C confirms this, T suggests exploring the incident in detail and C agrees to this.

At this point T and C begin a process of experiential search, in which attending to affect served two different kinds of information functions. From T4 until T9, the therapist is trying to get a feel for the point at which the reaction was triggered. This could probably have led to recognition of the salient features of the stimulus situation at that time. This search turns out to be complicated in this case because it seems to be a sort of additive effect, starting with dinner at home, increasing at the party, and becoming the real "heavy weight" when she was driving home, thinking about the party. T decides to focus on the party and at T9 checks whether or not the reaction (the sense of a heavy weight) was present when C entered the party. After C says it was not, T instigates a focus on the quality of C's inner experience, helping C to track when it began to shift as a function of the stimulus situation at different times. That is, T attempts to keep a sense of the stimulus situation alive and in focus while C checks internally to see if the really heavy feeling had yet been felt.

The second kind of information function of affect in this experiential search process focused more on the differentiated quality of the feeling and its message to the client. For instance in C12, C18, and C26, the client used such words as "detached," "overwhelmed," and "not even being there" to describe the feeling.

At C30 she identifies the time when the real weighted feeling hit her in its full intensity, and at C31 and C32 she begins to identify the things that were evoking the feeling. Then in C35 she begins to realize that the feeling is telling her something, that she really doesn't want to work with this family any longer, but is afraid of hurting the child if she discontinues.

C35 is the Meaning Bridge. She recognizes that this bodily reaction of "heaviness" is signaling something to her. She is also able to broaden this realization, recognizing that this weighted feeling descends on her in situations in which she is doing something she deeply doesn't want to do but feels helpless to change. In other words, she recognizes that the puzzling reaction comes in situations that she construes as "having to do something she doesn't want to do."

Continuation of the Transcript—Stage 5

T35: So you end up feeling sort of wasted and flat when you're doing something you don't want to do.

C36: Yeah. Like I . . . really . . . I put myself in a situation where I really don't want to be there sort of thing. So maybe it's sort of a way of getting out of it in a way.

T36: So when you force yourself to do something you don't want to do, you begin to feel this flat . . . blah . . . kind of way. Are you saying that that gives you an excuse to get out?

C37: Maybe. Or maybe it's just a . . . a sign that I shouldn't be doing that, or whatever.

T37: Is it like an alert system of yours, saying, "Hey, you know . . . "

C38: Sort of. Maybe I shouldn't be doing this or (*short pause*) or change things a little. I think there's a lot of things . . . you know, that I'd like to see change. But I shouldn't feel so helpless. Like I tend to sometimes feel a bit helpless as far as being able to change things for myself . . . even something like that. Maybe I should listen to myself . . . and say, "You know, maybe I'll stop this thing and do something different." And . . . it happens in other situations. That sort of feeling . . . it happens . . . that detached feeling.

T38: So the times when you feel you're being forced some place where you really don't want to be—you kind of get this detached feeling?

C39: Mmm . . . Hmm . . . I think so . . . I think that's when it happens (*short pause*) It doesn't happen all the time, you know. I just . . . once in a while. Like (*short pause*) I'm just trying to think of that weighted feeling though. It's once in a while that happens. And it's almost anger in a way too, I think. There's anger in there . . . like there's sort of . . . I start thinking about different things . . . about my family, and I think, you know, just little things. Even about my sister, which really shouldn't . . . like . . . bother me too much.

T39: So there's also glimmerings of some anger, and things start coming to you.

C40: Yeah. And somehow . . . um . . . Yeah. It's kind of weird. Yeah. There is definitely some kind of anger. There are some times, when I think about my sister and the way she is sometimes, I think . . . that sometimes it's directed towards her. Although I don't know how to express it, or I don't know how to tell her.

T40: Sometimes you really feel angry with your sister but there's no way of showing this, or changing it?

C41: Or intimidated sort of, in a way.

T41: You feel too intimidated to express your anger to her?

C42: Yeah. In some ways. And that's probably having something to do with not really wanting to hurt her. I don't know . . . And I think . . . the thing I notice . . . I don't know . . . It's kind of weird (*short pause*) I always make myself look sort of weaker almost. Although I know I'm stronger, but somehow I make myself look lower than her, or weaker.

T42: So, you're trying to put yourself down, next to her. So that she feels bigger and stronger . . . and more powerful.

C43: Sometimes I do do that . . . And I think . . . I feel that's pretty stupid actually.

T43: It seems stupid, but somehow it's just something at the time that makes you somehow feel you have to put yourself down. You have to pretend to be this weak little sister.

C44: Not all the time. But . . . I still feel like sometimes. It's as though I've got to, you know, paint a sort of picture of myself . . . which isn't really me at all.

T44: So you've got to pretend to be something else.

C45: Yeah, so she doesn't feel as threatened by me, because I feel in some way she's sort of threatened by me. Umm . . . and so I just sort of make myself look differently so that she won't be threatened. So, and I think that's exactly what happens.

T45: I see. So you've got to try and pretend to be someone else so that she won't feel threatened or hassled by you.

C46: Yeah, sort of alter myself or . . . when I'm around her. Which is kind of dumb because it's not really me. Like I find I'll be telling her things which aren't necessarily true. I sort of distort things a little bit just so . . . I don't make myself look too independent or too strong or something like that.

T46: So you're kind of caught between her seeing you as a threat and you not really wanting to be seen that way, so you kind of distort what you are so that you aren't seen as a threat.

C47: Mmm. I think so, yeah. I think also I do that some with my brother. I notice . . . like even yesterday, last night I walked in and he was sitting there. He knows that I'm about to get my BA. So he says "You're going into teaching, but that doesn't pay very much does it?" He just says things like that to make it look like it's no big deal, kind of thing.

T47: So you kind of feel he's putting you down.

C48: I guess maybe he's threatened or intimidated that I've got a BA and he hasn't.

T48: So you feel he is worried about your BA or that he is jealous?

C49: Yes, when he says that kind of thing to me.

T49: So you kind of feel he's trying to push you down and keep him on top.

C50: And maybe sometimes I choose to set myself up for that, or, you know, almost in a way as I do with my sister, pretend that I'm still, you know, still Judy, the youngest kid in the family sort of thing and still the little one.

T50: So sometimes you still play the baby and that you haven't really overtaken your big brother.

C51: In, in some ways, so he won't feel threatened, like I just sort of, almost like change again.

T51: There's something about his being threatened, something about you threatening him that worries you. You just don't like the thought of you threatening him . . .

C52: Yeah. And I think it's silly that I have to sort of act like I'm not intelligent. Why can't I just be myself and if he's threatened sort of thing, you know, big deal? (*short pause*) But he doesn't want to see me sort of grow up. I don't think he really wants things to change that much somehow.

T52: So somehow you're still feeling that he doesn't want you to change. He doesn't want his world disturbed.

C53: And maybe I act younger to make him feel better, that maybe things aren't changing. I . . . you know, I'm not changing that much.

T53: So you keep feeling that he doesn't want anything to change, including you.

C54: Yeah, I don't think he does. And . . . I've been learning an awful lot at school, and I realize that I don't want to be there, at home, for much longer. And I see other things that I really want to do in life rather than stay at home.

T54: So there's something . . . You really want to kind of revolutionize what's happening at home and kind of change and grow and leave.

C55: I do. But then at the same time I want to reassure him that things aren't going to change that much, that I'm still your little sister, you know. Why can't I just, you know, be myself and maybe . . . Like some of the things I've learned I could teach my family or something. (*short pause*) But really I just choose not to for some reason.

T55: So you'd really like to kind of show them this grown up, independent, mature Judy, but something stops you. Something holds you back.

C56: Yeah, and it, it's not even just at home. I think, you know, it can be generalized to different situations . . . (*short pause*) being afraid to let . . . people know who I really am, sort of, or what I really think.

T56: There's just something about revealing yourself . . .

C57: Or, yeah, letting people know who I am. And I tend to sort of change just a little bit, for some reason, when I'm around people . . . just sort of change you know.

T57: It sounds almost as if you become a chameleon, like if the environment's green, then you're going to take on that (C: Camouflage.) and camouflage yourself.

C58: I know it sounds like I'm a big victim here. That's just the way I've been feeling sort of (*short pause*) but it's, you know, it's just as much my fault, like really when I think about it.

T58: So it's not so much them. There's something in you that holds you back from showing them who you really are . . .

C59: In some ways, like . . . yeah, for some reason. But maybe it's not . . . maybe it's just the way I feel about myself sometimes, that makes me feel like I'm a threat, maybe. I'm not sure.

T59: It's something about the way you feel about yourself?

C60: I don't know if it has something to do with my, you know, my self-image or something, or just the way I see things. That somehow if I'm my real self, I'll hurt other people . . . that I'll be really damaging.

T60: That somehow seeing the real grown-up Judy would be absolutely devastating.

C61: But that's really weird. That's almost like I've got to protect them all from the real me. But that's stupid. I'm not that powerful . . . So maybe they'll be hurt a little. (*brief pause*) My brother and sister may have to change how they see me. But it won't destroy them. That's stupid.

T61: So I guess you're saying, "The real me isn't really powerful and destructive. It's safe to be me!"

C62: Yeah. The real me . . . I'm intelligent and I've learned a lot. I'm moving beyond being the little sister. I still don't want to hurt people, but somehow . . . I don't think I would.

Commentary on Stage 5

After the Meaning Bridge, the client continues to track the meaning of the weighted feeling, trying to sense the message conveyed by the feeling. At C38 she suggests that the message is that she needs to change things, and that there are a lot of things in her life that she would like to change. She has begun the process of deepening, broadening, and owning that characterizes stage 5.

During stage 5, the tracking of feelings and their meaning is still primary, but accessing this affective level serves a function that is somewhat different from those served in the earlier stages. For instance at C39 the client begins to engage in the process that we call "tasting" of opposing feelings. She deliberately evokes the weighted feeling and finds that there is "anger" in it, anger toward her sister, that she wants to express. T reflects this and C says she feels "intimidated" (C40). As C tastes this sense of being intimidated, she realizes that it stems from her fear of hurting her sister, and that she must protect her sister by putting herself down.

It is as if the conflicting aspects were being pitted against each other. She feels what she really wants for herself but then feels and explores the fears that are stopping her. She is alternating between getting a real sense of her own strength and what she wants and needs on the one hand, and then on the other hand experiencing the sense that this would be destructive and that she must not do it.

At C58 she begins to "step back" and own and examine her own agency in the impasse. She realizes that there is something in the way she feels about herself that makes her feel that she is a threat. She realizes that she fears that her "real self" would be very damaging, and when T reflects this as "absolutely devastating," she is able to reject it as absurd. She is not that powerful. Her real self would not be destructive.

In the tasting process in stage 5 the need is usually pitted against some other powerful feeling, such as a fear, a "should," or a negative evaluation of some key aspect of self. When the relative valences of these opposing affective states changes, "resolution" becomes possible.

Resolution is reached in C61 and 62. She realizes that there is a kind of grandiosity in her fear that she will damage her sister and brother. She realizes that it isn't going to devastate them, that they aren't really that vulnerable. After this resolution point she begins to think about what it would be like to be really herself. She still feels a sense of "I mustn't do this," but it seems to have much less force. The emphasis is on what she really wants for herself.

During the next session she continues this exploration. She also realizes that part of her bitter feelings toward her family stems, not so much from them directly, but from what she has felt she had to do to herself. In later sessions she does some exploring of the ways in which this self-schema of being potentially damaging developed within the family climate. This gave her some sense of closure, but was not necessary for resolution. In fact we find that reaching resolution of a problematic reaction does not usually require historical explanation, although it may come later.

CONCLUSION

Emotion and feelings are central in client-centered theories of personality and therapeutic change. As Seeman (1984) has pointed out, Rogers's view of optimal therapy process is much the same as his view of optimal human functioning in general. The "fully functioning person" (Rogers, 1963) is open to his/her own experience, both inner and outer, and experiences all his/her feelings without fear. Fully functioning people trust their own organismic experiences as the basis for choice and action.

The dimensions of client-centered therapy discussed and illustrated in this chapter involve two related aspects of optimal functioning. In the first place one is able to experience all one's feelings without fear. In the second place one is open to and trusting of one's emotionally toned experience as a basis for choice and action.

Although a single change event from each of these dimensions has been illustrated here, a number of other change events involving these dimensions could probably be identified and studied. In reading Leitaer's (1984) searching analysis of crucial issues in the concept of therapist unconditional positive regard, we were struck by several possible change events within the Affirmation dimension that would be fascinating to study. For instance, a potentially important marker could probably be identified at times when therapist congruence seems to be inconsistent with unconditionality of positive regard. Another marker that might signal an opportunity for a powerful affirming impact would be times when a client wants the therapist to speak from his/her own internal frame of reference. Within the Experiential Search dimension, Evocative Unfolding at problematic reaction markers and Gendlin's Focusing (1981) are only two of the many possible approaches. For instance, Clarke (1989) is investigating a change task she calls a "construction of meaning" event.

Responding to feelings in client-centered therapy requires real empathy, prizing, and therapist congruence. But to be maximally facilitative there should also be differential responding at different affect markers. Even at a particular marker such as a vulnerability or problematic reaction marker, there are moment-by-moment process markers of the client's experiential state. As we have shown in the evocative unfolding event, emotional experience plays a variety of different roles in the different stages of the exploration of a problematic reaction, and the therapist needs to respond differently to emotion at these different points.

An experienced, empathic client-centered therapist probably does respond differentially to different "feeling markers," without explicit awareness. But if we are to improve client–centered therapy and train our students to be maximally facilitative, it is important to learn more about different feeling markers, and to conduct research on how best to facilitate resolution of these underlying states. Rather than diluting the impact of the primary relationship, such awareness of ways to be maximally facilitative at different times should enhance the positive impact of the relationship.

REFERENCES

Anderson, W. (1974). Personal growth and client-centered therapy: An information-processing view. In D. A. Wexler & L. N. Rice (Eds.), *Innovations in client-centered therapy* (pp. 21–48). New York: Wiley.

Bower, G. H. (1981). Mood and memory. *American Psychologist, 31,* 129–148.

Butler, J. M., & Rice, L. N. (1963). Adience, self-actualization, and drive theory. In J. M. Wepman & R. W. Heine (Eds.), *Concepts of personality* (pp. 79–112). Chicago: Aldine.

Clarke, K. M. (1989). Creation of meaning: An emotional processing task in psychotherapy. *Psychotherapy: Theory, Research, and Practice, 26,* 139–148.

Elliott, R. (1986). Interpersonal process recall (IPR) as a psychotherapy process research method. In L. S. Greenberg & W. M. Pinsof (Eds.), *The psychotherapeutic process* (pp. 503–528). New York: Guilford.

Gendlin, E. T. (1962). *Experiencing and the creation of meaning.* New York: Free Press.

Gendlin, E. T. (1979). Experiential psychotherapy. In R. Corsini (Ed.), *Current psychotherapies* (rev. ed. pp. 340–373). Itaska, IL: Peacock.

Gendlin, E. T. (1981). *Focusing.* New York: Bantam.

Gendlin, E. T. (1984). The client's client: The edge of awareness. In R. L. Levant & J. M. Shlien (Eds.), *Client-centered therapy and the person-centered approach* (pp. 76–107). New York: Praeger.

Greenberg, L. S., & Safran, J. D. (1987). *Emotion in psychotherapy.* New York: Guilford.

Gurney, G. G. (1984). Contributions of client-centered therapy to filial, marital, and family relationship enhancement therapies. In R. L. Levant & J. M. Shlien (Eds.), *Client-centered therapy and the person-centered approach* (pp. 261–277). New York: Praeger.

Hart, T. J. (1983). *Modern eclectic therapy.* New York: Plenum.

Leitaer, G. (1984). Unconditional positive regard: A controversial basic attitude in client-centered therapy. In R. L. Levant & J. M. Shlien (Eds.), *Client-centered therapy and the person-centered approach* (pp. 41–58). New York: Praeger.

Leventhal, H. (1979). A perceptual–motor processing model of emotion. In P. Pliner, K. Blankenstein, & I. M. Spigel (Eds.), *Perception of emotion in self and others* (Vol. 5, pp. 1–40). New York: Plenum.

Leventhal, H. (1984). A perceptual–motor theory of cognition. In L. Berkowitz (Ed.), *Advances in experimental social psychology* (pp. 36–80). New York: Academic Press.

Maslow, L. H. (1954). *Motivation and personality.* New York: Harper.

Rice, L. N. (1974). The evocative function of the therapist. In D. A. Wexler & L. N. Rice (Eds.), *Innovations in client-centered therapy* (pp. 289–311). New York: Wiley.

Rice, L. N. (1983). The relationship in client-centered therapy. In M. J. Lambert (Ed.), *Psychotherapy and patient relationships.* (pp. 36–60). Homewood, IL: Dow-Jones Irwin.

Rice, L. N. (1984) Client tasks in client-centered therapy. In R. L. Levant & J. M. Shlien (Eds.), *Client-centered therapy and the person-centered approach* (pp. 261–277). New York: Praeger.

Rice, L. N., & Greenberg, L. S. (1984). The new research paradigm. In L. N. Rice & L. S. Greenberg (Eds.), *Patterns of change: Intensive analysis of psychotherapy process* (pp. 7–26). New York: Guilford.

Rice, L. N., & Saperia, E. P. (1984). Task analysis of the resolution of problematic reactions. In L. N. Rice & L. S. Greenberg (Eds.), *Patterns of change: Intensive analysis of psychotherapy process* (pp. 29–66). New York: Guilford.

Rogers, C. R. (1959). A theory of therapy, personality, and interpersonal relationships as developed in the client-centered framework. In S. Koch (Ed.), *Psychology: The study of a science: Vol. III. Formulations of the person and the social context* (pp. 184–256). New York: McGraw-Hill.

Rogers, C. R. (1961). *On becoming a person.* Boston: Houghton Mifflin.

Rogers, C. R. (1963). The concept of the fully functioning person. *Psychotherapy: Theory, Research, and Practice,* I, 17–26.

Rogers, C. R., & Skinner, B. S. (1962). *Education and the control of human behavior.* Debate held at the University of Minnesota.

Seeman, J. (1984). The fully functioning person: Theory and research. In R. L. Levant & J. M. Shlien (Eds.), *Client-centered therapy and the person-centered approach* (pp. 131–152). New York: Praeger.

Tulving, E. (1972). Episodic and semantic memory. In E. Tulving & W. Donaldson (Eds.), *Organization of memory* (pp. 382–402). New York: Academic Press.

Wexler, D. A. (1974) A cognitive theory of experiencing, self-actualization, and therapeutic process. In D. A. Wexler & L. N. Rice (Eds.), *Innovations in client-centered therapy* (pp. 49–116). New York: Wiley.

Wiseman, H. L. (1986). *Single case studies of the resolution of problematic reactions in short-term client-centered therapy: A task-focused approach.* Unpublished doctoral dissertation, York University.

Wiseman, H. L. & Rice, L. N. (1989). Sequential analysis of therapist–client interaction during change events: A task-focused approach. *Journal of Consulting and Clinical Psychology,* 57, 281–286.

9

Affect in Focusing and Experiential Psychotherapy

KATHLEEN N. McGUIRE
The Focusing Community, Eugene, Oregon

INTRODUCTION

This chapter represents Eugene Gendlin's experiential therapy as worked through this author's own personal emphasis upon the catharsis of emotion as a healing factor. I have asked Gendlin to write a free-standing chapter on his own view of emotion in psychotherapy. He was also generous enough to make detailed comments on my original draft of this chapter. His comments have helped the two of us to see the one area where we do have a substantial disagreement. This is in my emphasis upon catharsis as a change factor and almost as a *goal* of focusing. Gendlin sees catharsis as a repeating of emotion that often gets in the way of the less dramatic unfolding of body steps, which he sees as basic to focusing. A fuller description of this difference occurs at the end of my chapter.

ROLE OF AFFECT IN HUMAN FUNCTIONING

Distinction between Emotion and Felt Experiencing

It is important for the purpose of this chapter to begin by making a distinction between "sheer emotion" and "felt experiencing," as these concepts will be used in this chapter. Gendlin (1962) makes the distinction as follows:

Let us also compare "experiencing" with the common term "emotion." We said that "experiencing" is a felt datum, and this word "felt" may suggest that it must be an emotion. Often, some emotion is the most important aspect of some present "this" or experiencing. However, just as often, a client will refer to "this feeling" and when he comes to conceptualize it later it will turn out to be a complex of many meanings (such as "I know what is really at the bottom of it, it's that I feel so inferior in action and people will despise me because . . ." and so on at length). In this last-mentioned example, it is clear that the client has for some minutes been trying to "get at" just what the "feel" of what he is talking about is. This "feel" isn't just an emotion (in this case). It is a directly *felt* datum that *implicitly* means a great deal. Therapy is largely the process of directly referring to, "getting at," "feeling out" the feel of what the client first talks *about*. Thus, "experiencing" may be defined as the (directly referred-to) "feel" of some situation, concept, object, personal relationship, content, or the like. (pp. 243–244ff., n.9c)

In the general literature, the terms "affect," "feeling," and "emotion" are used indiscriminately and confusingly to denote these two different types of human functioning. It is usually "sheer emotion" that is talked about and studied, while "felt experiencing," and the subtleties of meaning that arise from attempts to articulate it, is overlooked. Yet, it is from contact with felt experiencing, not from sheer emotionality, that the possibility for change in psychotherapy arises.

Function in Human Living

Sheer emotion, as an automatic and visceral reaction to a stimulus situation, probably at the most primitive level functions to throw the organism into "fight or flight" as necessitated for the survival of the organism. These responses can occur outside of conscious awareness. In their function of alerting the organism to danger, emotions can be elicited by very minimal evidence of danger in the stimulus situation. This is adaptive in that "fight or flight" can be initiated quickly enough to avert possible danger. It can be maladaptive for human beings inasmuch as perceptual schemata that classify situations as dangerous and evoke an emotional reaction, once developed, become very difficult to change. A minimal stimulus evokes avoidant behavior, and the organism has no chance to be exposed to new information in the situation. It becomes difficult for the person to learn that, while certain stimuli signaled danger in earlier situations, there is no such danger in present situations and that emotional reactions are no longer adaptive.

While sheer emotion is a narrow, primitive, repetitive response, felt experiencing is a broader bodily sensing of the personal context, past, present, and future intending, as it is functioning in the present moment. Its role in human functioning is to give meaning. It is of felt experiencing that a person can ask: "Why does this particular situation make me so angry?" and find an answer in terms of personal history and personal values: "Oh, because this person reminds me of my father, and, when my father acted this way, I really was in danger of annihilation." It is in relation to felt experiencing that the person can re-evaluate the situation: "I'm not in danger now. I'm bigger. I can handle it." It is such re-evaluation that leads to personality change. Note that a re-evaluation arises from a change in felt experiencing, not a reconstrual, which can be arrived at through logic without reference to the preverbal.

ROLE OF AFFECT IN PSYCHOTHERAPY

Emotion, Focusing, and Catharsis

To the psychotherapist, sheer emotion signals the presence of a trouble spot—an area of unprocessed and repetitive response to pain. Tears in the eyes, anger in the voice, they say to the therapist: "Whatever we're talking about now is important. It evokes emotion and a defensive reaction of fight or flight to the pain."

The experiential therapist will want to go to the felt experiencing implicit in emotional areas so that bodily living can be carried forward. "Experiential focusing" is the technique used in going from sheer emotionality to felt experiencing: "Can you get a broader sense of that anger in your body?"; "Can you stop and sense into the meaning of these tears for you?"; "Ask your body: 'What's this anger all about?' and wait and see what comes." Emotionality, without this step of focusing upon the felt experiencing implicit in it and creating a new whole sense within which the emotion is newly experienced, will repeat and repeat without changing. Similar events will stir the same emotional response over and over again. If "catharsis" is just such a repetition of the original emotion without the step of deeper focusing upon the felt meanings implicit in the emotion and the creation of a new, bodily lived whole, then catharsis will not lead to personality change.

An example may help to delineate between the repeating of sheer emotion in an unchanging way and the carrying forward of experiencing as that emotion is experienced within the new whole created within the therapeutic situation.

A client talks about her anger at her partner for making the decision to leave his individual therapy without consulting her. This angry emotion is a familiar one, arising in an unchanging way in similar situations. It repeats and repeats and is not productive in terms of resolving the situations:

CLIENT: Yes. I felt both ways, and I said both things 'cause I didn't know how they fit. No, the process was rotten. When I made the decision about here: I'd come to the point where I was going to talk to you about changing what we were doing, I let him know. I didn't ask for his approval or, but I let him know how I got to it, and was willing to hear. And it definitely had to do with things that concerned him. So he said he could see how he did it really badly, and he was genuinely sorry . . . I was remembering the time about graduate school that he called up and told me what he was thinking of doing and I just said, "I don't want to talk to you." The thing just seemed so off the wall.

The therapist asks the client to focus, to try to get in touch with the larger felt whole that underlies the repeating emotion of anger:

THERAPIST: Could you just right now try to feel what all your feeling is about? It seems like almost this whole hour there have been tears right behind your talking, and I've been trying to figure out what they are and I haven't come up with it. It's like you're strained still with something.

The client comes up with a larger contextual whole. There are tears in her eyes; the angry emotion switches to sadness or hurt:

C: Well (*tears in eyes, voice cracking*), I know the hard places for me are being left out because I am one step away from being not wanted . . . (*voice fading*)

From touching upon the felt whole, she comes up with many more aspects of the situation:

C: And I said that it was the same thing about Linda [the other woman], the same thing about things happening . . . Losing somebody that you love and not being able to protect (*tearful, voice cracking*) them or yourself from it, (*crying*) (*long pause*) whether it's some accident or somebody deciding, (*crying*) you know, saying they're not going to do this [relationship] anymore. (*crying*)

The therapist asks her to focus upon the felt whole again:

T: Can we stay with the deciding one maybe for a while because we've done the, having someone die, but it seems like it's a different case to think, the feeling that the person could just decide to stop loving you or could push you out of his life . . . It seemed the second one is more of what it was like in your family, that they would just decide not to love you anymore, decide to leave you on the outside, that there wasn't anything you could do.

The client enters a deep state of grieving:

C (*long pause, crying*): I don't know how other people decide things. (*crying*)

Here she is not simply recycling the angry emotion but is feeling within the present new whole, which includes her capacity to look at herself empathically as well as the therapist's support, a sadness for her past pain and confusion.

With continual focusing instructions from the therapist, which ask the client to attend to the broader feeling under whatever emotion she is experiencing, the client goes through the following steps, often accompanied with deep sobbing and sometimes laughter (often after healing catharsis).

C: It has to do with losing people and it has to do with being lost myself.

T: Being lost yourself?

C: It seems to be two sides of it—one of losing people that I love and the other side of it is what it feels like to be lost and not wanted by people . . . I always—when we'd travel or we would do anything, I always thought—they were my parents and my sister, I always thought of them as three and me. My sister has said (*laughs*) that she thought of it in totally another way, that she never felt connected to them (*laughing*). I said, "No, it was you and them," "Oh no, it was you and them." (*laughing*) I always— I remember they would sit in the front of the car and I would always sit in the back so I talked to my reflection in the glass, (*laughs*) . . . ugh . . . and that must be a lonely isolated place to be. I really took that as meaning something very deep that I always was in the back by myself. So feeling left out and cut off and pushed away—those are very hard things . . . Or even unconsciously, but when people are around who do it, there's always the possibility that the next moment they will love you. That must be what battered kids—you know how they keep loving their parents because they think if they get through this, the next instant . . .

T: Can you feel that feeling, that there's always the chance that maybe they'll love you?

C (*laughing*): I don't want to. (*laughing*)

T (*laughing*): What a grim little feeling to go around with!

C: That's why it's so different when Frank is around, you know, and in one of his withdrawn places, or if he's at work, you know. I mean that's how it used to be those beginning years when he was around and just totally remote like on some ice cap, and I figured if I could just get through this, any minute he could be warm and loving. It amazes me how far people will go. Those were some of the hardest times in my life I think, waiting for things like that to change. (*pause, crying*) That's why I've tried to do it so differently with Will [her son]. A couple of nights ago, I was cleaning up after supper or something, and he said, "You know, I think I just need to be a little closer. I feel like we're too separate," (*laughing*) and you know we had been doing separate things, and for weeks it won't matter. I said, "OK, what do you need?" He said, "I just need a hug and just to be a little closer." . . . And what a wonderful thing, you know, (*voice cracking*) to be able to walk up to somebody and say, "I need to be closer," and they say, "Oh terrific. I'll be closer then." Can you imagine? (*laughs, sighs*)

T: Can you imagine what that would have been like in your situation?

C: (*laughs*) I'd feel like it was a miracle. (*crying, pause*)

T: But in your case, you felt that way—"I need to be closer" and there wasn't anything you could do except wait for them to change.

C: It was so hostile and so cold and so punitive—that's what I remember. (*crying*) It comes from such terrible places. (*crying, pause*) I see this mouth just shouting and judging and judging and shouting.

T: That was your mother?

C: (*nods*) (*crying, pause*)

T: And there wasn't anywhere to go for warmth?

C: My uncle _____. He was very erratic. Sometimes we saw him once or twice a year.

T: That's not much warmth!

C: But I don't know any other place. (*sighs, long pause*) I'm really glad I came out (*laughs*) being able to do what I can do. You know, having it and being able to give it away. (*pause*) And seeing how different it can be for somebody else when they get it (*voice cracking*). I was really determined that I would never do that to anybody, and that it would be different for Will. (*pause*)

T: Do you have a sense of whether that place in you can ever be healed or what it would take to ever heal it?

C: I think to be with somebody (*voice cracking*) for a long time, and just to—be safer—I don't think it would take it away, but I think it would probably make it as good for me as it could be, and I'll make my peace with it, you know.

The therapist continuously brings the client back to the "sore spot," encouraging more tears, anger, and laughter, but in the context of focusing upon the broader felt sense and finding a word or image that can carry the experiencing further. It would be "sheer emotionality" if the therapist had encouraged the client to beat a pillow in her anger or simply to "cry as much as you can" without asking for focusing ("What is that anger?"). The client comes to a moment of resolution, of being able to imagine a next step that would heal the old hurt. She is slightly changed in her entire bodily way of living the issue.

The bodily felt whole within which the client is living in the moment includes past painful experiences, connections with present painful situations, comparisons with more positive outcomes in how she deals with her son Will, the client's capacity to feel for her past self and to imagine a future solution, as well as the therapist's nurturing attention. Gendlin points out that it is inadequate to label this a reliving of past experiences. It is a new living, a carrying forward. However, he does not give value to the changing, healing quality of the tears, sobbing, and laughter that accompany the bodily shift in the way the issue is lived. He equates this kind of catharsis with the nonproductive repeating of the emotion of anger with which the client started. This author would like him to give more attention to the qualitatively different nature of these two forms of "emotion."

Direct Reference to Felt Experiencing

Gendlin, in his seminal work *Experiencing and the Creation of Meaning* (1962), and in many later articles (Gendlin, 1965, 1965/1966, 1966) is the theorist who has best delineated the realm of felt experiencing and its relationship to cognitions, emotions, images, and other symbolic phenomena. Gendlin distinguishes among the many forms of human symbol making (behavior, emotions, cognitions, images, environmental situations, perceptions) and the presymbolic ground from which symbolizations emerge and in reference to which symbolizations acquire their meaning. "Felt experiencing," or the preverbal, preconceptual ground of being, exists independently of symbols and can be referred to directly (Gendlin, 1965). It is in such moments of "direct reference" to felt experiencing that the possibility for the creation of new meanings, and, thus, of personality change (Gendlin, 1964) resides. Direct reference includes those moments when one sets aside symbolizations and stops to attend directly to the experiential feel of a particular symbolization.

If someone is asked, "What's the meaning of 'democracy'?" he/she will probably pause for a moment, refer to the bodily felt experiencing that contains every nuance of meaning of that word acquired through years of personal, lived experiencing, and then begin to respond by forming words and images out of that felt experiencing. If I ask you, "How are you today?" and you stop for a moment and tune into your bodily feel for the day, then you will form an answer that arises as an accurate symbolization of the wealth of information preconceptually accessed in that moment of pause.

If a client is asked, "What makes you so sad?" the therapist does not want him/her to answer with pat intellectualizations that are ready to hand. Instead, the therapist hopes that the client will refer directly to the felt sense of the experience of the sadness in this moment and only then attempt to form words or images for expressing it.

There is a distinction between these moments of direct reference and sheer emotion as outlined above. The literature on the felt side of human functioning ignores this distinction between well-defined emotions, such as anger, sadness, joy, and the bodily sensed, unclear whole, which Gendlin calls the "felt sense."

Gendlin's Theory of Personality Change

In his "A Theory of Personality Change," Gendlin (1964) describes the following process in which change occurs. It is a process that moves back and forth between symbols and the presymbolic, felt ground of meaning. Here is this author's summary of that process, especially as it applies to therapeutic work with emotion:

Direct Reference

First, there must be a moment of direct reference to a "felt sense," the preconceptual bodily feel of an issue, which is without words or other symbols. Such direct reference may be asked for explicitly through a focusing instruction ("Can you stop for a moment and just get in touch with the feel of this whole issue?") or it may be stirred up indirectly by any number of therapeutic techniques aimed at the arousal of emotion (Gestalt role-playing, Freudian interpretations, Rogerian reflection of felt meaning, Lowenian bioenergetics, Jungian dream analysis, etc.). If emotion is stirred by the latter array of techniques, then the focusing step must still be taken. "It seems emotion has been stirred by what we have done. Can you stop for a moment and just sense into the broader whole of that feeling?" Galvanic skin response tests show a drop in anxiety with direct reference, even if the content focused upon is of a seemingly upsetting nature (Gendlin & Berlin, 1961).

Explication of Felt Meaning

After direct reference to a felt sense, comes "explication of felt meaning," or the careful crafting of words, images, or gestures that are exactly right in expressing the felt sense that has been referred to. Explication may involve several attempts at symbolization, each reflected by the therapist and checked against the felt sense.

Felt Shift

When explication reaches the point where the symbolizations created are exactly right in capturing the nuances of the felt experiencing, then the client may experience a "felt shift," a moment in which there is a bodily experience of release and change in the felt referent. Electroencephalographic recordings show changes in wave patterns, both during direct reference and during felt shifts (Don, 1977). The felt shift, whether it is a barely perceptible release of tension or a dramatic cathartic unfolding, is the crux of personality change. It is as if the issue has been turned 180° and can suddenly be seen from a different perspective. The felt shift is a *physical* event, again, preverbal. While words, images, and emotions follow immediately, it is the physical event that is healing. While a felt shift is often marked only by a sigh, or a relaxation of tension in the shoulders, it is also often accompanied by a much deeper kind of physical catharsis in the form of intense sobbing, often mingled with laughter at how good it feels for this sadness to be releasing. It is this kind of catharsis, as distinguished from the repetitive stuckness of sheer emotion, that is part of the deepest kind of healing on a bodily level.

Global Application

After the felt shift, there may be some moments of "global application," as a flood of symbolizations and memory follow upon the bodily release. The person may make many connections between different areas of conflict or between past and present situations. There is a quality of truth to these "emergent insights," of "Oh, yes, this is how it is; I know it now," as opposed to the hypothetical nature of much earlier exploration: "Maybe I feel this way because of how my father treated me." It is important to note that global application follows upon and is almost a by-product of the felt shift. It is a symbolization of change that has already occurred at the bodily level. Global application, though it may occur, is not necessary to personality change. It is the felt shift in the way the issue is carried in the body, rather than any intellectual insights, that determines the changes in behavior, emotion, and cognitions that will be manifested as "personality change." Intellectual understandings, unaccompanied by a bodily felt shift, do not cause change. So we have the client who arrives in therapy, often after a "successful" analysis, saying, "I know that I can't be sexual with women because of my mother's symbiotic and suffocating relationship with me but nothing has changed. I *still* can't be sexual with women." The healing step in therapy will be to go back to the bodily feel of the interaction with the mother and to carry forward that experiencing through many small steps of direct reference and explication of felt meaning.

THERAPEUTIC TECHNIQUES

Focusing and Direct Reference

While the felt shift, when accompanied by a cathartic bodily process, is a dramatic moment of personality change of special interest to this author, it is the often less dramatic moments of direct reference to felt experiencing that are the true catalysts of personality change. The work of the experiential therapist is to produce such moments of direct reference. If direct reference can be facilitated, felt shifts in experiencing will eventually follow, often in their own unpredictable way.

As mentioned above, Gendlin emphasizes the slow steps of direct reference and not dramatic moments of catharsis. Felt shifts may be (but are not always) dramatic. Gendlin might even say that such deep catharsis could happen without there also being a felt shift in the way the issue is carried in the body, although this author disagrees. However, it would be easy for attention to become focused upon such dramatic happenings. Felt shifts, dramatic and subtle, are a product of many small steps of "focusing" upon felt referents, and it is upon this focusing that Gendlin wishes to place emphasis.

Focusing is a technique for setting aside already known symbolizations and attending to the fresh, bodily experience of an issue. Gendlin invented the focusing technique when research on the process of psychotherapy (Rogers, 1967; Gendlin, Beebe, Cassens, Klein, & Oberlander, 1968) showed that the success of clients in verbal psychotherapy could be predicted within the first few sessions of psychotherapy, and predicted more accurately on the basis of the client's own capacity to focus upon and to speak from bodily felt experiencing than on the basis of particular therapist interventions. Clients who started therapy high in this capacity for direct reference, as measured by the Experiencing (EXP) Scale (Klein, Mathieu, Gendlin, & Kiesler, 1969), more often succeeded in therapy, while clients who could not refer to felt experiencing most often failed.

Focusing Training

Gendlin decided to concentrate his energies on teaching clients to refer to felt experiencing. He developed the skill called focusing (Gendlin, 1981), which basically instructs clients to set aside existing symbolizations and to refer to the felt sense of the entire situation. As in the steps of personality change outlined above, focusing proceeds through a process of steps:

1. Clearing a space.
2. Finding the felt sense of the problem.
3. Finding a "handle" word or image (a symbolization).

4. Resonating the handle against the felt sense until the symbolization is just right for the felt sense.
5. Asking open-ended questions of the felt sense, ("What's the worst of this?"; "What's in the way of this being all OK?"; etc.) and waiting for symbols to come from it.
6. Receiving whatever has come in a gentle, accepting manner (see Gendlin's book for an in-depth presentation of the focusing steps).

When practiced alone or in the company of another, focusing can lead to felt shifts in experiencing and, thus, long-term changes in cognitions, emotions, and behavior. Gendlin has developed a focusing workshop where focusing is taught as a skill, outside of the context of ongoing psychotherapy. Trainees work in small groups and one-to-one sessions practicing each step of focusing. An entire day is spent just learning to "clear a space," a first step. Clearing a space involves learning to "put down" issues that are being carried as bodily tension until the body can be experienced relatively free of tension for at least a few moments. Trainees are instructed to lie or sit in a comfortable position, to close their eyes if they wish, and to relax their bodies. Many different kinds of relaxation exercises and guided imagery techniques may be used, and some trainees might have to spend hours or weeks simply learning to relax and to tolerate the bodily sensations and images that arise from a relaxed body. Other trainees, who can quickly go into a very deep meditation or hypnosis-like state, may have to learn to relax *less*. Focusing is only possible in an in-between state where attention can still be placed upon various inner processes.

Once trainees have entered this in-between state of focused attention, they are instructed to clear a space, using any one of a variety of images for making a list of issues and setting them aside one by one. For instance, trainees may be told to imagine that they are sitting on a park bench with a big sack full of parcels (Neil Friedman, personal communication). The parcels represent the issues they are carrying as physical tensions that day. They are instructed to imagine taking the parcels out of the bag, one at a time, each time describing the parcel as a particular issue and getting a feel for the way they are carrying that whole issue in their body. After a moment of feeling the bodily quality of that issue, they are instructed to imagine placing that particular parcel on the park bench at a comfortable distance from themselves and, using that image, to put that bodily feel outside of the center of their body for a while. The point now is not to attempt to solve the issue, but to have the bodily experience of "setting it down" for a while and being able to feel what the body feels like when it is momentarily free of carrying this issue.

Within Gendlin's theoretical framework, a person cannot work on an issue when he/she is totally immersed in it in a bodily way. The person must be able to get a little bit separate from the feel of the issue, and then to relate to that feel in a focusing way, asking it "What are you all about?" or "What is the worst of it?" or "How are you stuck?" and waiting until words, images, or gestures arise directly out of the bodily feel. These symbols are then checked or resonated against the bodily feel and modified until they are "just right." "Just right"-ness is experienced as a bodily shift in the tension associated with the issue.

In a focusing workshop, after learning how to relax and how to have the experience of a "cleared space," trainees continue guided practice in the other steps of focusing: (1) choosing one of the issues, or "parcels," to work on; (2) bringing the feel of it back into the center of the body and getting a felt sense for the whole of it; (3) finding symbols that seem accurate in expressing the felt sense; (4) resonating, checking, and modifying the symbols until they are "just right"; (5) gently receiving whatever feeling or information arises during the felt shift; (6) checking with the felt sense of the issue again, seeing how it has changed, and starting another cycle of focusing upon it if desired. This is the barest outline of the focusing steps. For further understanding of the focusing process, the reader is referred to Gendlin (1981) and McGuire (1981).

Experiential Psychotherapy

Focusing can be practiced alone or in a peer context. It is a careful process for learning to discriminate among several different inner processes. However, many clients would balk at the introduction of such extensive instructions for making distinctions in inner space. Clients who have a lot of fear and resistance around feeling things in the body (this author has seen this to be especially threatening to some who have been physically or sexually abused, but it is also difficult for many others who have simply been told that feelings are bad, weak, or useless) may need a longer-term combination of focusing instruction with other techniques of verbal psychotherapy. In "experiential psychotherapy" (Gendlin, 1973, 1974, 1983; McGuire, 1984), intervention with focusing instructions happens more subtly within the flow of ongoing verbal psychotherapy. As the client describes a recent event and shows signs of emotion or implicit meaning at some point in the description, the therapist says, "Can you stop and just feel into the sense of that whole upsetness?" or "Can you just sense into the meaning of that argument for you?" and so on. When an interpretation, a reflection, or the use of an image stirs some sign of emotion, the therapist again asks for focusing: "Can you see what all of that feeling is about? Don't answer from your head. Just stop for a moment and let your body tell you."

If the client is continuously far from any present experiencing and caught in abstract intellectualization, the therapist may intervene more strongly in a focusing way: "Wait. Let's just stop for a moment and see if you can feel this issue in your body. Can you just check and see if you can feel it anywhere in your body? Is it in your throat or your chest or your belly? Stop and sense into the tension there . . . Can you imagine relating to it in some way . . . putting your arms around it gently . . . receiving it in some way? . . . Try asking it gently, 'What do you have to say to me? What's hurting you?' and see what words or images come from it . . . Just stay with it gently for a while."

The therapist's task, when working experientially, is to produce moments of direct reference, of sitting with or being in touch with felt experiencing (*not* emotion, but the broader, felt whole underlying emotion). If direct reference happens, eventually this relatedness to stuck, frozen-off aspects of experiencing will enable them to unfold.

While a client is focusing and attempting to come up with fresh symbolizations for bodily felt experiencing, the therapist's most important other tool is Rogerian reflection of feeling, or more precisely, *reflection of felt meaning*. As the client grapples for words or images or gestures that are just right for capturing the felt sense, the therapist reflects these attempts at symbolization. As the client hears the reflected symbols, he/she can check them, or resonate them, against the felt sense, refining them until he/she hits upon the "just right" symbols that release a felt shift. For the experiential therapist, focusing instructions and reflections of felt meaning alternate with now and again the use of another technique to facilitate access to a felt sense that can then be focused upon (Gendlin, 1974; McGuire, 1984).

TRANSCRIPTS

The Model for Change

The following transcripts illustrate the focusing process when it happens successfully and when it is circumvented in therapy. The basic model is that of Gendlin's theory of personality change (Gendlin, 1964):

1. An emotion or image arises or the client chooses an issue to focus upon;
2. *Felt Sense*: the client attempts to get the broader felt sense of the issue, image or emotion by "focusing";
3. *Explication*: the client looks for symbols (words, images, or gestures) to convey the felt sense;
4. *Checking*: as the therapist reflects these symbolizations, the client checks them against the felt sense, refining them until they are "just right" in capturing the felt sense;

5. *Felt Shift*: when symbols are found that are "just right," the client experiences a felt shift, indicated by a visible release of bodily tension and sometimes by a deep catharsis of tears and sobbing;

6. *Global Application*: Verbal expressions of an "Ah hah!" nature sometimes follow upon the felt shift in the process of emergent insight called global application. It is an *application* of the changed bodily living to many areas. The seeming insights are a by-product of this bodily change. The "insights" are not the cause of change but one of the effects.

7. *Felt Sense*: At the end of such a cycle, the client again attends to the felt sense, noting any changes, and beginning a new cycle of focusing, if desired.

An Example of Successful Focusing

This is a 10- to 20-minute vignette of focusing therapy that happened in a classroom demonstration situation. The client is a 30-year-old woman, a graduate student in counseling psychology. The therapist is Neil Friedman, author of *Experiential Therapy and Focusing* (1982). (Dr. Friedman trained with Dr. Gendlin, as well as others.) Dr. Friedman combines Gendlin's empathic listening and experiential focusing techniques with other interventions, especially those from Gestalt therapy. (The step from the model that is illustrated appears in brackets.)

C: Um . . . what I want to talk about a little bit is a feeling that I'm . . . um . . . just beginning to recognize or that's just beginning to be there. I-noticed-it-yesterday kind of thing, so I thought "Great . . . work on it." [Felt Sense]

The client starts already talking about a felt sense—an unclear, bodily feel for an issue that is in need of explication.

T: So, it's kind of like a brand new bud that you noticed there yesterday.

The therapist reflects the meaning.

C: Yeah . . . but I knew it was coming, as well, 'cause it's all around terminating . . . from here . . . um . . . with clients . . . internship . . . so a lot of termination. [Explication]

The client knows intellectually that the feeling is related to termination, but such intellectual knowledge doesn't help. Her bodily living in relation to the experience needs to be carried forward. A focusing question would be, "How is this termination issue being carried in the body?"

T: So, like, you knew it was on the way and you started feeling it just yesterday.

The therapist simply reflects again, giving the client space for the attempts at explication that she is making.

C: Yeah . . . um . . . hm . . . (*long pause*) [Felt Sense] And it's . . . there's sadness there. That's not what's on top right now, but there's a lot of sadness with it, and I'm just kind of checking in and seeing if there's stuff around, like, after that, if I'm questioning . . . [Checking] what's going to be there after that. But it doesn't seem like it's that . . . all of this ending . . . It's everything, like . . . I've been here a long time and . . . um . . . though this year I'm in the graduate program and doing it in one year, it's intense . . . um . . . it's kind of like my whole life is here in a lot of ways, and it's like . . . it's all going to be over really soon. [Explication]

During the long pauses, the client stops all talking and just tries to feel into the felt sense that is there. After some moments of this direct reference, she finds words for a new aspect of the felt sense: "There's sadness there." She tries out various symbolizations for the felt sense, checking or resonating them against it to see if they fit. She thought, intellectually, that maybe "I'm questioning . . . what's going to be there after that." But she checks this intellectualization against the felt sense, and it doesn't produce a bodily response of resonance: "But it doesn't seem like it's that . . ." She tries out various other symbolizations, trying to close in on the felt sense: "I've been here a long time . . . it's intense . . . my whole life is here . . . it's all going to be over really soon." These verbalizations are in the ball park, but there is not yet an "Ah hah!" experience as the body responds to the "just right" symbols. There is still a sense of vague reaching for symbols.

The therapist reflects again and then asks for direct reference, or focusing, again: "just let yourself be quiet now and see what's there." He asks her to suspend thinking and sense freshly exactly what is there in the felt sense.

C: (*sigh*) (*long pause*) (*sigh*) [Felt Sense]
T: Just give yourself time. Let your attention go down inside your body . . . Just breathe into it, just in a friendly way . . . think of all of it . . .

The client cooperates by focusing deeply upon the bodily feel of the issue. The sighs, in relation to the pause, indicate some beginning of a felt shift in the way the body is carrying the issue. Direct reference, in itself, begins a change. A part of experiencing that has been cut off and held static as a bodily tension is now being touched with focused attention. The simple act of attempting to relate to it and to make symbols for it lets it start to change. The therapist facilitates this relatedness with more focusing instructions that emphasize simply being with the bodily feel in a relational way: "Just breath into it, just in a friendly way."

C (*long pause*): [Felt Sense] I can really feel the loss (*tearful*) and somehow it has to do with when my mother died . . . um . . . and that loss. [Explication; Felt Shift]

Again, the client cooperates with a pause for direct reference. She finds new words for the feel of this issue: "I can really feel the loss and somehow it has to do with when my mother died." This is the beginning of a bodily carrying forward. The events around termination at school had touched upon the unresolved grief around the mother. The client had not been conscious of this connection at the beginning but only conscious of the vague, bodily felt discomfort around the ending. The new symbolization about the relationship to the mother's death has also not been offered as an intellectual connection made either by the therapist or the client. It has emerged directly from the bodily carrying forward. It is important to note that the client might have started out with the intellectual connection but not been able to go anywhere with it until focusing upon the bodily feel led to a change in the body's way of carrying the issue. She might have said: "I'm upset about ending here, and I think it has to do with my mother's death, but I don't know exactly how." Again, the "how" would have had to come from direct reference to the *feeling* of upsetness and explication of it. The explication would be a carrying forward of the way that issue is lived in the body and would change every aspect of the client's experience of that issue.

T: So the loss of school brings up the loss of mother.

C (*sniffling, tears*) [Felt Sense]: Yeah. There's real similarities there. Like she had cancer, and I knew, and I began here right after she died.

T: Um.

C: And I guess it's almost . . . when you said the words "Loss of mother" or "Loss of school brings up loss of mother," somehow, I had this whole other sense of how (*tearful*) nurtured I've felt here.

T: Un huh.

C: (*tearful*)

T: The school has been like a mother to you.

C: (*tearful*) Yeah . . . (*very tearful*) I'm not ready to lose another one. (*sobbing*) [Felt Shift]

T: (*softly*) Not again. Not another one.

Client and therapist continue the process of focusing and the issue of termination is experienced as part of a new whole. The client experiences the unresolved grief for her mother in the context of the nurturing presence of the therapist and the awareness of school as a nurturing place. The process of grieving is carried forward on the bodily, lived level. Tears and deep sobbing accompany the bodily shifting of the felt sense.

C (*sobbing, sighs*): Oh, God . . . now I'm getting more and more connections, like, I realize, I'm graduating in August and I don't know the exact date, but it's within 4 days of when she died.

T: So, it's in August.

C (*tears*): I see more and more connections coming out. I think that, um (*tears, pause*) losing my mother felt like I also lost my family. I'm the only (*tearful*) female really left, and she was the link, and kind of, without her, it's really dissipated . . . and (*inaudible*) . . . um and being here has been a family as well (*tearful*) . . . um . . . and . . . oh . . . that will dissipate. [Global Application]

The client refers to the experience of global application: "Oh, God . . . now I'm getting more and more connections . . ." New conceptualizations continue to emerge, accompanying the bodily felt shift and unfolding of the felt referent.

T: So it's not just the loss of school, or even the loss of mother, but the loss of family. That she represented family, and the school represented family.

C: Yes . . . in a way I haven't been aware of.

T: Uhhm.

C: And, when she died, that was a loss I hadn't anticipated . . . I knew I was losing her, but I didn't know until afterwards that I was losing family as well. [Global Application]

T: Hm . . . that was a part you didn't anticipate.

There is particularly the new realization that loss of mother/school = loss of family, again, not a connection made intellectually but one that emerges as she lives out of a new bodily whole.

At this point in the transcript, we have reached the end of a cycle of focusing. The therapist senses that there is more work to be done and initiates another cycle by asking the client to focus: "Can you just go back inside and see what you feel there?" The client finds more grieving for her mother. The therapist works with this emotion through a combination of reflective listening, focusing, and Gestalt techniques. We will skip about 5 minutes of this exploration and go to a final, focusing question that the therapist asked as he sensed the time for the session coming to an end:

T: What does it need? What can help things? Go inside.

C: Well, I got immediately, I need to start therapy again. And to do that now would have something nurturing . . . sustaining . . . that would be . . . it wouldn't relate to the ending, it'd be happening now. [Explication]

T: Yes, yes.

C: And I really want to do that. Um . . . So it really surprised me that it popped up.

T: It was pretty clear.

C: Yeah.

T: Does it feel OK to stop here? Do you know where to go?

C: Yeah. Yeah.

The therapist again gives a focusing instruction, this time suggesting that the client ask the felt sense "What can help things?" and, instead of answering from her head, find an answer that resonates with the felt sense. The client answers that she has found an action step that fits: She will start a new nurturing for herself by entering therapy.

The client began by reactively responding to the situation of leaving school with the same emotional reaction that was appropriate to her mother's death. She then focused upon the felt whole underneath this emotional reaction and experienced the painful past experience within the new whole created in the nurturing therapeutic interaction. She becomes able to imagine an action (nurturing herself through going into therapy) that is an appropriate resolution of the present situation. Gendlin points to the importance of describing change as a *new* living, rather than a re-experiencing of past pain:

> I get upset when you talk about insights. Who needs them? She does not re-experience her grief, it only looks like that. She has her mother-experience in midst of having the therapist there, *this* time it is different, she has time to work it out, she can tell the mother-person about it, etc. She gets "connections" she's never had, but that means the whole is being experienced from a felt sense, as it was not then. She won't resolve her mother-grief by re-experiencing it over and over, but by experiencing this past within and as part of a wider present, thus not re-experiencing *it*, but—as she says—the nurturance that's going on now, here. And that's why the past can change in how it functions in her body. It's not changing because she sobs it over and over. I know *she says* it's the connections that are doing the thing, but we know it's the whole in her body changing in the present living process. That's why the connections come. They're only signs of what's physically happening. The excerpt is just right!! It shows her changing physically through *new steps in the present, not* through re-anything. (E. Gendlin, personal communication, 1987)

An Example of Less Successful Focusing

The episode takes place in about the middle of an hour-long therapy session. Therapist and client have been working together for more than 30 sessions at this time. The client is very intellectualized and has great difficulty locating a bodily felt sense. He also seems to be afraid of approaching feelings. He is 40 years old. The therapist is the author, again trained by Gendlin but incorporating Gestalt and other techniques.

The client started the session by saying that a friend of his thinks there's "one major block and not a whole bunch of complicated things" keeping him from choosing a career and being able to commit to a relationship. The therapist has tried in a variety of ways to help him to get a bodily feel for what's blocking him. In the following excerpt she makes another attempt at focusing instructions:

C: It may be like I can't practice an instrument very easily. But I mean, I can understand the music. I'll sit and listen to someone perform it and I realize that I know exactly what I have to do to do it. But I won't . . . and it's . . . (*pause*)

T: And why is that? Don't answer from your head. You're looking for the block. It's just like you and your friend M——— talked about. It's a block. It's like this. (*holds hands in front of abdomen as if holding a stone*) It's like a big blob down here.

C: Well, maybe it's something as simple as discipline . . .

T: You can't start out with "maybe" . . .

C: My mother always said it was discipline.

T: Anything that starts with "maybe" is more like thinking. I want you to see if you can feel the blocked place in your body.

Unlike the client in the first transcript, this client doesn't start with an unclear bodily feel but with intellectual hypotheses about his situation. The therapist tries to help him to find how he is living the issue in his body. She tries to provide very concrete bodily images. But, instead of referring to his body, the client immediately answers from his head, with more hypotheses: "Maybe it's something as simple as discipline." The therapist directs him away from thinking and toward his body.

C: No. I can feel a tension in through here. (*points at upper chest*) (*pause*) [Felt Sense] I can't paint a word picture of it.

T: Just sit quietly a little longer and see if you can—just ask yourself, just see if you can come in touch with the block. We all agree that there's some one small block in your life that if you can get over it—now see if you can feel it as a block. The stuckness.

C: I feel a kind of defiance. [Explication]

T: What are the words for that? (*pause*) Is that in relation to me?

C: No. Well, maybe. It might come to that 'cause you're making me do it.

T: Right. (*laughs*)

There is an emotion ("I can feel a tension in through here") and, as the client focuses upon the broader felt sense, he finds words for it: "I feel a kind of defiance." One can hypothesize that the present situation is bringing up painful past experiences that had to do with being asked to do something. The therapist asks the client to focus upon the broader felt sense of the "defiance": "What are the words for that?" But the client edges away from the bodily feel and back into "maybe": "Well, maybe. It might come to that 'cause you're making me do it." His words are not a fresh symbolization of the present bodily feel, but an intellectual guess. The therapist continues to try to go either to the felt sense of the block or of the defiance, but instead is caught in a transferential power struggle. She suspends focusing for the time being and works at interpreting the transference. Later she will attempt focusing again.

The client circumvents the focusing instruction by a variety of defenses (changing the subject, positing intellectual hypotheses, engaging the therapist in a power struggle). There are some tiny moments of direct reference and explication when he names the emotion of "defiance" and then pauses when asked to find words for that feeling. However, he never really stops very long to focus upon the felt sense, allowing words or images to arise from it. He seems afraid of discovering something new and keeps tight control with his intellectual analyses.

RESEARCH DIRECTIONS

EXP Level as a Research Variable

Fortunately, Gendlin's concept of "experiencing" has been well researched. During the ground-breaking research (Rogers, 1967), which led Gendlin to describe the focusing process, Klein, Mathieu, Gendlin, and Kiesler (1969) created the Experiencing (EXP) Scale as a measure of a client's ability to refer directly to felt experiencing. The EXP Scale is a seven-point ordinal measure that describes qualitatively different manners of relating to felt experiencing. At the lowest end, clients make no reference to their own inner experiencing and feelings but talk in completely externalized terms. By level 3, clients may demonstrate some emotional involvement through gesture and voice ("sheer emotion") but still they refer to emotion only as part of the narrative story ("I saw him coming down the street and I hit him. I was mad. He had it coming for the way he treated me."). The person doesn't yet describe the event from an internal perspective. At level 4, clients begin to show some sign of inner reflectivity. Emotions are described, not just behaviorally, but from an internal perspective ("I hit him because he made me so angry. I've never been so angry. It makes me mad when people treat me that way.") At level 5, true focusing begins as clients begin to ponder upon the causes of their emotions or other issues, struggling with a murky, preverbal sensing of the concern ("I want to figure out why I respond so angrily to such situations. It's a mystery to me. It seems so automatic and intense.") Stage 6 captures the moment-to-moment flux of felt experiencing and symbolization as clients make words freshly for changing and shifting felt referents. Stage 7 measures the height of the felt shift and the following global application, the moment-to-moment reintegration of experiencing as it is lived into as a new bodily whole.

The EXP Scale can be used to measure the difference between successful and unsuccessful attempts at focusing and even to predict which clients will be successful. Klein, Mathieu-Coughlan, and Kiesler (1986), Mathieu-Coughlan and Klein (1984), Rice and Saperia (1984), and Greenberg (1984) have written detailed chapters showing how EXP can be used to measure the effectiveness of various therapeutic interventions. In the transcripts above, the client in the successful vignette started out at level 5 EXP, posing a problem about feeling and beginning immediately to struggle with articulating it: "I want to talk about . . . a feeling that I'm . . . just beginning to recognize or that's just beginning to be there. I noticed it yesterday . . . so I thought, 'Great . . . work on it . . .' it's all around terminating . . ." With a little bit of reflection and a brief focusing invitation from the therapist ("Just let yourself be quiet now and see what's there . . ."), she moves into level 6 EXP, as she makes new words for feeling as it emerges and shifts in the present moment ("I can really feel the loss and somehow it has to do with when my mother died . . . and that loss . . . There's real similarities there . . . whole other sense of how nurtured I've felt here . . . I'm not ready to lose another [mother]."). She moves into level 7 as more and more connections arise ("I see more and more connections coming out. I think that . . . losing my mother felt like I also lost my family . . . and being here has been family as well . . .") and a new step arises ("I got immediately, I need to start therapy again. And to do that now would have something nurturing . . .").

The client in the unsuccessful vignette spent almost the entire session at level 2 and 3 EXP, with brief breakthroughs to level 4 after persistent attempts at focusing by the therapist. He starts at level 2. ("It may be like I can't practice an instrument . . . I can understand the music . . . I realize that I know exactly what I have to do to do it."). When the therapist tries to deepen EXP level through focusing instructions, he comes back with level 2

("Maybe it's . . . discipline . . . my mother always said it was discipline".).
After more therapist-induced focusing, he breaks into level 4 for a moment
("I feel a kind of defiance.") but then drops immediately back to level 2
hypothesizing ("No. Well, maybe. It might come to that."). Repeated
attempts at focusing brought him no deeper than level 4 EXP. He did not
experience the kind of felt shifts and reintegration of experiencing described by levels 6 and 7 EXP, and it can be hypothesized that his deep
personality structures were little changed by this session.

Sheer Emotion, Catharsis, and the Felt Sense: Three Distinct Processes

Gendlin was kind enough to provide commentary on my original draft for
this chapter, as well as to write his own free-standing chapter on emotion
in therapy. I was surprised to find in his commentary that he took quite
strong exception to my emphasis upon the cathartic process as basic to
focusing. Until that time, I had assumed that we did basically the same
thing as therapists. However, here is a sample of some of his reactions to
my chapter:

> re-experience, re-evaluate, re-process, and the emphasis on *pain*—that's
> all *your* stuff. Just label it as such. . . . If you want it to be me, do not move
> from emotion to felt sense. The hardest way to get a felt sense is from
> emotion—one has to put the whole thing out first, usually, *pull out of the
> emotion*, then get a felt sense directly, or from an image of the whole
> thing. . . .
>
> I would ask you to please differentiate between a felt shift and catharsis.
> . . . A felt shift is a way in which the whole thing, as a felt sense, shifts—
> *often very slightly*, FROM WHICH THEN little further steps come. . . . Cathar-
> sis is usually intense, a discharge. . . . Throughout: divide catharsis and
> re(experiencing) from citing me. The "slow steps" of direct reference
> don't go at all with sobbing, and *cathartic bodily unfolding* is just using
> my word "unfolding" in a way that it isn't meant to do. (E. Gendlin,
> personal communication, 1988)

The discovery of this difference indicates the need for the creation of a
new conceptual category, one that distinguishes between emotion that
repeats in an unchanging fashion and emotion that is seen as part of a
healing change process. This author suggests calling the former "sheer
emotion" as in Gendlin's usage (Gendlin, 1962), reserving the term "catharsis" for the latter. Gendlin is most concerned with a third, nonemotional felt event, which he calls the "felt sense" or "bodily sensed whole":

> You would pinpoint exactly what is little known and little understood, the
> bodily sensed whole, always unclear, but which has a life of its own so that

one cannot "define" it, until one hits upon what carries it further and opens it . . . *rather than* recognizable classifiable affect like sad, glad, scared, or mad. (E. Gendlin, personal communication, 1987)

Using this distinction I have delineated the following areas of similarity and possible difference between Gendlin and myself on the issue of affect in psychotherapy:

1. We are both agreed that the repeating of sheer emotion is *not* a change process.

2. We are agreed that, when sheer emotion is present, the change-producing intervention is to instruct the client to step out of the emotion and to focus upon (sit quietly with) the broader felt sense underlying the emotion. It is in the articulation of new symbols from this broader felt experiencing that change will occur.

3. Gendlin indicates that he is likely to steer away from arousing emotion, since he feels that it interferes with the focusing process. He indicates that he is more likely to ask clients to focus upon an image or to go directly to the felt sense of an issue. While I also use images and direct focusing instructions, I am also likely to use role-playing or Gestalt techniques to arouse an emotion and then to ask the client to focus upon the broader felt sense underlying the emotion. I am also likely to stop the client when I see signs of emotion (tears in the eyes, trembling voice, anger in voice) and to ask him/her to find and to focus upon the broader felt sense. I am not sure whether this is a difference in theory or in practice. I would find it very surprising if Gendlin does not intuitively use signs of emotionality as a guide in choosing areas to focus upon.

4. Gendlin indicates that he would interrupt catharsis, have the client "pull out of it," and focus upon the felt sense. I would not interrupt catharsis, since I see it as a healing process, which, in itself, leads to new steps in experiencing. I have seen some Gendlin-trained therapists interrupt catharsis and instruct the client to pull back and focus with a greater distance, and I have felt that was a mistake, that it violated a natural healing process. However, when I have been in the client role with Gendlin himself, or when I have seen him work, I have not seen him interrupt the process but wait until its natural conclusion and then ask for focusing upon the deeper felt sense. So, I need clarification from Gendlin here: We are agreed that one would interrupt sheer emotionality to ask for focusing. Does he mean to say that he would also interrupt catharsis? If so, we are in disagreement.

It seems more likely to me that we have a difference in theoretical emphasis, while in practice we may do much the same. We are usually agreed upon which transcripts are powerful examples of the focusing process. Gendlin places emphasis upon the moment in focusing when the client takes a "breath of fresh air," experiences something he/she has never experienced before. In the first example above, this would be at the end when the client is asked to focus upon "What would it take to heal it?" and answers: "To be with somebody for a long time and to be safer." I am more drawn to the actual process of catharsis. I see in catharsis a way in which the client attends in a loving, empathic way to his/her own former hurt and grieves for him/herself. This is a healing, new experience. While I place my theoretical emphasis upon this part of the process, in practice I go back and forth between this grieving for one's own past hurts and the articulation of the new steps that arise out of this grieving process: "What would it be like if it were all OK? Can you feel that?"; "Can you sense into this new way that you are loving yourself right now? What are the words or images for that?"; "It seems what's new is this sense of rightful anger for yourself. Can you really feel what it's like to stand up for yourself that way?" I imagine that Gendlin's work shows the same back and forth between healing the past and articulating the new.

In terms of research, a measure should be created that can distinguish among sheer emotion, catharsis, and direct reference to a felt sense. Then the research question becomes: Does catharsis add a dimension to the change process facilitated by focusing or is it unnecessary for the deepest change?

REFERENCES

Don, N. S. (1977). The transformation of conscious experience and its EEG correlates. *Journal of Altered States of Consciousness, 3*(2), 147–148.

Friedman, N. (1982). *Experiential therapy and focusing.* New York: Half Court Press. (Available from the author at 11 Donnel Street, Cambridge, MA 02140)

Gendlin, E. T. (1962). *Experiencing and the creation of meaning.* New York: Free Press.

Gendlin, E. T. (1964). A theory of personality change. In P. Worchel & D. Bryne (Eds.), *Personality change* (pp. 100–148). New York: Wiley.

Gendlin, E. T. (1965). Expressive meanings. In J. M. Edie (Ed.), *Invitation to phenomenology* (pp. 240–251). Chicago: Quadrangle Books.

Gendlin, E. T. (1965/1966). Experiential explication and truth. *Journal of Existentialism, 6*(22), Winter, 131–146.

Gendlin, E. T. (1966). Existentialism and experiential psychotherapy. In C. Moustakas (Ed.), *Existential child therapy.* New York: Basic Books. Reprinted (1970) in J. T. Hart & T. M. Tomlinson (Eds.), *New directions in client-centered therapy* (pp. 70–94). Boston: Houghton Mifflin.

Gendlin, E. T. (1973). Experiential psychotherapy. In R. Corsini (Ed.), *Current psychotherapies* (pp. 318–352). Itasca, IL: Peacock.

Gendlin, E. T. (1974). Client-centered and experiential psychotherapy. In D. A. Wexler & L. N. Rice (Eds.), *Innovations in client-centered therapy* (pp. 211–246). New York: Wiley.

Gendlin, E. T. (1981). *Focusing*. New York: Bantam Books.

Gendlin, E. T. (1982). *A process model*. Unpublished manuscript.

Gendlin, E. T. (1983). *Experiential psychotherapy*. Unpublished manuscript.

Gendlin, E. T., Beebe, J., Cassens, J., Klein, M., & Oberlander, M. (1968). Focusing ability in psychotherapy, personality, and creativity. In J. M. Shlien (Ed.), *Research in psychotherapy* (Vol. 3, pp. 217-241). Washington, DC: American Psychological Association.

Gendlin, E. T., & Berlin, J. I. (1961). Galvanic skin response correlates of different modes of experiencing. *Journal of Clinical Psychology, 17*(1), 73-77.

Greenberg, L. S. (1984). A task analysis of intrapersonal conflict resolution. In L. N. Rice & L. S. Greenberg (Eds.), *Patterns of change: Intensive analysis of psychotherapy process* (pp. 67-123). New York: Guilford.

Klein, M. H., Mathieu, P. L., Gendlin, E. T., & Kiesler, D. J. (1969). *The Experiencing Scale: A research and training manual*. Madison, WI: University of Wisconsin Extension Bureau of Audiovisual Instruction.

Klein, M. H., Mathieu-Coughlin, P. L., & Kiesler, D. J. (1986). The Experiencing Scales. In L. S. Greenberg & W. Pinsof (Eds.), *The psychotherapeutic process: A research handbook* (pp. 21-71). New York: Guilford.

Mathieu-Coughlin, P. L., & Klein, M. H. (1984). Experiential psychotherapy: Key events in client-therapist interaction. In L. N. Rice & L. S. Greenberg (Eds.), *Patterns of change: Intensive analysis of psychotherapy process* (pp. 213-248). New York: Guilford.

McGuire, K. (1981). *Building supportive community: Mutual self-help through peer counseling*. (Available from the author)

McGuire, K. (1984). *The experiential dimension in psychotherapy*. (Available from the author)

Rice, L. N., & Saperia, E. P. (1984). Task analysis of the resolution of problematic reactions. In L. N. Rice & L. S. Greenberg (Eds.), *Patterns of change: Intensive analysis of psychotherapy process* (pp. 29-66). New York: Guilford.

Rogers, C. (Ed.). (1967). *The therapeutic relationship and its impact: A program of research in psychotherapy with schizophrenics*. Madison, WI: University of Wisconsin Press.

PART III

THEORETICAL COMMENTS

10

On Emotion in Therapy

EUGENE T. GENDLIN
University of Chicago

I am concerned with three questions:

In focusing we find that a bodily sense can know a great deal about situations. How is it possible for the body to have all this information?

We find not only old information. Focusing on a bodily felt sense can bring creative steps of new development and resolution. How can the body lead to something new to the culture, and more intricate than we could deliberately invent? In other words, how are the steps we get in focusing possible?

Thirdly, how do emotions differ from a felt sense, and how are the two to be dealt with, to bring therapeutic change?

I will first discuss these questions theoretically, and then turn to practice. I distinguish emotion from "felt sense." A felt sense is a vague, implicitly complex, physical feeling that can come in your body in regard to any situation or any aspect of life. I will try to show why in psychotherapy we must focus on the felt sense. To do so seems unpromising at first. A felt sense seems vague and also much less intense than an emotion. We must surely welcome all emotions during therapy, especially blocked ones that have not been felt. But, the felt sense is needed to reach what gives rise to emotions, as well as for new steps.

This chapter was written in response to the chapter by Kathleen McGuire and then revised and expanded to include what I learned in further conversations with her.

THEORY

The First Question: How Does the Body Know so Much?

Body and environment together make up one interactional process. The body is made of environmental materials. Every living body contains (implies, is with, is of, is in, is . . . . .) the environment. Of course, your legs are made for walking; but also, all the way up into your body your organs are arranged so that walking is possible and implied to happen. If you sit too long, a need to walk develops in your whole body. Animals that climb trees have differently constructed bodies, not just different limbs. An aquatic creature differs from us in every bit of it. From one bone of a prehistoric animal one can infer not only the whole of its body, but also the whole environment, and what its body does in it. The concrete body develops from one cell—it is a product of life processes. These are all interactions with an environment. Interactional information about the environment is therefore implicit in body structure and in every bodily process.

A sentient body not only is, but also feels its interactions with the environment. We must not think of feeling only as emotions. Emotions are narrower and more specific. I will discuss them below. They come sometimes, but animals (including humans) sense their interaction with the environment all the time. This bodily sensed interaction implicitly contains the complex information I just mentioned. A vast amount of information is sensed—not in separated facets—but as a global, bodily sentience.

In the history of thought, this bodily sentience is a crucial, forgotten dimension! We have been accustomed to assume that only the five external senses give us information about the environment. Such sense data are then supposedly arranged by association and thought. Feelings were said to be mere "reactions to" the facts—after the facts are given by the five external senses and reason. For two millennia feelings were said to contain no information about one's situational reality. How could this have been believed?

Almost the only feelings that were considered were the emotions, that well-known list of recognizable, definable feelings such as anger, fear, sadness, joy, and triumph. But, the emotions had a bad reputation because they can get in the way of dealing with the external things. That gave feeling a bad reputation.

There is a more basic sensing: sentient tissue process and sentient behavior. Animal bodies sense the complex environment with which their tissues interact, and with which they behave. An animal body does not just react to external stimuli. It prefigures and implies its own continuing life process. It is born with a highly structured set of tissue and behavior processes. At every moment it prefigures and implies a next step of these processes. Behavior sequences are inherited along with bodily structure. Animals have inherited mating dances, nest building, infant care, and intricate food search, all part of their bodily sentient processes. And, we, too, inherit not only the lungs, but also the breathing behavior, not only the sex organs but also the sexual intercourse sequence. Human infants need to, and soon do crawl; they don't learn that from the adults around them.

Of course there is also fresh perception, but it occurs into (and modifies) an already highly structured, bodily implying of next steps of life process.

In humans this bodily implying is elaborated (not newly created) by culture and learning. Much of human brain expansion happened after culture already existed. Culture elaborated our bodies and brains, and made the environmental interaction even more complex. But we sense this elaborated environment physically, with our bodies.

Your situation is not just what the five senses give you. Consider: Does your sense of a situation consist of bits of color, sound, and smell, arranged by your thoughts? No, a situation doesn't consist of sense bits. Nor does it consist of separate bits of any sort. You can think of a few special factors, but you cannot think all of the parts of a situation separately. But you speak and act from a sense of the whole situation. That sense guides how you act and what you say, think, and need, in the situation. You would be lost without that bodily sense of the situation.

How could psychology have missed this for so long? To be sure, we were said to feel our bodies "kinesthetically," but that word means the sense of motion when we move. Similarly, the "proprioceptive sense" was said to be the sense of our posture. It seems not to have been known that we have a bodily sense of each situation in which we live and act.

How could that have been missed? I think it was because this bodily sense is not usually a direct, inner datum. We don't notice it, because usually no "it" comes inside, unless we first pay an odd kind of attention in the body. Only then does it come. When it comes as an inner datum, inwardly sensed, we have a new term for it: "a felt sense."

People rarely have a felt sense. We usually act and speak sentiently, but without stopping to let that sentience come to us as a datum of inner attention. We attend to the people, and the things. Inwardly there are emotions, thoughts, images, memories, usually not a felt sense.

In all ages people must have had this type of body sense, but only at rare times. Some people, for example poets, had it more often. But, even today it is not yet widely known.

At rare times, perhaps when we are in difficulty, we might pay direct attention to how the body feels in the situation. Then a unique body sense of this situation can come, in response to attending in the body. Sometimes it is already there, but not usually. For most people some learning is necessary, before they can attend so as to let such a direct object of reflective attention come in their bodies.

From a felt sense we can obtain much more intricate and better information about the situation, and how we are living in it. The great amount of preseparated information I mentioned earlier is implicit in the felt sense. But at first, when a felt sense comes, it is an unclear, murky sense, and seems quite unpromising. One does not know what it is one feels. To spend time attending to such a concrete sense of something, without quite knowing what it is, that is what we call "focusing" (Gendlin, 1981).

So far I tried to answer my first question, how our bodies can "know" so much about our situations. It is because bodies are interactions, because much of that is sentient, and because the sentience can also come as an inward datum, a felt sense.

The Second Question: How Are New and More Intricate Next Steps Possible?

In focusing we find not just old information, but new steps. Before we discuss that, we have to understand that even old information is not just static—not like a state. Rather, it is always a bit of ongoing process, and its coming then always implies next bits of process. Let me first make that clearer:

Bodily sentience always implies a next move. We should not say of sentience that it just is; rather, it is-for a next move. Inhaling brings an implied exhaling. Feeding implies digestion and defecating. Only as one bit actually happens, does the next one become implied. So these are not items of information next to each other, as in a file. You must actually inhale, to get the implied exhaling.

In focusing it often seems as if the next step contradicts the previous. I felt bored, and then, focusing on the whole felt sense, I find I am angry, and then, focusing on that changed felt sense, I find I am really afraid I can't handle the situation, and then further, that I can handle it but I have this odd sense that I'm not supposed to be able to handle it, and that, in turn, is because . . . . . hmm. After more such steps, perhaps now I can. These steps were not already there, waiting, separated and next to each other. To get the last one, I had first to live in each of the others. The actual coming of each has the effect of changing the whole, so that the next one can actually form—and imply a further step.

Each bit of life process is always also a further implying. The body's sentience is not a mere perception of how things are, as if what to do about it were a different question. It is not like a committee report, which has a first section on the facts, and a second on recommendations. And, even that distinction doesn't work: The committee members fight about how to construe the facts, precisely because that will imply what needs to be done. Bodily sentience is an implying of next moves. You don't first feel hot, and then, after that, feel a desire to be cooler. The sense of "hot" is the wanting to be cooler, and moves to cool off are implicit.

Values are not external additions to facts. Nor are meanings added on, as if attached later. Bodily sentience is intricately meaningful, but it isn't a static meaning. Rather, it is the implying of further events and next moves.

Hunger is not just a static state. It "means" food, and food means something to a hungry animal. But means is not a static relation of one thing merely representing another. Rather, food means, by changing hunger to satiation, rest, and the need to defecate. Bodily sentience means the next body-environment event.

Lower animals are engaged entirely in life-necessary moves. Higher animals also explore and play. This must not be thought of as involving less of the body. Compared with the most essential life processes, exploration and play involve a wider bodily sentience, the sentience of a wider environment and many more possible next moves. Human situations now involve much that was once the result of play and exploration.

Bodily sentience totals all possible moves into one actual, unique next move. As I said earlier, many facets are totaled, which were never previously separated. We need the concept of a preseparated multiplicity here. Much that can be separated, has never been separated. We must not think of it as a lot of separate facets, lying next to each other, unconsciously sensed separately. Rather, the body is this sentient totaling, without first having each one.

For example, I walk into a room full of people, greet some of them, and sit down in an available chair. In a few short moments my face has interacted with several individuals. Some got a warm look, others a different fitting acknowledgment. My face does that. I don't usually control my face, and when I try, I can't be sure of it. I don't need to recall my internal feelings as separate things about these people. My body knows my history with these people implicitly. Consciously I may be thinking only that I wish I weren't late.

We are all familiar with this wise bodily sentience *in-interaction*. It can drive the car, do much of our work, and act more or less appropriately most of the day, without forming into distinct things like an emotion or a felt sense.

After I sit down, if I wish, I can find what it was, in me, which greeted each person. I would have to attend in my body, to let a distinct felt sense of each of them come. It is not already there, and yet, what greeted them was not just unconscious in me. I can sense a continuity between this felt sense which just came, and what my face did with each. What it did now seems quite understandable, given this felt sense—and yet both my felt sense and my facial expression were quite new. I haven't seen this person since last week's events, and these were totaled in along with past history. What a lot of complexity there is in a little half-smile!

Quite new next steps are really commonplace, aren't they? And yet our theories make novelty a puzzle. They assume that explanation must show that what happens was only some rearrangement of earlier experience. Actually most any moment is a new totaling, more than past experience. The past functions in any present, certainly. But, we notice that something is wrong when we get the past itself, rather than the new present.

So the current theories are not right, to assume that the past functions like numbers in a math problem, which remain the same and are only rearranged, to produce the answer.

Especially, it is wrong to consider the body as a fixed system that can change only over the millennia of evolution. Quite the contrary!

The fact that different species do evolve shows that the living body is not a fixed thing. But didn't we say that behavior like breathing and walking comes along with the individual's body structure? Isn't inherited behavior pretty well fixated? No, in a moment a new bodily totaling can change it. Put an ant on a fuzzy rug: Now it crawls quite oddly, a new more intricate crawl that was never part of its repertory. What happens is an interaction with the rug. The ant need not first learn this new crawl—it comes out new—and more intricate than its usual crawl. A body's capacity for behavior does not consist of fixed repertory units. When either body or environment change, that implies and shapes the next move, which can be new and more intricate.

Emotions Narrow the Sentient Context

The cat's body ongoingly senses many things around it. It explores each thing, and hears the slightest noise. But at certain cues (for example, a strange cat on its territory) the cat's body suddenly gets ready to fight. There is a huge physical change: Its tail is suddenly thick, its heart pounds, and the cat hisses. Its whole body is taut. Now it ignores much of the surroundings to which it usually attends so sensitively. Only with difficulty could its attention be distracted from the other cat. The scope of its attention is narrowed.

The emotions of animals are just as valid as ours. Animals also feel ours: When someone cries, the dog or cat will come and try to lick the person's face. The only difference is that animals have their feelings only in-action, not as inward things in an inward space.

In-action, the higher animals have both the wide, and the narrowed interactional sentience. Human inner things get made from both of these.

Inner emotions are made from the narrowed sentience. The felt sense is made from the all-inclusive sentience.

Even narrowed, the cat still knows *what it was, that made it* angry and ready to fight. It was the other cat. But if it wants to find out just how the other cat could have got in, that will have to be done later when our cat is calm again. The cat will then remember where it first saw the other cat, and it will search that spot suspiciously many times. It will also look in other spots, when it is again sensitive to the slightest thing. But right now it cannot sense all that, because its body has experienced a large change; it has become *fight-ready*. We say it is angry. The cat's emotion is just as valid, even though its fight-readying does not form as an inner datum, attended to as something within the body, or in an inner space.

For animals it is adaptive that their sentience narrows and zeroes in on what is relevant for fight, flight, or on whatever special interaction suddenly comes to be implied by the body. Animals fight physically. For humans, such anger is obviously adaptive in a brawl, or for foot soldiers in bayonet charges. But, for much of modern warfare, or in boxing under rules, and in our daily battles, anger is not always adaptive. Mostly we fight not just physically, but by means of the complexities of a human context. When we are angry, we miss some of that context. All of it is not totaled by bodily fight-readying. Therefore we may fight better when we have cooled off. And yet, we would not want to be without anger. Without it coming in us, we may also fail to find a way in a situation. It is often anger that must do it for us, by breaking up a situation, or by changing it, or stopping someone (Gendlin, 1962, 1970, 1971).

Similarly, our working, eating, and sexual situations have all been elaborated so that our next moves must form from the wider sense of the wider environment, and yet we need our emotions and appetites for these situations. It is frequently their failure to come at the needed times that brings people to psychotherapy. Also, some of the most important aspects of life involve emotions. After all, it is just because of that importance, that nature narrows the interaction down to them so suddenly and greatly, when these parts of living come by.

So it cannot be a question of preferring the felt sense over emotions, or vice versa. Obviously we need to understand the relations they have to each other.

So far we saw one relation between them: Emotions arise out of the wider context, which their coming then narrows. This has not been well understood. One cannot recover the origin of an emotion by sensing only the emotion itself.

Nor can one finish with an emotion just by feeling it over and over again. Some therapists assume a finite quantity of past "garbage" in the body. They think that, if all if it could come out, none of it would be left inside. But emotions cannot be exhausted. They are not things that lie in us, as if we could "get them out." Rather, emotions are freshly generated, each time they come. We can let an emotion come, over and over again, just by bringing home to ourselves some situation that did—and will again—make us have that emotion. Once it comes, we no longer sense all of the situation that made it come. And, also, before it came, we sensed the wider context only in action, not as a felt sense. To let the wider sensing come as a felt sense may be the only way to then get steps of change in the wider context that gives rise to the emotion.

Let us look more closely at when emotions come: Emotions come at certain distinct spots in a story of events. Only certain event sequences can make you angry or guilty. Similarly, fear and shame come just at certain spots in a story of events. Culture has elaborated our situations, and that largely determines when a human will have a given emotion. All sorts of things that an animal would not stand for, can be done to you without your becoming angry—it depends on the story of events. You are insulted only when others do or say—certain things.

Emotions are a short list. I mentioned anger, fear, guilt, shame, and of course joy, triumph, sorrow, jealousy, and awe. There is no agreement on which further ones should be included, and one can see why. There is a very wide range of "feelings" that are not all called emotions. Some of these do have names (e.g., hope, disappointment, helplessness, longing, depression, being overwhelmed, missing someone, embarrassment, looking forward to something, feeling as if someone is always about to criticize you)—these too are feelings. So it was always absurd to think of human feelings as only emotions. These others do at least have names, but there is a vast gamut of other feelings, that we all know, yet have no names. To tell about them, we need to devise a new phrase, and sometimes we need to tell a whole story. The story might be the actual events, or an as-if story: "I feel as if I were in a prison, and as if it were up to that person whether I can ever get out."

Those we are inclined to call "feelings" have more of the context with them, even if they have a name. Those that require telling a whole story have even more context. We see that when we focus on them. Sometimes the texture of the context goes on and on: For instance, "It feels like if I do anything, it will be wrong and make things worse; I'll have spoiled it; if I hadn't touched it, it could have been wonderful, and—I won't be able to fix it because I never was, which is all that sadness, that's still there. And always, what I do is. . . . . and that doesn't work because. . . . . and that makes me angry [note the several emotions embedded in this texture of a feeling], whew, what a lot of anger, hm; it sort of protects me from seeing, uhm. . . . . if I saw I would. . . . . and that would be bad because. . . . ." On and on.

To sense all of that texture at once, would be a felt sense, but that texture is no static fact—the whole texture changes, the quality of the parts changes, the felt sense changes, shifts, as each new bit emerges.

The common feelings that have no name and need a story approach the texture width of a felt sense, and it is not difficult to get to a felt sense from them.

As we just saw, such a "feeling" contains, or rather, can generate or regenerate a number of emotions, as we enter into it. Emotions are embedded within such a texture! So emotions only seem to have less context, because they come in certain recognizable spots in a very regular and short story (like the other cat invading this one's territory). Actually the emotion is part of two stories: the short one and the whole context.

Very traditional people sometimes frustrate a therapist. If one asks, "Why did you get angry?" they tell only the event. On further questioning they are puzzled: "What are you asking me? Wouldn't anyone be angry in my spot?" Indeed, anyone in the same culture would get angry then, but we know from therapy, and especially from focusing, that the wider context is involved also in the coming of emotions. That seemingly endless wider context was there, and does have much to do with how the emotion arose, but only the emotion forms as an inward datum. Then the context is missing except when one is in action again. In order to sense the whole context that gave rise to the emotion, it would have to come as a felt sense.

We saw, first, that emotions are not things by themselves. Emotions are only part of a story, usually a narrow story. But, secondly, we saw that this narrow story is itself only part of the story. The wider context was involved in giving rise to the emotion, although then the emotion seems to have come only in its narrowed story. A strange cat came in, and must be fought. Just where and how is not part of fighting it now.

PRACTICE

We saw that humans have two kinds of inner things. The wide sentience can become an inner datum as a felt sense. In contrast to animals, our narrowed zeroing-in can become an inner datum, something we can hide, and carry on in self-responding in an inner space—an emotion. But obviously we still also retain the animal's capacity to be sentient in action, both with the wide sentience, and emotions in action.

Being human involves both the spontaneous rolling out, and the inward self-responding. If we lack the self-responding, we feel much of ourselves only when we act. But we also lose too much, if we lack the spontaneous moving out. We need both.

Let me first discuss what other modes of therapy, especially those that move outward, may add to focusing, and then turn to how focusing adds something that they miss.

What Focusing Misses

In a real sense focusing misses every other useful avenue of therapy. It needs to be combined with them all.

Focusing is an entry into a crucial mode of sensing. Every other method of therapy works much more effectively, when focusing is added. But, one cannot gain this advantage if one uses only focusing and not the other methods! Focusing improves other methods by letting them work as they are intended. For example, no psychoanalyst ever says, "I intend my patients to have only cognitive insights." Rather, the interpretations are intended to reach a deep level. By focusing, patients take interpretations down to that deep level; they try them out there, just as interpretive therapists intend. Similarly, focusing enables clients to do Gestalt role playing as Gestalt therapists intended, not as a play that is first thought up and then acted, but as arising directly from sensing the body. And so it is with all the methods. They intend and wish for it, but they lack the specific, differentiated steps to find the felt sense. All therapists intend their methods to be used on the deep level that a felt sense makes possible, and their clients sometimes do that. They can do it more often, if focusing is added to each method.

On the other hand, if we use only focusing by itself, we lack almost everything. I have never proposed focusing as a method of therapy by itself. Why miss anything that is helpful? It may seem daunting to combine hundreds of therapies, but most of them do not really differ, except in the global conceptions in which they are advertised. We need to look for real differences. Some of these concern what I call "the avenue" on which a therapy takes place. I think we want to combine all the avenues.

For example, interpersonal interaction is a main avenue of therapy. Focusing has to be understood as happening best *within* an interaction. Even when silent throughout, focusing is usually deeper in the company of a partner, than alone. To resolve some things, one needs a steady person on the other end of the process. But interaction is much more than the wider context of focusing. The events of the interaction itself can bring therapeutic change.

Some other avenues of therapy are dreams, imagery, role playing (as in Gestalt reversal), dance movement, action steps during the week, and catharsis. It may seem hard to relate these avenues, but they are already unified in every human being, since each person has them all. Why tell a client "I work only with your feelings, not your dreams," or "Here we only go inside, we ignore our interaction"? Why exclude any major human dimension?

It is true that some avenues fit some clients *more easily* than others, but it is wrong to limit people to just those dimensions that they have already developed. For example, jogging is good also for sedentary people, not just for athletes. A little of what a person lacks can make a lot of difference. We should neither force, nor preclude any avenue of therapy for a client.

Rather than arguing these against each other, let us look for the specific processes that are actually used on each avenue. These go very well together in practice. Each makes us responsive to a range of observations, and that sensitivity stays with us when we practice the others, and improves them.

Focusing is like a motor. It powers all the other methods like a motor powers the car. Wheels and chassis don't move without it. But who can drive anywhere in just a motor?

This analogy overstates the case for focusing. No single way can be the only way for human beings. It also overstates the need for other methods; one can go far with focusing alone. But let us always ask, "What can we learn from the other method?" as well as "How would that method work better with focusing?"

Completing an Expressive Sequence

Many events, especially in childhood, generate strong emotions and at the same time block their expression. If a child can cry, shake, and scream, it is sooner done with a painful event. But, along with bad events, children are usually also prohibited from expressing anything. One meaning of "completing" an incomplete experience is to let these long-missing expressive sequences happen.

Another kind of completion concerns the interaction: what one could not tell the original people, how one could not fight back. Incomplete interactions need to be completed. A great deal of old anger can sometimes be best completed if the client directs to the person a single sentence stating the truth (Jackins, 1962). But, in therapy there needs to be room and welcome to cry the uncried tears, to sob, shake, or move to express old pain and fury in more than words.

But it is not a question only of completing old, blocked expressions, but also of developing new and freer ways of being.

Welcoming—Not Stopping—Any Expressive Rolling Out

Cathartic therapists are right to tell other therapists not to stop expressive discharge, however intense it may be. Clients find it hard to stop a discharge for some minutes, until it completes itself. Trying to stop it gives inexperienced therapists and clients a scary sense of being out of control. Then the client may remain unnecessarily afraid of some half-known thing for years. Instead, stay right there with the client. If the client is pounding the wall, put a pillow between. That's all that's necessary.

The reason inexperienced therapists stop catharsis is because it can look awful. That is because you are on the outside; waves of emotional expression are coming *at you*. If you have experienced catharsis from within, moving outward, then you know it feels precious, life-forwarding, not something you would want stopped.

A person's body may shake, there may be sobs and runny noses, but it feels good from inside. A pillow between the wall and hands or feet is all you need to worry about. I have dents in my file cabinet and bashed-in plaster in my wall. I am pleased with both.

I welcome discharge when it has already come.

The next question is whether it should be deliberately engendered, and if so, with whom and when. On that question agreement is not so easy, and I am not as sure of the way I have chosen.

Indicating That Catharsis Is an Open Possibility

My way is not to decide for someone whether or not catharsis should happen. But I do indicate that it might come, and that it will be welcome if it comes. At some point, early, I say, "You know, you can scream into one of these pillows, if that ever feels right to you." I might even demonstrate it, if the client doesn't believe that such a thing could be. Or, I might say, "You can tip that mattress up against the wall, and kick it" and actually show how the mattress tips up, and demonstrate the motions. "That may feel right to do, sometime, or, it might not."

This opens many possibilities. It shows that one doesn't have to sit still all the time. Some clients know other modes, for instance Gestalt or movement therapy; now they know they can get up and move here, if they wish. It tends to free the space for what might come to a client to do, that would be like pounding the couch.

I believe that catharsis should be an open, known, and included possibility. Beyond that I don't believe I should engender it.

Currently, one client, after having used catharsis extensively and I think helpfully, went on to a much further, deeper process in which it has not reappeared. Perhaps she will need it again. She knows it well, and knows I welcome it. Another client is now using it as a helpful, but quite small part of a much wider process.

On the issue of pushing or not pushing, I know where I stand. But, we need more specific ways to practice catharsis well.

Moving Outward

If therapy deals only with inward data, whether emotion or felt sense, it misses a crucial dimension of the process of change. Therapy must involve more than focusing on inner data in reflective inner space. There also needs to be a movement outward, into interaction. Focusing as such does not sufficiently provide the moving out.

For example, Gestalt provides for spontaneously rolling out. I have already said how focusing helps this come from deeper, but with focusing alone this rolling out may not happen at all.

In the theoretical part of this chapter I said that animals have emotions and the wide sensing, but only in-action, not as reflected-upon inner things. I did not mean that humans have them only as inner things! We have emotions and the wide sensing in both ways, both as inner data and in-action.

In inner and outward modes, the content can seem to be the same, but the whole manner of being alive is different. To change in a major way, both are necessary. To add this to focusing, I advise, not specifically catharsis, but any of the modes of therapy that move outward. Most frequently I recommend Gestalt, which I have also included in working with dreams ("Question 8," Gendlin, 1986a).

This dimension is more general than discharge, or role playing, or action steps. It is constantly available in every interaction. A knowledge of this dimension lets therapists welcome it, when clients move outward, in the interaction with us.

The knowledge of this dimension also enables us to bring it into the room ourselves. Without thinking about it, we instance it. For example, when I have very shy student-therapists, I instruct them to interrupt every client very often—for a week or two—until they can move through that habitual shyness and fear. Then it becomes easy, and they can distinguish their real sensitivity from mere shyness. Some experienced therapists, while not shy or afraid, are habitually so quiet and controlled that the client cannot move out to encounter a solid person.

None of this is meant to return to the popular prejudice that unreflective behavior is more real than inner space. Inward process develops and widens the inner source of moving out, but the moving out does have to happen. This dimension of therapy can be implicit in any other method, without taking up extra time. Moving out, rolling out, is an essential dimension of therapeutic change that is not provided by inward process dealing only with inner data.

How Would the Rolling-Out Methods Work Better with Focusing?: How Catharsis Misses the Felt Sense

The straightforward "discharge" or "catharsis" of emotions is certainly valuable, especially where certain emotions have been blocked. Rolling out, unreflectively, can be a way to find, and release such blocked modes of the body. But it is also important to attend inwardly, to find the emotion as an inner referent. Experienced Gestalt clients seem not to know what I mean at first, when I say, "Now that this has rolled out, can you sense the inner place that it comes from?" After someone has cried, I may say, "There is a crying place there—can you feel it inside?"

So that is one distinction: From inside moving outward is not the same thing as moving inward and letting inward data form. Both are important.

To feel something as an inner object is a change. People who "act out," lack, but can discover that emotion inwardly. To do so is a change, not just a representation; feeling something makes a change in it. It becomes different from how it was in acting out.

Another distinction is between emotions we have often felt, and one that could not come before, so we feel it now for the first time at its full depth. Every emotion is a major bodily change, as we saw. Those that are familiar make the same change in us again and again. But an emotion we have not fully felt before, or have not expressed into outward action before, brings about a change in what and how we are. This may have to be repeated a number of times, so that we change. But once that has happened, feeling and discharging the same emotion brings no more change.

For therapy, emotions that have never been expressed or have never been inwardly felt before need to be distinguished from having the same familiar emotions over and over again. That doesn't mean we dismiss long-familiar emotions. In therapy there must be respect and room for whatever comes, and it may also soon lead to something new. But we know that no more therapeutic change can be expected from just feeling and expressing just this emotion again.

Some therapists seem to know only the one fact, that feeling something fully, all the way, brings change. So, if a troubling emotion can still come, they assume that it must not have been felt fully enough. But it is not mysterious that the emotion can still come. That does not indicate anything wrong. It can be regenerated indefinitely from deeply entering into the past events that made it.

But what if it still comes also at troubling times, and prevents a fresh experience of the present? What if the evidence is clear that something is still wrong in regard to it? Then I argue that discharging it over and over won't help. We need the felt sense of the wider context to form, and lead to new emotions that have not yet formed, and we need the series of steps that can come from a felt sense.

Like the coming of an emotion, the coming of a felt sense is a great bodily change. Even if it leads to no further steps, just its coming is a change in the whole body. The whole sentience which just was in-action, rolls itself into a datum, so that there is now also an "I" who senses—"this."

Yet its coming may seem a slight change—everything just a shade different. The felt sense may seem to be only a slight wisp. Without a trained
sensitivity for how the body feels from inside, one can miss it. That its
coming was a change is more evident, when the little steps of change begin
to come from the felt sense. These may be quite intense.

New and old intense emotions can emerge from a felt sense. It is
important to understand that even the old emotions have already somewhat changed, when they come in the context of a felt sense. The ensuing
steps soon show that change.

"Ah," one says, "there is that old sadness . . ." as if it were no different
than ever. And yet, one is breathing differently, sensing it as part of its
whole context, and this old context itself part of the wider present moment, now. Soon little steps that are quite new can come.

A felt sense is always in present time, and in the present interaction.
Much of the past is in a felt sense, but totaled in along with the present
situation.

Of course, the present interaction, a friendly person present, makes a
huge difference when one is only reliving something from the past. How
can we clarify this distinction? We all agree that present interaction is
always important, and affects how the past is experienced. In addition to
this, I am arguing that the formation of a felt sense is still another way in
which the present can affect how the past is experienced. That is because a
felt sense is always a fresh, present totaling in which the parts do not retain
their old quality.

When people accustomed to catharsis have a feeling, they move
immediately to a narrower—and more intense—mode in which there is
only the past. And which past? Usually a familiar past. Then the same
emotions will be discharged, over and over. That is not usually the intention of the therapist or the person. The issue is not that the therapists of
cathartic methods don't know that repetition doesn't help after a while.[1]
But a new training is needed, to let a felt sense come, to recognize it when
it does, and to stay with it, so that new emotions and new steps can come.
One must know that a felt sense is less intense than an emotion. If one
always seeks for intensity one will miss the felt sense, even if it is already
there. The felt sense is often slight, at first, and easily passed up, even if it
has already come. And, usually, to let it come, one must be willing to
attend quietly to inward physical sentience for a while, when as yet,
nothing much is there.

Most people require certain special instructions to let a felt sense
come. One has to place one's attention into the center of one's body, and
sense what comes there in relation to some problem, situation, or aspect
of life. The client can also ask certain verbal questions inwardly, such as
"What does that whole thing make . . . . . there, in the middle of my
body?" Sometimes it helps to pretend, ironically, "That whole thing is just

fine; it's all solved. Isn't it?" Usually the body quickly responds with the not-fine quality of that problem: "Oh—there it is—uh . . . . ."

Sometimes the felt sense comes without a therapist's deliberate and sensitive effort to help it come. But usually the therapist must know and work for a felt sense.

The felt sense is a physical quality. But intense emotion is physical too. One difference is that the felt sense does not at first fit a recognizable category. Its hallmark is that it is unclear, fuzzy, murky. Yet it has a very precise character, as one discovers if one tries to say what it is: It resists. It has a life of its own. It is already just so, "symbolized" *in-interaction*, and it does not budge unless one finds those rare words, images, or moves that "fit." But a fit is a carrying further, a slight change one can feel. Quality words fit best, such as, "heavy," "sticky," "fluttery," "jumpy," "tight," or some odd phrase. An image can do even better. But words or images are important only to help hold on to the felt sense. Whether anything fits or not, we go on to ask, "What is it about that problem, which makes my body feel this way?"

A whole science has developed, consisting of little moves to get a felt sense, and to engender the little steps that can come from it (Gendlin, 1981, 1986b, 1987; Grindler, McGuire, & Gendlin, 1982–1983). The instructions are needed because there is usually no felt sense. It must come, like emotions, appetite, sleep, and other bodily comings. We cannot control, but we know how to help, its coming, and how to make the ensuing change steps more likely. Each time what comes must be received, but then one lets a fresh felt sense come. After a step there is a different one, and from it another step becomes possible.

Too much didactics robs clients of the open space of their hour. That space is needed if a therapeutic process is to arise. A therapeutic process comes from deep, under the client's conscious content; nothing we do substitutes for that process. If the therapist grabs the initiative too often or too long, then it does not come (and if it has come, it stops). Small bits of instructions may or may not succeed, but they do not derail the client's impetus. They can be inserted often.

Two Needs for the Present

Here I am concerned with two misunderstandings:

1. To process the past, it is not enough just to re-experience the past as it was. A new present experiencing is needed, to process the past.

2. Processing the past is not all we need. There also needs to be a processing of present life.

Present Processing of the Past

It is really an odd assumption, that repeating the past would change it. Why would it? Where would the change come from? And yet, therapy is often spoken about that way. For example, Freud said that transference is the vehicle of psychoanalysis. But how can the transference itself be the change vehicle? It cannot very well be the transference that brings about the "resolution of the transference." What does, then? The cognitive interpretation doesn't make the change, either, as Freud pointed out in *Beyond the Pleasure Principle* (Freud, 1940). He also said that the "alliance with the analyst" shifts the energy balance in favor of the ego. This is true; one can do more when one has a supportive ally. But just what more does one do when one has the ally?

Of course, no one really thinks that just repetition changes anything. But why is therapy so often formulated that way? It happens even in descriptions of therapy in detail. One becomes aware of the repressed; one digs out the past; one finds what went wrong. And then?

Clearly it cannot be that digging up and repeating the past is what brings change. Something is constantly missed here. There is something about how this digging up is done, so that the past changes in the very process of being seemingly only "dug up." It changes in the present act of being brought up. But, we all know that it changes sometimes—and sometimes not. To understand psychotherapy would be to understand *how the present process can change the past*, and can change our trouble as it comes up.

To change the past means a change in how the past affects us, how it functions in our present experience. We work on the past because it is implicit in our present experience and throws it off. But all present experience implicitly contains and is guided by past experience. Examine any present moment, and you will find a vast amount of the past implicit in it. When does it "guide," and when does it throw us off? The difference is: Most of the time this past functions seamlessly. That means the past is not here in the old pieces. The past guides by being changed and fitted into the present, so that you actually experience the present, not the past. But, in some respects the past fails to function in this good way. Rather than becoming part of the new present, you experience the past instead, just as it was. It refuses to let itself be modified so as to become part of a present.

Therapy can be understood as designed to let the past function differently, not as the shaped piece that it was, but part of a present process. Obviously, then, there has to be a present process, and the dug-up past has to be made a part of this present process, so that it can come to function as all other past experience functions.

I have pointed out that the context was probably not experienced as a felt sense in the past. So the felt sense cannot come just from repeating the past as it was. Not only is the felt sense not there, in the past, but the wider sensing which was there, just before the traumatic events, is also missing; this is because once an emotion comes, it narrows that context. For both reasons it is necessary, at some point, to move from an emotion to that wider context, the felt sense.

I have already mentioned, that a felt sense is always in present time, and it brings both persons' present attitudes into the totaling, so that it affects the past directly, as an experience. In contrast, when past emotions are relived as such, the present interaction provides only a (very important) outer rim.

Therapists of all orientations prize their patients. A close, gentle, and supportive interaction always matters. But it can remain separate, if no felt sense is engendered, and the client's body is given over to the past experience as such. Instead, if the client begins with the felt sense of a problem—some aspect of present life—the past will often emerge, too, but as part of present living. But many therapists don't know how to help a felt sense to come.

Of course, one is the present adult even while re-experiencing the past child. But if one physically re-experiences only the intense emotions of the past, then one brings one's present adult in only afterward. Then one has the probem of "integrating" what one has relived, but this is a wishful word. What is the procedure for integrating? No single procedure, rather the traditional modes of therapy are usually cited for the integrating, after all. Focusing provides integration as it goes along.

At least sometimes, the past needs to be part of a felt sense, if it is to change. It is not enough to relive it as it was, and then return to the present time at the end of a session. Moments of reliving need to come out of a felt sense, and moments later, again part of a changed felt sense, through many such steps. That is how the present changes the past.

Why is it, that a felt sense is always in present time? Is this true? It seems so. It is my whole sense, now, of all that happened long ago and since, and how it all affects me now. It is a new totaling made by the present body. The past exists in it, and can be found in any felt sense. But it is how that past is carried now, in the wider present body. If that present totality implies the next steps, they will be different from what would come if the past is segmented off, and lived as such.

Present Processing of Present Life: New Steps

One needs to experience not only how one was, but also how one needs to become—how one has never been!

One must not always go into the past from the felt sense. The past will always be there, still implicit in any present experience. But if the therapist insists on always going back into the past, then certain crucial new steps cannot come. Of course, processing the past has indirect results in present life, but there is also a felt-sense processing of present life. Indeed, that needs to be the overall context even while reworking the past, as I argued above. But surely we must be able to process present concerns as well!

A whole population of patients has developed, who are expert at deep processing of the past, but cannot process present events. From any present difficulty they go instantly to their childhood, and then process that instead.

Always going to the past involves assumptions we would never accept, if we saw them written out. It is as if nothing in the present can ever be difficult, as if reworking the past will automatically provide us with the development we missed over the years, as if we never needed or wanted new and further developments for ourselves, as if new steps were not constantly needed.

If permitted, the therapeutic process will bring something new, which will alter how the past is experienced. For example, a client feels something very sore from the past, and a strong pull to die. She says that she badly needs rest, but resting is impossible, because something in her will not rest.

(*silence*) This needs to rest, and it can't. If it lets down and rests, it will die. (*silence*)

Now suddenly, it feels like a house on stilts. It is lifted off of this sore place. Now the sore place is like a layer, and it can breathe. Do you know those steel posts they put into the ground, to hold up a building? These stilts are like that. (*silence*)

Now that sore place can breathe.

Later she said, "When I was little, I played a lot with stilts. I used to go between the power wires on them. It was dangerous, but it was play! Stilts! I haven't thought of those for years. And play, and danger. How does this process do that? It uses all these things to make something that wasn't there before."

I often find such things in people's dreams. For example, one person was touching something that could not be borne. Just touching it made everything slide. Earlier, she had reported a dream in which there were other children. I knew enough to say, "Let's bring them in with us. Children are safe. They're always good things. They could help us." Doing so felt better. Soon she said, "I think there were *lots* of children." Then she said, "*Oh, yes—a whole army of children!*" Now she could touch what had been untouchable before.[2]

Tears

Let me illustrate some of the above by discussing tears, and different kinds of crying.

First of all, the importance of tears does not lie only in the tears themselves. If tears are suppressed, all that would come with them may be held back as well.

Whenever I notice that clients force back the tears, I work to make crying welcome. If that isn't possible, I ask to hear what is in the way. And I bring the question up periodically, if I see tears being forced down. I say that I believe tears should be welcomed. I ask the client to decide to welcome the tears when they come again. I would like the client to send an inward message to the tears, that they are welcome to come—or not to come—not stopping them, or pushing them.

I think the message and attitude of inward permission (the same as in focusing generally) is one thing focusing can contribute. Letting is better than forcing. The new forcing (I *must* cry) is the same oppression as the old forcing down. But I do not look only for a freeing of the crying. I also look for new steps of another kind. When crying about the past is implicit, one need not always go there — again and again. About certain past events it never stops being possible to cry. That one can still cry in the same places does not mean one must keep going back to them. Nor does all past-processing come before new present growth steps. Each can help enable the other. The present person must often get much stronger, before some past events can come and heal. I look for present growth steps from the start. Sometimes present steps, too, can bring tears.

Tears can be about life now, and not only when it is sad. A certain kind of tearfulness comes with the stirring of one's need for living *now*.

There are also quiet, gentle tears. The deepest tears are not always uncontrollable sobbing. Very gentle tears can be deeper still. They can come when people are deeply touched, or when they touch a deep part of themselves. Tears can come when something new stirs, and comes alive for a moment.

I welcome all kinds of crying, but it seems important to point to this, easily missed kind: When something *new* stirs, it may bring quiet tears. Then it would be foolish to try to convert that into something old. If the past were always deeper, life would be mostly over.

Such quiet, present crying can also be *about* the past. For example: "I tried so hard . . . . . " (*quiet tears come*) The person is inwardly touched; something stirs, senses itself, and cares for itself in a new way.

Such crying also comes with steps of present life. For example, someone long labeled "crazy" says, "When I hear you say that back to me, it seems to me almost like — I *do* make sense" (*tears*).

Or, a person developing a new way of caring for herself says, "Oh . . . . . I gave up my part of the program because I didn't feel there was time (*tears*) . . . . . for me."

Another example: In response to something I said, one client said, "No. That's just wrong. (*long silence*) Just then, when I pushed you back, I felt myself! There *is* a me, behind all that stuff!"

Such new life-steps can happen with or without crying. That does not indicate their depth. Crying may not go with a new forward energy, but that energy may be a present life-step.

When steps are allowed to come freely, they may be either about the past or the present. The past is always implicit, but the step can be one of present life. Such steps are often more intricate than the common vocabulary, and provide new alternatives one could not possibly have predicted or invented.

Therapy does not consist only of present experiencing of the past. It includes present experiencing of the present.

From the felt sense one needs to ask not only "What is wrong?" but also "What needs to happen? In what direction is development? How do you need to be? What would a right step feel like?" It might be a forward energy, or a playfulness, or a needed new way that has no name.

If one always expects tears or some other emotional manifestation, and if one is set always to work with the past, one may fail to recognize new steps, and one will also fail to engender them. Then one processes only what was wrong, and not what has never yet been and needs to develop.

We all have to rework the past. But when new forward-moving life stirs in the client, that isn't the moment to reassert the past.

When a new step comes, receiving it needs no special skill. But it does need the therapist's company and welcome, so that the new step has time fully to come in, and be.

Therapists are in the habit of always looking for what is wrong. But when a new step comes, it is the new step that needs to be responded to. One needs to respond to anything new that might be better, more hopeful, more alive, more assertive, freer, gentler, any new move. One need not always look for something wrong with it. There is time to do that later, if it turns out to be necessary.

Similarly, I hope it is obvious that when a step brings a new shape, the therapist would not want to push the client back into a past shape. In our earlier example, the client at a crucial juncture, in relation to the desire to die, got a quite new step. She felt her usual self lifted up, as if on stilts, so that a deep layer underneath could breathe. Surely one wouldn't want to respond with: "Does that feel precarious?" or "When did you ever use stilts?" At that moment, when she is alive in a new way, we wouldn't want to return her to an old way.

The client played with stilts as a child. In a dangerous game she often went on them between the power wires near her home. It was then clear that this past experience was part of her present new step. It retained the sense of moving in a dangerous place. But look how this past was freshly reworked in a step from this felt sense, now — a step she never had before. Old ways remain possible; she could easily be back in them. One could ask about the past pain that made her tempt death then. I would do that later, if she had not often felt that already. But a new step is easily lost; one easily falls back into an old shape. No therapist would want that.

CONCLUSION

When two methods integrate in the body of one therapist, the sensitivities trained by each method come to be implicitly present in how one practices the other. Then the usual words no longer have the same meaning. Kathleen McGuire (see Chapter 9, this volume) has the sensitivities of both methods. Therefore much of my critique of "cathartic" methods is addressed to others, not to her chapter, where catharsis now has a more specific and informed meaning. For example, she says she "hardly ever lets people pound for very long." She often stops "a hollow acting out" and gets the person to focus, so that something "more basic" comes. When she sees tears in clients' eyes, she asks them to get a felt sense in that place. So focusing is implicit in how she practices "catharsis." She distinguishes between "repetitions of the past" and "deep processing" (her term). Clearly, the latter is no longer just what I have been calling catharsis above.

She also practices focusing itself, of course. She uses focusing when emotional discharge becomes repetitive. She emphasizes the present felt sense about the past. She receives what comes, so she would not constantly send clients back into the past, when a present step has come. Perhaps all I had to add is an equal emphasis on such felt-sense steps of present life.

Room for emotion and felt sense can be made within any method.

NOTES

1. In a review of *Focusing*, Keith Borden (1988) points out:

> In *Primal Man* (*1975*) and *Prisoners of Pain* (*1980*), Janov warns against what he calls "abreaction" . . . with great intensity but without a deep connection. Also . . . Janov warns that even a genuine primal . . . may not lead anywhere because it is being used as a defense against feeling move superficial pains. [Finally] it is possible to wallow in the pain of an event again and again without achieving anything more than the masochistic indulgence of bathing ourselves in pain.

> Another way of characterizing . . . these therapeutic missteps is to say that they lack two key elements of . . . focusing: discerning the body's message at a deep feeling level, and letting this discernment lead to a body shift, a shift in the organism's inner stance toward a situation or itself. . . . When "false primals" occur, it is focusing which is lacking.

Evidently, these pitfalls of reliving have been known for a long time, and the experienced reviewer cited here finds focusing to be the missing element.

In the same review Borden also writes: "However . . . focusers do not primal. . . . Gendlin . . . counsels keeping a certain distance from the feelings which emerge. Deep feelings are witnessed, questioned, and listened to, but not entered into."

I hope this chapter clarifies this impression. If an emotion has been felt over and over again, we might do something like he describes, to keep from falling into the same place one more time. Usually, we would fully receive and respond to an emotion at the intensity at which it came. But, we would not work to intensify it artificially either. We would welcome it at its own intensity, and certainly we "enter into" it.

Yes, we often counsel finding "the right distance" — where one can feel "the whole thing," because that is where a felt sense comes. Perhaps focusing can be used to avoid emotional directness and intensity. If so, what Borden says needs to be quoted and pondered. But, it is important to emphasize that one must step back, to let a felt sense come. If that is always understood as an avoidance, and if every familiar emotional tonality is always heightened, then one will necessarily repeat the same emotions over and over.

Borden knows from experience that focusing makes for a deep connection, and that then a bodily shift comes. But he does not recognize that focusing is not only deeper, but also *wider*. In contrast to an emotion, a felt sense *forms from more of the present body*, and that is probably why a felt shift comes.

2. Peter Levine (1991, 1990–1991) has developed a new method, working from neurological sources. He writes:

> Just as the driver, enjoying the countryside, actively "becomes unaware of" and constricts the periphery of his environment when another car comes rapidly towards him on the same side of the road, constricts his visual field, becoming unaware of events in his visual periphery, so the individual experiencing anxiety loses touch with the sea of his sensations and body awareness.

Levine's therapeutic method is based on the neurological theory that

> if a person preparing to escape a threatening situation by running, will, if this attempt is thwarted, have those responses . . . diminished in future situations. . . .

The individual may suffer a pervasive deficit in a whole class of defensive behaviors. In this sense . . . [this] is profoundly disembodying.

. . . re-enactment . . . leads to a seemingly bottomless hole . . . of despairing repetition of the original traumatic episode. . . . It is suspected that endorphine levels are increased upon traumatic re-exposure and therefore patients may feel relief . . .

Levine works with the events that led up to the trauma, but not until he first prepares a number of ways to *restructure* the neurological sequence of events so that it comes out as it should have, rather than as it did.

In order to avoid retraumatization, reworking must occur . . . gradually . . . from the periphery of the sequential events surrounding the trauma towards its center.

Also:

As it is most often useful to approach traumatic events "peripherally" with positive aspects, I ask [the patient] to tell me more about the pants [which in the example gave him] pleasure, pride, and excitement.

Levine's method requires training. I cite it here because it shows some of the considerations I mentioned, but in quite different terms.

David Grove (1989), working with adults who were abused as children, similarly warns against retraumatization. His valuable method can be learned from available audiotapes. He also works gently from the periphery inward, and also emphasizes certain positive aspects which can come newly in bodily felt imagery. For example, something suddenly appears and wraps itself protectively around the client-as-a-child.

REFERENCES

Borden, K. (1988). [Review of *Focusing*]. *Aesthema*, No. 8, June.

Freud, S. (1940). *Beyond the pleasure principle*. London: Imago.

Gendlin, E. T. (1962, 1970). *Experiencing and the creation of meaning*. New York: Free Press–Macmillan.

Gendlin, E. T. (1971). A phenomenology of emotions: Anger. In D. Carr & E. Casey (Eds.), *Explorations in phenomenology*. The Hague: Nijhoff.

Gendlin, E. T. (1981). *Focusing*. New York: Bantam Books.

Gendlin, E. T. (1986). *Let your body interpret your dreams*. Wilmette, IL: Chiron.

Gendlin, E. T. (1986b). What comes after traditional psychotherapy research? *American Psychologist, 41* (2), 131–136.

Gendlin, E. T. (1989). A philosophic critique of the concept of narcissism. In D. M. Levin (Ed.), *Pathologies of the modern self*. New York: New York University Press.

Grindler, D., McGuire M., & Gendlin, E. T. (1982–1983). Clearing a space. *The Focusing Folio, 2*(1).

Grove, D. (1989). *Healing the wounded child within* (Eight tapes). (Available from the author, 20 Kettle River Drive, Edwardsville, IL 62025)

Jackins, H. (1962). *Fundamentals of co-counseling* (manual). Seattle: Rational Island Press.

Levine, P. (1990–1991). The body as healer: Revisioning of trauma and anxiety. *Somatics, 8*(1).

Levine, P. (1991). Revisioning anxiety and trauma: The body as healer. In M. Sheets-Johnstone (Ed.), *Giving the body its due*. Albany, NY: SUNY Press.

11

Perspectives on Emotions
in Psychotherapy

CARROLL E. IZARD
University of Delaware

Throughout the cognitive revolution of the past 25 years and even during the half century that psychology was dominated by behaviorism and cultural relativism, a few theories continued to emphasize the role of emotions. In the past decade, emotion concepts and variables have become part of the mainstream of social, personality, and developmental psychology, and they are steadily becoming more prominent in psychophysiology, neuroscience, and psychopathology. This volume is evidence of their presence in the theory and practice of psychotherapy.

In describing what he called the emerging mentalist paradigm in psychology, the neuroscientist Roger Sperry (1988), said: "Instead of excluding mind and spirit, the new outlook puts subjective mental forces near the top of the brain's causal control hierarchy and gives them primacy in determining what a person is and does." In my view, the emotions are the organizing and motivating mental processes ("subjective mental forces"), and their effects are realized through their influences on cognition and action. A number of the contributors to this volume are essentially in agreement with this position.

In an effort to place emotions and psychotherapy in perspective, I shall comment on the emotion processes that might occur in the personal experience of the psychotherapist, the implications of the therapist's choice of a particular emotion theory, and a possible functional division of emotion processes and cognitive processes in consciousness that could significantly influence approaches to psychotherapy.

THE EMOTIONS OF THE PSYCHOTHERAPIST

The role of emotions in psychotherapy depends in part on the therapist's conception of emotions. The therapist's conception may be simply a set of beliefs about emotions or a particular framework dictated by specific theoretical premises. Because the therapist functions both as a scientifically trained professional and as an emotionally responsive person, his/ her basic beliefs about the place and significance of emotions and his/her own emotional makeup are part of the therapeutic process. Thus one's own emotions, emotional responsiveness, and beliefs about emotions have to be factored in with intellectual commitment to a formal theory of emotion.

Only a few general remarks can be addressed to therapist-specific differences in emotional responsiveness and beliefs about emotions. Therapist emotion responses consist of three parts: the emotions experienced by the therapist, the emotions expressed verbally and nonverbally, and emotion-related behavior (i.e., responses resulting from the influence of emotion experience on cognition and action). Therapists, like everyone else, have different thresholds for emotion activation, and even within the individual therapist the threshold for one emotion may be markedly lower than the threshold for another emotion. Although most of the evidence for individual differences in proneness to experience a particular emotion (such as sadness, anger, or shyness) comes from studies of early emotional development (Hyson & Izard, 1985; Izard, Hembree, & Huebner, 1987; Kagan, Reznick, & Snidman, 1988), there is reason to believe that these are biologically based differences that characterize personality throughout the life-span. Given therapist differences in responsiveness to emotion-eliciting verbalizations and actions of the client, the same client response will elicit a different emotion or a different level of emotion in different therapists. Thus because both sadness and anger (including inner-directed hostility) characterize depressed adults and children (Blumberg & Izard, 1985, 1986; Izard, 1972), it can be expected that some therapists will respond more emotionally to the sadness, others to the anger.

This difference in therapist emotion response might result in real differences as well as client-perceived differences in therapist empathy. All of this suggests that the therapist's theoretical orientation alone cannot account for all the variance in the therapist's emotion responses and that therapist's knowledge, acceptance, and keen awareness of his/her own emotion dispositions probably facilitates the therapist–client relationship and the therapeutic process.

Experimental evidence (Rusalova, Izard, & Simonov, 1975) suggests that the therapist, like anyone else, may experience emotions but not express them. However, once an emotion is in consciousness, whether expressed or not, it influences a variety of cognitive processes, including person perception, memory, and empathic/altruistic behavior (Forgas & Bower, 1987; Isen, 1984; Izard, Wehmer, Livsey, & Jennings, 1965).

THE EMOTION THEORY OF THE PSYCHOTHERAPIST: BIOSOCIAL OR CONSTRUCTIVIST

The particular emotion theory adopted by the psychotherapist should have an impact on how he/she influences the therapeutic process. Indeed, theoretical propositions, especially insofar as they become part of the therapist's beliefs about emotions, may make a greater difference than findings from empirical studies of psychotherapy (Morrow-Bradley & Elliot, 1986). For this reason, it may be helpful to place emotion theories in perspective by briefly noting their positions on major issues that have implications for psychotherapy.

For the purposes of this synopsis, the numerous theories of emotion will be considered as two groups: biosocial and cognitive or constructivist. Many of the differences between biosocial and constructivist theories stem from differing assumptions regarding the role of genes and biological processes in emotions and personality. Biosocial theories assume that important features of emotions and emotion-based personality characteristics are rooted in our biological makeup and that the genes we inherit are significant determinants of the threshold and characteristic intensity level of each basic emotion. On the other hand, cognitive theories assume that genetic factors are inconsequential and that emotions are cognitively constructed, that emotions derive strictly from interactions of the person with the environment, particularly the social environment.

The Activation of Emotions

Constructivists argue that emotions are determined solely by the cognitive processes of appraisal or evaluation. Essentially, their explanation of causation is unidimensional. Biosocial theorists opt for a multifactor causal model. They recognize that evaluative processes lead to emotion and that cognition is a very important determinant. However, they hold that emotion may be activated by several additional processes: physiological drive states, changes in brain levels of hormones and neurotransmitters, and uninterpreted sense data. Evidence shows that acute pain can activate anger in infants before they are capable of evaluating and interpreting the agent of harm or of making causal attributions (Izard et al., 1987). There is a considerable body of evidence showing that adults develop feelings and preferences before they make the discriminations necessary for recognition memory (Zajonc, 1980).

Functions of Emotions

Constructivist theories of emotion tend to treat emotions as transient responses, and they continue to look to cognitive processes as the determinants of behavior. Biosocial theorists see emotions as the primary organizing and motivational forces in cognition and action and in the development of personality. In their view, cognition adds specificity to motivation, thus helping to define affective-cognitive structures—goals, values, and action strategies. The evidence supporting this view has been increasing over the past two decades. It has been shown that emotion expressions communicate internal states and motivate others to respond (Izard, 1990; Izard & Malatesta, 1987). Several studies have shown that mothers' emotion expressions actually guide and direct specific behaviors of their infants. An infant will cross a modified-visual cliff if his/her mother stands on the opposite side and smiles, but none will cross if she expresses fear (Klinnert, Campos, Sorce, Emde, & Svejda, 1983).

Numerous studies have shown that induced-emotion feelings influence perception and cognition. For example, subjects made happy and angry saw more happy or angry faces in interpersonal scenes when the contrasting stimuli were presented in a stereoscope. The results suggested that the induced emotion actually influenced the unconscious cognitive processes involved in the resolution of the binocular rivalry set up by the stereoscopic presentation (Izard et al., 1965). A number of other studies have shown that positive-emotion feelings facilitate empathy and altruism and increase creativity (Isen, 1984). Indeed, the salubrious effects of positive emotion suggest the usefulness of techniques for their induction, during and between therapy sessions.

Emotion–Cognition Relations

Constructivist and biosocial theories of emotion generally agree on the following aspects of emotion–cognition relations.

1. Cognition (appraisal, evaluation) activates emotions.
2. Beliefs, social roles, cultural rules, and individual-specific life experiences influence both the quality and intensity of emotion experiences and emotion expressions.
3. Once activated, emotions influence cognition (perception, thought, memory).

Most biosocial theorists agree that the following factors influence emotion–cognition relations. Cognitive or constructivist theories are generally not concerned with these factors or tend to discount them.

1. There are biologically based individual differences in emotion thresholds or proneness to experience particular emotions. There is substantial evidence that positive emotionality and negative emotionality are relatively independent factors that show trait-like stability over time (Diener & Emmons, 1984; Tellegen, 1985; Watson, 1988). There is also firm evidence that specific emotions, such as shyness, are biologically based yet modifiable through experience (Izard, Huebner, Blumberg, & Phillips, 1988; Kagan et al., 1988; Suomi, 1987).

2. Emotions can be activated by changes in brain chemistry and neural activity and by increases or decreases in hormones and neurotransmitters. Such changes are not always due to learning, experience, or the stress of life events. They may be due to genetic factors, the unfolding of genetic material with development (aging), diet, drugs, or disturbances in circadian rhythm.

3. Emotions can be activated by changes in physiological states. As already noted, unanticipated pain can activate anger in infants. It is commonly observed that intense hunger and fatigue lower emotion thresholds.

4. Evidence from neuroscience (e.g., LeDoux, 1987) shows that emotions can be activated by automatic, unconscious processes in subcortical pathways, without cognitive mediation. This research describes the neural basis for a functional division of emotion and cognitive processes and is consistent with the concept of noncognitive feeling states that influence cognition, action, and the processes of psychotherapy.

The Regulation of Emotions

Constructivist theories see the regulation of emotion as largely a matter of cognitive processes. Hence psychotherapists who follow cognitive theory depend more on cognitive and cognitive–behavioral techniques than on affective and expressive techniques. Both constructivist and biosocial theories recognize that emotion regulation is in large measure a function of developmental processes and that a number of basic mechanisms of emotion control are a function of biological maturation, attachment processes, and socialization.

Biosocial theories also recognize the role of expressive behavior in emotion regulation. A number of studies have shown that emotion experiences can be activated by the manipulation of facial expressions. The weight of the evidence suggests that these techniques are effective in influencing the broad classes of emotion (positive, negative), but the effects have not been convincingly shown to be emotion specific (Laird, 1984; Matsumoto, 1987; Winton, 1986). Even more impressive evidence comes from studies in which subjects are motivated to manage emotion expressions that result from naturally occurring or stimulus-induced emotion. In general, these studies have shown that when subjects exaggerate or suppress stimulus-induced emotion expression, both physiological responding and self-reported emotion experience increases or decreases accordingly (Izard, 1990). Research has also shown that other types of expressive behavior, such as posture, influence emotion and emotion-related phenomena (Riskind, 1984). These data have direct implications for the use of expressive behavior in therapeutic techniques.

THE RELATIVE INDEPENDENCE OF EMOTION AND COGNITION AND THE SIGNIFICANCE OF NONCOGNITIVE FEELING STATES

Research shows that people may respond emotionally before they reason why (Zajonc, 1980). This has important implications for recognizing and dealing with emotion feelings in psychotherapy. For example, the biosocial view allows for the possibility that emotions activated via automatic, sub-cortical processes (Izard, 1990; LeDoux, 1987) may be represented in consciousness as unlabeled and unarticulated feeling states. This suggests that the therapist needs to attend carefully to all forms of expressive behavior and not rely solely on language as a means of identifying and dealing with emotions. It also implies that automatic emotion responses may precede and influence the cognitive appraisal of the event.

Cognitive theories see emotion and cognition as inseparably intertwined in consciousness, whereas biosocial theories define the subjective experience of emotion as a feeling state and describe mental phenomena involving both feeling and thought as affective–cognitive structures. Defining subjective emotion strictly in terms of feelings allows for the possibility of examining the various ways in which feelings and cognition relate and influence each other. It also allows for the possibility that feelings may be unlabeled and unarticulated. Such uncognized feelings may be conceptually equivalent to "unconscious motivation." But what is inaccessible to consciousness is the verbal material and action strategies associated with the emotion, not the emotion feeling. Feeling is by definition a phenomenon of consciousness. Such a conceptualization of emotion experience also allows for the possibility that distorted relations may develop among feelings, thoughts, and memories, and that a particular feeling may become dissociated from appropriate cognition. This position is similar to the one enunciated by Freud (1915/1957) in *The Unconscious.*

Although the elements of consciousness are highly interrelated, it seems particularly important for psychotherapists to consider conscious experience in terms of functional units or separate processes. Actually, clinicians were the first to emphasize the possibility of the independent operation of conscious processes. In particular, they observed that thought and feeling may not always be appropriately connected and that poor connections or dissociation may lead to psychological disorders. With the renewed interest in emotions as factors in personality and psychotherapy, it seems prudent to re-examine the issue of functionally distinct emotional and cognitive processes in consciousness. I have already referred to some of the research that supports such a division of mental functions (Isen, 1984; Izard et al., 1965; Izard & Malatesta, 1987; Zajonc, 1980).

Emotion feeling versus emotional experience. Perhaps it would be helpful if I try to make a clear distinction between a feeling state—the subjective experience of an emotion—and an emotional experience or affective–cognitive process. (The distinction is being made from the standpoint of a biosocial theorist.) The subjective experience of an emotion is best conceived as a feeling or feeling state. An emotional experience or affective–cognitive process is a blend, or network, of feelings and cognitions. The nature of emotion feelings is determined by evolutionary-biological processes. Cognitions are based on representations derived from learning and experience. If we accept these definitions, then we can delineate the characteristics of emotion feelings that have implications for their management (by therapist and client) in the psychotherapy process.

An emotion feeling defines a particular quality of consciousness. A given emotion feeling is inherently adaptive by virtue of its motivational and cue-producing properties. Emotion feelings become involved in psychological disorders when they become associated with inappropriate images, thoughts, and actions. This results in maladaptive affective–cognitive structures. Thus the challenge to psychotherapists is not to change the nature of emotion feelings as defined by their particular cues, action tendencies, and motivational states, because all of these features are basically adaptive and integral to the human personality. The challenge is to free emotion feelings of "excess baggage"—their connections to inappropriate cognitions and behaviors.

An emotion feeling gives rise to or includes action tendencies. Just as biosocial theory excludes cognition from the subjective experience of an emotion, so does it exclude actions or instrumental behaviors. Thus aggressive behavior is not a part of the subjective experience of anger. The tendency to act out in some way (verbally or physically) is a part of the subjective experience of anger, but action tendencies can be suppressed or modified through learning and experience.

Emotion feelings provide cues for cognition. As discussed in the foregoing paragraphs, induced emotion influences what is actually perceived, what is remembered, and what is done. As is the case with action tendencies, the cues inherent in emotion feelings can be suppressed or modified in ways that may become maladaptive.

An emotion feeling may be brief (emotion state) or enduring (mood). Some biosocial theories maintain that some level of emotion feeling is always present in consciousness. If we accept this assumption, then we have to acknowledge that appraisals of emotion eliciting events and situations—all evaluative processes—are influenced by ongoing emotion (as well as ongoing cognition and action).

The subjective experience of an emotion (feeling state) can be present in consciousness and influence perception, cognition, and action even though it remains unlabeled and unarticulated. As already noted, such unlabeled emotion feelings may account for what is commonly considered unconscious motivation. In unconscious motivation, feelings are actually operating in awareness, but the verbally labeled memories associated with the feelings are inaccessible.

CONCLUSION

The contributors to this volume have generally been attentive to those factors in emotion–cognition relations that are generally agreed upon by both biosocial and cognitive theorists. Not all of the contributors have recognized the factors involved in emotion–cognition relations that have been primarily the concern of biosocial theories of emotion.

The chapters of this volume testify that leaders in psychotherapy and psychotherapy research are concerned with the role of emotions in therapeutic relationships and the therapy process. Many of the gains from the theories and research of constructivists and some of those of biosocial theories have been incorporated in the study and practice by psychotherapy. Continued efforts by psychotherapists to integrate the gains from the cognitive sciences and from the emerging science of emotions appears to be highly profitable.

REFERENCES

Blumberg, S. H., & Izard, C. E. (1985). Affective and cognitive characteristics of depression in 10- and 11-year-old children. *Journal of Personality and Social Psychology, 49*(1), 194–202.

Blumberg, S. H., & Izard, C. E. (1986). Discriminating patterns of emotions in 10- and 11-year-old children's anxiety and depression. *Journal of Personality and Social Psychology, 51*(4), 852–857.

Diener, E., & Emmons, R. A. (1984). The independence of positive and negative affect. *Journal of Personality and Social Psychology, 47*, 1105–1117.

Forgas, J. P., & Bower, G. H. (1987). Mood effects on person-perception judgments. *Journal of Personality and Social Psychology, 53*(1), 53–60.

Freud, S. (1957). The unconscious. In J. Strachey (Ed.), *Standard edition of the complete psychological works of Sigmund Freud* (Vol. 14, pp. 159–215). London: Hogarth Press. (Original work published 1915)

Hyson, M. C., & Izard, C. E. (1985). Continuities and changes in emotion expressions during brief separation of 13 and 18 months. *Developmental Psychology*, *21*, 1165–1170.

Isen, A. (1984). Toward understanding the role of affect in cognition. In R. Wyer & T. Srull (Eds.), *Handbook of social cognition* (pp. 179–236). Hillsdale, NJ: Erlbaum.

Izard, C. E. (1972). *Patterns of emotions*. New York: Academic Press.

Izard, C. E. (1990). Facial expressions and the regulation of emotions. *Journal of Personality and Social Psychology*, *58*(3), 487–498.

Izard, C. E., Hembree, E. A., & Huebner, R. R. (1987). Infants' emotion expressions to acute pain: Developmental change and stability of individual differences. *Developmental Psychology*, *23*(1), 105–113.

Izard, C. E., Huebner, R. R., Blumberg, S. H., & Phillips, R. D. (1988). *Infants' interest in the human face predicts their emotion expressiveness and emotion decoding ability at age five years*. Unpublished manuscript.

Izard, C. E., & Malatesta, C. Z. (1987). Perspectives on emotional development: I. Differential emotions theory of early emotional development. In J. D. Osofsky (Ed.), *Handbook of infant development* (2nd ed. pp. 494–554). New York: Wiley-Interscience.

Izard, C. E., Wehmer, G. M., Livsey, W., & Jennings, J. R. (1965). Affect, awareness, and performance. In S. S. Tomkins & C. E. Izard (Eds.), *Affect, cognition, and personality* (pp. 2–41). New York: Springer.

Kagan, J., Reznick, J. S., & Snidman, N. (1988). Biological bases of childhood shyness. *Science*, *240*, 167–171.

Klinnert, M., Campos, J., Sorce, J., Emde, R., & Svejda, M. (1983). Emotions as behavior regulators: The development of social referencing. In R. Plutchik & H. Kellerman (Eds.), *Emotions in early development: Vol. 2. Emotion: Theory, research and experience* (pp. 57–86). New York: Academic Press.

Laird, J. D. (1984). Facial response and emotion. *Journal of Personality and Social Psychology*, *47*, 909–917.

LeDoux, J. E. (1987). Emotion. In F. Plum (Ed.), *Handbook of physiology—The nervous system IV* (pp. 419–459). Washington, DC: American Physiological Society.

Matsumoto, D. (1987). The role of facial response in the experience of emotion: More methodological problems and a meta-analysis. *Journal of Personality and Social Psychology*, *52*(4), 769–774.

Morrow-Bradley, C., & Elliot, R. (1986). Utilization of psychotherapy research by practicing psychotherapists. *American Psychologist*, *41*, 188–197.

Riskind, J. H. (1984). They stoop to conquer: Guiding and self-regulatory functions of physical posture after success and failure. *Journal of Personality and Social Psychology*, *47*, 479–493.

Rusalova, M. N., Izard, C. E., & Simonov, P. V. (1975). Comparative analysis of mimical and autonomic components of man's emotional state. *Aviation, Space, and Environmental Medicine*, *46*(9), 1132–1134.

Sperry, R. W. (1988). Psychology's mentalist paradigm and the religion/science tension. *American Psychologist*, *43*(8), 607–613.

Suomi, J. (1987). Genetic and maternal contributions to individual differences in rhesus monkey biobehavioral development. In N. A. Krasnegor, E. M. Blass,

M. A. Hoffer, & W. P. Smotherman (Eds.), *Perinatal development: A psycho-biological perspective* (pp. 397–419). New York: Academic Press.

Tellegen, A. (1985). Structures of mood and personality and their relevance to assessing anxiety, with an emphasis on self-report. In A. H. Tuma & J. D. Maser (Eds.), *Anxiety and the anxiety disorders* (pp. 681–706). Hillsdale, NJ: Erlbaum.

Watson, D. (1988). Intraindividual and interindividual analyses of positive and negative affect: Their relation to health complaints, perceived stress, and daily activities. *Journal of Personality and Social Psychology, 54*(6), 1020–1030.

Winton, W. M. (1986). The role of facial response in self-reports of emotions: A critique of Laird. *Journal of Personality and Social Psychology, 50*, 808–812.

Zajonc, R. B. (1980). Feeling and thinking: Preferences need no inferences. *American Psychologist, 35*(2), 151–175.

12

Emotion Theory and Psychotherapy

RICHARD S. LAZARUS
University of California, Berkeley

INTRODUCTION

It has long been an accepted tenet of psychology that the emotional life offers the best source of information about how clients think they are faring in the adaptational agendas of their lives. As Rice and Greenberg (Chapter 6, this volume) put it, "Tracking the quality of the feeling reaction enables clients to become aware of the meaning the stimulus had for them, their 'experienced reality' at the moment when the reaction was triggered."

More than any other source of information, clinicians have traditionally used emotions to grasp, and help the client grasp, what is personally important to them (motivation), what the client assumes about him/herself, the world, and life (beliefs), how the client appraises the significance of what is happening in relationships with others and the physical world, how the client copes with troublesome relationships, the action tendencies that flow from all this, and how observable actions are responded to by important others.

There is a good statement in Rice and Greenberg (Chapter 8, this volume) that emphasizes the personal meanings involved in emotion as follows: "we are always 'angry at' or 'afraid of' and . . . it is the meaning of the feeling in context that is of greater signficance than the emotion of anger and fear itself." And Butler and Strupp (Chapter 4, this volume) make a similar point in stating that "the problem is not the passive experience of certain emotions, but the distorted, maladaptive *meaning(s)* attributed to particular affective situations by the individual and his/her significant others."

Most books on psychotherapy offer strategies for bringing about change. Three important points about therapeutic change flow from my cognitive-relational theoretical analysis of emotion: First, emotions are organized motivational-cognitive-adaptational configurations, and the component constructs of this configuration are usually fused and interdependent. It follows that if one construct, say thought or motivation, is truly changed in more than a superficial way, all others are changed, whether therapy is concentrated on the *motivational pattern*, the *way of thinking*, the dysfunctional *emotional reactions*, or the counterproductive patterns of *action* in given environmental settings (Lazarus & Folkman, 1984).

Second, the specifics of what has gone wrong vary with the client. They may be manifest in faulty appraisal, inept coping, unserviceable goal commitments, or in counterproductive actions, which are all part of the emotion process gone wrong. Often, as a result of the client's efforts to deal with conflict and threat by means of defensive strategies, such as denial or detachment, there is a lack of integration among the main constructs of the client's mind, namely, cognition, motivation, and emotion. To pursue the treatment it would be well for the psychotherapist to make some sort of diagnosis of what seems to have gone wrong, a suggestion that takes us back to a time when diagnosis—not as labeling but as understanding of the pathogenic process—was fashionable.

Third, changes in cognition without the simultaneous involvement of motivation, emotion, and action are apt to be minor and intellectual, as Wachtel (1977) points out in his distinction between intellectual and emotional insight. In therapy, one must try to involve the emotions as well as thought, and vice versa, clients must achieve an understanding of their emotional life. Therapists seem to agree that it is necessary for clients to confront the sources of their emotions—including their goals and assumptions—to act, and to discover something different about the pattern of relationship with the environment than was previously recognized. In this process, all the constructs of the mind must be engaged, motivation, cognition, and emotion, and to make therapeutic advances the person must live out his troubles in action in a relevant environment.

This is surely what Guidano (Chapter 3, this volume) had in mind when he wrote:

> In the first place . . . the client must experience during the therapeutic process some affect-laden event able to exert pressures toward a reorganization. Throughout this process, the therapist must be able to provide tools of analysis and self-observation which, by increasing the flexibility and plasticity of the client's levels of awarenes, will enable him/her to accomplish gradually a progressive reorganization, one where the problematic perturbation is assimilated and understood in a more abstract and integrated conception of self and world, not involving any particular intense emotional distress.

I am struck by the consensus in the chapters of this book that the living connections between thought and emotion constitute the center of therapeutic attention, and that what is being said sounds like the psychotherapeutic writing of 40 years ago in the emphasis on emotional insight and the necessity of working through or relearning. The consensus is found whether the writer had adopted a dynamic, client-centered, cognitive-behavioral, or some other perspective on treatment. Elsewhere (Lazarus, 1989) I cited evidence of this consensus from the writings of Arnold Lazarus (1981), Meichenbaum (Meichenbaum & Cameron, 1983, p. 141), Ellis (1984, p. 216), in spite of his emphasis on rationality, Beck (1987, pp. 161–163), and Foa and Kozak (1986, p. 20), who cited Lang (1977, 1979). It appears that we have finally reached the point at which psychotherapists are less interested in denigrating each other's views and have become willing to seek points of agreement about emotional dysfunction and the principles underlying treatment.

EMOTION IN PSYCHOLOGICAL THOUGHT

Only the other day academic psychologists were talking about the cognitive revolution, and now only a few years later a remarkable upsurge in interest in emotion has occurred, and it is spawning large amounts of theory and research. This renewed interest, by the way, restores psychology to its proper focus on human adaptation, which has always been a central concern in clinical work. Unlike other psychological processes that reflect partial or limited—though important—psychological functions such as cognition and motivation, the topic of emotion expresses the adaptational struggles of a whole person who is trying to manage the tasks, opportunities, and problems of living in the social and physical world. Analysis of the emotion process could help restore the partnership that once existed between academic theory and research and clinical practice.

What I think happened in academic thought is this: First, there was a loosening—in the good sense—of an epistemology that had imprisoned theory, speculative thought, and research within behaviorism and logical positivism. With this loosening we could again talk about the classical constructs of mind. It began in the 1960s with *cognition* and returned us to an ancient, commonsense outlook that says that the way a person thinks and understands the world has causal significance for emotion and adaptation. However, modern cognitive psychology seems to have left out meaning, motivation, emotion, and adaptation from its purview (cf. Norman, 1980). It is necessary to turn to *emotion* to make sense of how the person struggles, successfully or unsuccessfully, to actualize personal agendas by dealing with an often refractory, hostile, and dangerous world.

Given the new focus on emotion, it also became necessary to re-emphasize *motivation*, since emotions make no sense without a grasp of what people want and do not want. And as it becomes obvious that the business of emotional encounters depends on what people desire and fear, we are about to have a motivation revolution, too. As the ancients recognized, to understand emotional reactions requires a grasp of motives and thoughts and how a person confronts environmental demands, constraints, and resources in the daily adaptational encounters of living.

When motivation and cognition are examined in the context of how individual persons pilot their lives, we also speak of an *ego* or *self* as the unifying principle of mind. This brings to mind Hilgard's (1949) throughtful argument that goal commitments, or what is most and least important to us, are organized within a self, which is in essence a motivational concept. Furthermore, there can be no concept of defense mechanism without a self, with its individualized pattern of values and goals, to defend. I note, too, that Lewis and Michalson (1983) have taken the position that there can be no emotional life before a rudimentary sense of self has developed.

The following is a working set of propositions about emotion, which provides a sense of how the full-blooded cognitive-relational theory might ultimately look:

> Emotions are organized psychophysiological reactions to news about ongoing relationships between the person (or animal) and the environment. "News" is colloquial for knowledge or beliefs about the significance for personal well-being of the person-environment relationship. The quality (e.g., anger versus anxiety) and intensity (degree of mobilization or motor-physiological change) of the emotional reaction depends on subjective evaluations—I call these cognitive appraisals—of this knowledge about how we are doing in the short- and long-run agendas of living, and on the action tendency that points to the terms of the relationship. This significance depends on the interplay of a person's goals and beliefs, or personal agendas, and a provoking environmental context. Emotions are, in effect, *organized motivational-cognitive-adaptational configurations* whose status changes with changes in the person-environmental relationship as this is perceived and evaluated (appraised).

Among the most important issues that need to be addressed is the role of cognition in the emotion process. There has been much debate about this, some of it misleading. Because I believe clarification of this issue will help in the task of developing a comprehensive theory of emotion, in the remainder of this brief essay, I analyze some widespread misunderstandings about cognition-emotion relations.

MISUNDERSTANDINGS ABOUT THE
COGNITION–EMOTION RELATIONSHIP

I concentrate on four basic misunderstandings. They have to do with (1) the failure to distinguish between two kinds of cognition, knowledge and appraisal, (2) the idea that the concept of cognitive causation makes emotions cold and bloodless, (3) the assumption that there is only one way cognition can affect emotions, and (4) the uneasiness about the idea that cognitive mediation is a necessary condition of emotion. I shall discuss each of these in turn.

Knowledge and Appraisal

Both are important in emotion. *Knowledge* consists of what the person believes about the way things work in general and in a specific context. *Appraisal* consists of an evaluation of the significance of this knowledge for personal well-being. Without a personal stake in a transaction, knowledge is cold or nonemotional; it becomes hot or emotional only when the person senses that what is happening has implications for personal values and goals and requires action.

Butler and Strupp (Chapter 4, this volume) have also emphasized the importance of action as well as personal meaning in emotion, writing that "affect is simply one type of action that can emerge as a problem for the person. Furthermore, as with all actions considered within a dynamic perspective, the action is considered to have meaning, to fit into the context of a particular patient's life. . . ." It is, of course, an overstatement to speak of affect—or, as I prefer, emotion—as a type of action; rather, emotion always involves action tendencies or impulses, even though they may be inhibited and not acted out. When we are angry, we have the impulse to attack; when we are afraid, we have the impulse to flee; when we feel guilt, we have the impulse to atone or undo the damage; when we feel ashamed we have the impulse to hide what has led to the shame; and so on for each emotion. A growing number of cognitive and relational emotion theorists emphasize the importance of action tendencies in emotion (e.g., DeRivera, 1977; Frijda, 1986). These tendencies are what produce the physiological changes in emotion and make emotion hot and embodied rather than cold and detached.

Although knowledge is the cognitive stuff of which personal meaning is made, and therefore is *necessary* for emotion, it is *not sufficient* to produce emotion until its personal significance is appraised. On the other hand, appraisal is a necessary and sufficient condition of emotion. Much theory and research on cognitive factors in emotion draws on knowledge—not appraisal—in the form of attributions about causality (see Lazarus & Smith, 1988, for a review and analysis). The foremost advocate of an attributional analysis of emotion, Weiner (1985), has himself acknowledged this:

> A word of caution . . . is needed. . . . Given a causal ascription, the linked emotion does not necessarily follow. . . . Hence, the position being espoused is that the (attributional) dimension-affect relations are not invariant, but are quite prevalent in our culture, and perhaps in many others as well. (p. 564)

When I say that appraisal is a necessary and sufficient cause of emotion, I am asserting that without an appraisal that an encounter has been or might be personally harmful or beneficial, there is no emotion. Each kind of emotion, anger, anxiety, guilt, shame, happiness, pride, or whatever, represents a particular kind of harm or benefit, which is what emotions are always about.

Cognitive Causation Makes Emotion Cold and Bloodless

This is a baseless charge, a straw man, though it was one of the reasons for widespread interest in Zajonc's (1980, 1984) position that emotion and cognition are separate systems governed by separate anatomical structures of the brain. This idea is particularly appealing to those who like to reduce mental activity to neurophysiology. Tomkins (1981, p. 306) has used Shakespearean imagery for this charge, writing that "a remedy [is needed] for affect 'sicklied o'er with the pale cast of thought.'" The oversimple notion that emotion *is* cognition is encouraged by Solomon's (1980, p. 271) comment that "emotions are akin to judgments," and Sartre's (1948) statement, usually taken out of context, that "emotion is a certain way of apprehending the world."

Emotion, of course, is not merely cognition, and I don't believe any cognitivists have ever really suggested this. To say that emotion has cognitive causes, and that these causes remain an integral feature of the emotional state, is very different from saying that emotion is merely a form of cognition. An emotion is not only based on, and contains, knowledge and appraisal, but as I noted above it also includes other hot components, especially when there is mobilization to deal with harms and benefits.

My earlier statements about the role of cognition in emotion have led to some misunderstandings because I allowed myself to be entrapped by the ambiguous phrase, "primacy of cognition." This led some writers in this volume and elsewhere to defend the importance of emotion on the assumption that cognitivists downplay it. For example, Guidano (Chapter 3, this volume) writes that emotionality is involved in every aspect of mental processing, with which I agree, and that "the primacy of affect is equally evident throughout the entire course of an individual's life-span development." Butler and Strupp (Chapter 4, this volume) also write that "Artificially removing affective experience from meaningful contexts will most likely lead only to inconclusive disputes in the literature, such as the recent attempts to establish the 'primacy' of affect or cognition (e.g., Zajonc, 1984; Lazarus, 1984)." I consider unfortunate the implication that has been drawn from the debate by some that this relegates emotion to secondary importance.

Two points need to be emphasized: First, as Rice and Greenberg (Chapter 8, this volume) state, "Feelings are a cognitive–affective functional unit, a higher-level integration of emotion and meaning." Without cognition there is only activation or drive, and no direction or regulation. Therefore, to speak of cognition as causing emotion is to state a part–whole relationship between the two; cognition causes emotion and is also an inextricable feature of the total emotional state. Emotion, in turn, is never divorced from cognition, even when it is said to affect subsequent cognitions and emotions.

Second, to speak of one construct as causing another requires a temporal perspective, with thought or meaning preceding emotion, and emotion, which is the union of thought and motivation in a transaction, preceding subsequent thought and emotion. When this temporal perspective is adopted, it makes sense to say that emotion also causes thoughts, if by this we mean subsequent ones in the behavioral flow.

To say that appraisal causes and is part of an emotion is not to say that it is more important, but only that personal meaning is an essential aspect of emotion. Thoughts, action impulses, or somatic changes affect subsequent thoughts, action impulses, and somatic changes. It seems to me that most of the writers of this volume agree. Those who regard the term primacy as implying importance are not reading me correctly. When the issue is cast in terms of which comes first, there is inevitable confusion between the causality and the temporal relationship among the variables in the process.

There Is Only One Mechanism Whereby Cognition Can Cause Emotion

This misunderstanding is pernicious because it leads many psychologists to reject the proposition that appraisal is a necessary condition for emotion on the grounds that emotions are often instantaneous reactions and are found in infants and in relatively simple mammals, which have limited cognitive capacities and skills. Indeed, if we assume that conscious and deliberate judgments are required in the appraisal process, or that cognition is the serial scanning of meaningless bits of information (which is the dominant computer-based model of information processing) then appraisal could not possibly be *the* proximal cause of emotion.

The answer, of course, is that there is more than one mechanism of appraisal. Many writers have suggested at least two: one high-level, abstract, and dependent on deliberate and complex reasoning, the other primitive, rapid, and concrete. A similar position is found, for example, in Buck's (1985) distinction between analytic and synthetic cognition. In the analytic version, meaning is built up in the standard linear scanning of digital, computer-like analysis. In the synthetic version, which is similar to Gibson's (1966, 1979) analogue detection of ecologically significant information—often referred to by the term affordances (cf. Baron & Boudreau, 1987)—adaptational meaning is achieved instantaneously and without reflection, and is well within the cognitive competencies of infants and mammals. Leventhal (1984) makes a similar distinction between schematic processing and conceptual processing.

In the same vein, a neuropsychologist, LeDoux (1986), suggests that there is a primitive, subcortical pathway for evaluative activity that goes from the thalamus to the amygdala and which can stop short of the cortex. This permits an animal to make a rapid, crude, and hasty judgment about danger, a defensive reaction that can be aborted later if it proves false in more detailed cognitive (cortical) analysis. In other words, it is adaptive in an evolutionary sense to be safe rather than sorry.

We need not reject the proposition that appraisal is necessary for an emotion merely because it connotes to some—incorrectly—a time-consuming and complex decision process. Though a complex cognitive process is often entailed, it need not be. As is suggested by Guidano (Chapter 3, this volume), appraisal can draw on tacit knowledge; to this I add that it can be automatic and unconscious, and involve a simple, undifferentiated contrast between harm and no harm, or benefit and no benefit. These automatic cognitive appraisal processes are certainly available to very young children and relatively simple mammals, and are used even by adults (Hoffman, 1986), along with the more advanced forms of cognition.

Emotion Can Occur without Cognitive Mediation

Although this is a widely held position, I think it is wrong. Emotion is always about something of personal significance, and the fact that the probability of its occurrence in any given encounter is increased by purely physical states does not obviate the importance of personal meaning in the emotion generating process in specific encounters (cf. Gordon, 1987). How otherwise can we explain that the person gets angry, anxious, guilty, happy, prideful, or whatever, not just simply emotional in a diffuse way. Each is a different emotional state, implies a different relationship with the environment, and brings forth different action impulses. We have to explain not only the occurrence of emotion, but the specific emotion that is generated.

Superficially, the position that appraisal is necessary in emotion seems to be challenged by observations of the effects on mood of drugs such as lithium or other antidepressants, cocaine, or caffeine. Cocaine offers a nice illustration. Microbiologists say that cocaine induces euphoria by flooding the synapses with chemicals such as dopamine and norepinephrine, which facilitate neural transmission. The change in neural transmission is said to explain the mood changes, which is a half-truth because it is limited to the neuropsychological level. However, cocaine is also said to enhance self-confidence, provide a sense of security, and give the subjective impression of personal power in transactions with the environment, all of which also change the person's appraisal of relationships with the environment. Should we say that first the person experiences the mood changes, that is, euphoria and then appraises the implications of things differently? This would make the peripheral response, mood, a cause of the appraisal rather than an effect. From a cognitive-relational theoretical perspective, I think it works the other way around, with the person first experiencing and appraising the significance of improved functional ability and then feeling secure and happy. Drugs change our momentary appraisals and, thereby, our moods.

Since the changed neurophysiological process is *always* accompanied by the changed sense of efficacy (to borrow from Bandura, 1982), in sensate beings the events at both levels of analysis are confounded, and the only way to decide which way the process goes is to separate them for study, which is difficult if not impossible to do. This is, I believe, a key point. I note also that the euphoria is a phony high because nothing has actually changed in the person-environment relationship, except subjectively and for the moment. When the cocaine wears off, the person crashes, often becoming emotionally depressed, probably because the sense of increased efficacy has been lost. I would like to argue that changes in emotion can only come about when appraisal has changed, whether or not the chronic or recurrent person-environment relationship is also changed.

In any case, because we cannot separate the effects of drugs on mood from the cognitive changes produced by the drugs, the proposition that appraisal is a necessary condition of the emotional response is not undermined by the observation of drug effects on mood. The proposition that appraisal is a necessary condition of emotion is, in my view, the most parsimonious, nonreductive, and internally consistent conception of how things work.

TOWARD A COMPREHENSIVE THEORY OF EMOTION

The power of a well-developed emotion theory is that it specifies the variables and adaptational processes bringing about an emotion so that we can reason forward to predict emotions from their causal variables and processes, as well as backward from an emotion or emotion response pattern to the emotion-generating processes.

Emotion theory must do two things, at the very least. First, it must offer general propositions about the emotion-generating process and identify the important variables. Second, consistent with the general theory, it must offer specific propositions about the diverse kinds of emotion, such as anger, anxiety, guilt, pride, and so on. No theory at present does this thoroughly and programmatically, although several have made important steps in this direction (e.g., Frijda, 1986).

I do not have the space here to offer an adequate analysis of emotion generation from a cognitive-relational, transactional, process, and systems theory perspective. In my unpublished and ongoing efforts, hinted at in earlier writings (e.g., Lazarus & Folkman, 1984; Lazarus & Smith, 1988), I identify a number of *antecedent* variables in the adaptational encounter, such as goal hierarchies and stakes, beliefs, and situational demands, constraints, and resources, *mediating process* variables, such as appraisal, coping, core-relational themes, and action tendencies or impulses, all of which are important in the emotion process. The adaptational encounter is the basic unit of analysis of an emotion; it may be an immediate confrontation leading to an acute emotion that is based on some provocation, or an existential relationship with the environment leading to a diffuse mood that is based on an overall assessment of how the person is faring in life.

Core relational themes provide a molar concept of the essence of the relationship with the environment in each emotion. For example, the core relational theme for anger is, in brief, offense to me and mine; for anxiety it is an ambiguous threat; for guilt it is having thought or done something that offends internalized standards and has harmed another; for shame it is having done something that fails to live up to the standards of others and for which one fears rejection or abandonment (H. B. Lewis, 1971).

The core relational themes for each emotion are generated from a number of molecular *appraisal components*, for example, a goal that is compromised or facilitated, an external or internal object held responsible or blameworthy, a future expectancy of stasis or change, and the coping potential inherent in problematic relationships. These appraisal components form the cognitive basis for each core relational theme. Thus, in anger the sense of offense to me and mine, which is the core relational theme for anger, depends on a threatening provocation that is appraised as arising from an external source; when, however, the provocation is seen as internal, and there is apt to be self-blame, the core relational theme results in guilt or shame, or anger at the self.

Whatever the reader might think of the details of my cognitive-relational theory of emotion, a viable and comprehensive theory would be of great relevance to the practice of psychotherapy. Therapists, in turn, are in a very good position to contribute to a more sophisticated theory. The explicit recognition of the importance of emotion in psychotherapy in this volume bodes well for further gains in basic knowledge about the emotion process, which could also inform the development of more powerful treatment strategies to change dysfunctional emotional patterns.

REFERENCES

Bandura, A. (1982). Self-efficacy in human agency. *American Psychologist, 37,* 122-147.

Baron, R. M., & Boudreau, L. A. (1987). An ecological perspective on integrating personality and social psychology. *Journal of Personality and Social Psychology, 53,* 1222-1228.

Beck, A. T. (1987). Cognitive therapy. In J. K. Zeig (Ed.), *The evolution of psychotherapy.* New York: Brunner/Mazel.

Buck, R. (1985). Prime theory: An integrated view of motivation and emotion. *Psychological Review, 92,* 389-413.

DeRivera, J. (1977). A structural theory of the emotions. *Psychological Issues, 10,* 9-169.

Ellis, A. (1984). Is the unified-interaction approach to cognitive-behavior modification a reinvention of the wheel? *Clinical Psychology Review, 4,* 215-218.

Foa, E., & Kozak, M. J. (1986). Emotional processing of fear: Exposure to corrective information. *Psychological Bulletin, 99,* 20-35.

Frijda, N. H. (1986). *The emotions.* Cambridge, England: Cambridge University Press.

Gibson, J. J. (1966). *The senses considered as perceptual systems.* Boston: Houghton Mifflin.

Gibson, J. J. (1979). *The ecological approach to visual perception.* Boston: Houghton Mifflin.

Gordon, R. M. (1987). *The structure of emotions: Investigations in cognitive philosophy.* Cambridge, England: Cambridge University Press.

Hilgard, E. R. (1949). Human motives and the concept of the self. *American Psychologist, 4,* 374-382.

Hoffman, M. L. (1986). Affect, cognition, and motivation. In R. M. Sorrentino & E. T. Higgins (Eds.), *Handbook of motivation and cognition: Foundations of social behavior* (Vol. 1, pp. 244-280). New York: Guilford.

Lang, P. J. (1977). Imagery in therapy: An information processing analysis of fear. *Behavior Therapy, 8,* 862-886.

Lang, P. J. (1979). A bio-informational theory of emotional imagery. *Psychophysiology, 16,* 495-512.

Lazarus, A. A. (1981). *The practice of multimodal therapy.* New York: McGraw-Hill.

Lazarus, R. S. (1984). On the primacy of cognition. *American Psychologist, 39,* 124-129.

Lazarus, R. S. (1989). Constructs of the mind in mental health and psychotherapy.

In A. Freeman, K. Simon, L. E. Beutler, & H. Arkowitz (Eds.), *Comprehensive handbook of cognitive therapy* (pp. 99–121). New York: Plenum.

Lazarus, R. S., & Folkman, S. (1984). *Stress, appraisal, and coping.* New York: Springer.

Lazarus, R. S., & Smith, C. (1988). Knowledge and appraisal in the cognition-emotion relationships. *Cognition and Emotion, 2,* 281–300.

LeDoux, J. E. (1986). Sensory systems and emotion: A model of affective processing. *Integrative Psychiatry, 4,* 237–248.

Leventhal, H. (1984). A perceptual motor theory of emotion. In K. R. Scherer & P. Ekman (Eds.), *Approaches to emotion* (pp. 271–291). Hillsdale, NJ: Erlbaum.

Lewis, H. B. (1971). *Shame and guilt in neurosis.* New York: International Universities Press.

Lewis, M., & Michalson, L. (1983). *Children's emotions and moods.* New York: Plenum.

Meichenbaum, D., & Cameron, R. (1983). Stress inoculation training: Toward a general paradigm for training coping skills. In D. Meichenbaum & M. E. Jaremko (Eds.), *Stress reduction and prevention.* New York: Plenum.

Norman, D. A. (1980). Twelve issues for cognitive science. In D. A. Norman (Ed.), *Perspectives on cognitive science: Talks from the La Jolla Conference.* Hillsdale, NJ: Erlbaum.

Sartre, J.-P. (1948). *A sketch of phenomenological theory. The emotions: Outlines of a theory.* New York: Philosophical Library.

Solomon, R. C. (1980). Emotions and choice. In A. O. Rorty (Ed.), *Explaining emotions* (pp. 251–281). Berkeley: University of California Press.

Tomkins, S. S. (1981). The quest for primary motives: Biography and autobiography of an idea. *Journal of Personality and Social Psychology, 41,* 306–329.

Wachtel, P. L. (1977). *Psychoanalysis and behavior therapy: Toward an integration.* New York: Basic Books.

Weiner, B. (1985). An attributional theory of achievement motivation and emotion. *Psychological Review, 92,* 548–573.

Zajonc, R. B. (1980). Feeling and thinking: Preferences need no inferences. *American Psychologist, 35,* 151–175.

Zajonc, R. B. (1984). On the primacy of affect. *American Psychologist, 39,* 117–123.

13

Emotions, Development, and Psychotherapy: A Dialectical-Constructivist Perspective

JUAN PASCUAL-LEONE
York University

Emotions are no accident. They are a mode of existence of consciousness—one of the ways consciousness comprehends (in Heidegger's sense of "Verstehen") its being-in-the-world.
—SARTRE (1939/1960, p. 62)[1]

As soon as one thinks that the finger is the moon itself, one no longer wants to look in the direction the finger is pointing.
—THICH (1974, The Sutra of "The Perfect Awakening," p. 48)

The general aim of this chapter is to raise the possibility of an explicit, dialectical–constructivist, interpretation of affects/emotions that can help to integrate useful theory found or suggested in the other chapters.

The essay reflects four influences: other chapters in this volume, my early experience in medicine and psychiatry, 20-plus years doing neo-Piagetian research, and as many years of supervising graduate apprenticeships of university students. I list first some controversial issues evoked by my reading of other chapters in this volume. Then I present a process–analytical model of affect and emotions, which may help to clarify these issues. This model systematizes much thinking about affects/emotions in terms of a set of affective/emotional systems—affective systems evolved, via evolution, into an all-encompassing organismic signal system that informs and regulates cognition. The key ideas of this model of *affects* can be condensed in five points:

A1. Affects evolve from *a primary set of purely affective processes* which, as Wallon (e.g., 1954, 1938/1982) emphasized long ago, serve to ready the organism—via the hormonal/endocrine and the muscular tonus/ postural systems—for oncoming expected kinds of experiences. I say that these primary affects are functionally and neuropsychologically different from cognitions, although they may be cued by cognitive processes. They are dynamic processes that generate unconscious goals and unconscious evaluative expectancies in the organism, which lead to conscious, more elaborated, cognitive-and-affective plans and expectations. Freud anticipated this function of primary affects with his dialectics between "primary processes" (i.e., pure affects) and "secondary processes" (i.e., ego processes). Affects are a signal-and-readiness system of the organism for the organism, but at the same time, Wallon insisted (cf. Jalley, 1981; Wallon, 1954), affects are a signal system that communicates to other members of the species these global expectations, so as to recruit them for the task set by affects' often tacit goals.

A2. *Primary affects*, from which secondary affects and complex emotions evolve, are independently innate and different in content from cognition, but they *share with cognition the form (not the content!) of organization into psychological units.*

A3. *Affective processes*, whether primary or secondary, are organized into relatively autonomous but dialectically *interacting systems.*

A4. *Affective/emotional processes and cognitive processes are in dialectical interaction*: The goals of cognition are always ultimately set by affect, and affects/emotions become differentiated and developmentally evolved with the support of cognition, which provides both releasing signals and more or less automatized instrumental actions.

A5. Dialectical interactions among affects, emotions, and cognitions often lead to the emergence of new blends/strands of affect/emotion, which result from unconscious and automatic *dynamic syntheses of the organism*—syntheses that create more refined and complex affects/emotions that serve and reflect the organism's needs.

One theme that recurs in the chapters, and in writings of other current experts (e.g., Frijda, 1987; Lewis, 1987; Malatesta, Culver, Tesman, & Shepard, 1989), concerns the nature and function of affects and/ or emotions. I will thus start with four important points or informal postulates (cf. Safran & Greenberg, Chapter 1, this volume):

P1. Affects and/or emotions are not reducible to cognition. They constitute neuropsychologically independent means of both informing the organism, and other members of the species, about initial evaluative reactions (positive or negative affective valences) *vis-à-vis* experiences, whether external or internal, and of readying the organism, and other members of the species, for the expected oncoming kinds of experiences (see above). In contrast, cognitions inform the organism about the content and structure of the experiences themselves.

P2. Since the organism can neither create nor develop a new function without using some innate support (in the case of affect this machinery seems to be the brain's limbic organization), experts agree that affects and emotions have their own innate biological roots. Supporters of biosocial theories such as differential emotions theory (Izard, Chapter 11, this volume; Malatesta et al., 1989) stress that these roots are manifold: There must be distinct innate roots for every affect/emotion that is truly primary, in the sense of not reducible to combinations or adaptations of other affects/emotions. By contrast, cognitive-developmental theoreticians have often followed Piaget's style of theorizing by saying that the number of qualitatively distinct innate affects is quite small, and from this limited basis the full flower of children and adults' affective repertoire develops via differentiation and integration (e.g., Sroufe, 1979; Case, Hayward, Lewis, & Hurst, 1988). While taking a strong developmental position, I shall side with the view of differential emotions theory—a view that is consistent with much post-Piagetian research on infancy (e.g., Trevarthen, 1986, 1987, 1989; Lewis, 1987; Davidson & Tomarken, 1989). My reasons for believing in multiple innate roots of affect are epistemological, in the post-Kantian tradition: Development cannot be expected to produce something out of nothing; all constructively irreducible and qualitatively distinct affects must have an innate root. The fact that very young infants exhibit only a restricted number of affects does not preclude the possibility that there are other innately determined affects that emerge when development and learning make their manifestation possible.

P3. All researchers, irrespective of their persuasion, now agree that we must add, to the basic repertoire of innate primary affects, an acquired repertoire of emotions, constituted by affective-cognitive structures, whose essence is to integrate, within the same psychological processing units needed for adaptation, one or more primary affects along with relevant cognitive units. The socialization of emotions, the emergence of "defense mechanisms" and affective controls, the constitution of personality, of complex (positively or negatively) valued objects, the motives and goals, the emergence of the self and its world (as different from the actual immediate environment), these all require a structural blending of affects and cognitions created by a dialectical interplay of development and learning. But the distinction between primary affects (i.e., the constructively irreducible innate roots of emotions—Buck's [1985] "primes") and secondarily developed emotions (i.e., affective-cognitive structures) often is not clear among theoreticians, as shown in the common use of the terms "affect" and "emotion" as interchangeable. I shall maintain this important distinction, using *affect* to refer only to the noncognitive innate roots—simple or complex—of an emotion, or (in the expression affective feeling), to denote its distinctive subjective quality or qualities. I shall use *emotion* to denote either affective-cognitive structures, acquired through development, or the manifestation in performance of affects and/or affective-cognitive structures.

Since performance is always multidetermined (overdetermined!, as Freud emphasized) by both affective and cognitive determinants, affects take the form of emotions (i.e., affective–cognitive structures) when manifested in performance. Note that from a process-analytical perspective the difference between affect and emotion, as defined here, is as follows: Whereas emotions are constructed by the blending of pure affects (affective units) with cognitive units; affects are pure affects, in the sense that they do not (need to) contain more "cognitive" information than strictly needed for an automatized and innately transmitted "appraisal function" (e.g., Arnold, 1960; Lazarus, Chapter 12, this volume; Buck, 1985; Frijda, 1987; Safran & Greenberg, Chapter 1, this volume). The *appraisal or cue function* of an affective (or cognitive!) unit is the mechanism (in my theory a "releasing component," see below) that tells the unit when and where—in which context—to be activated and, perhaps, apply to produce performance. Further, consistent with the use generally found among contributors to this volume, I shall call *feeling* the qualitatively distinct subjective experience that activation of affects and/or emotions evokes in the subject, whether or not they apply to generate an actual performance.

P4. Affects and emotions frequently have dialectical relations (i.e., tradeoffs) with cognition. Cognition may provide cues for the releasing of affects and emotions, but affects and emotions constitute the goals toward which cognition and action strive. In addition, activated affects/emotions, and their feelings, can tacitly (without awareness) set the organism into specific processual formulas, or ways of processing and reacting, that are rooted in innate action dispositions (e.g., escape with fear, approach and perhaps imitation with love, etc.). These processual formulas become more manifold, more complex and refined, with learning and development. *Processual formulas* are specific ways (modes) of functioning in which the organism can be set by suitable combinations of activated affects/emotions (cued by context and/or cognitive units), which propitiate the production of certain types of (overt or covert; e.g., imagery) performances (cf. Wallon, 1954, 1938/1982). The origin of cognitive styles, from Witkin's field dependence-independence (Pascual-Leone, 1969, 1989) to Kagan's impulsivity–reflectivity (Kagan, 1966; Shafrir & Pascual-Leone, 1990), to the many *processual styles* (ways of coping, defense mechanisms, temperament, etc.) making up a person's personality, could—I believe—be traced to processual formulas frequently adopted due to affects and emotions (cf. Kagan, 1989). Much evidence, clinical and experimental, shows that processual formulas biasing cognitive growth in stipulated ways are induced by affects or emotions; and this can already be found in infants (e.g., Lewis, Sullivan, & Michalson, 1984; Lewis, 1987; Sullivan & Lewis, 1989; Bloom & Capatides, 1987; Bloom, Beckwith, Capatides, & Hefitz, 1988; Marc Lewis, 1989; Meng, 1989).

In the following three sections, I discuss three other important points about affect and emotion prior to presenting my dialectical constructivist model of affects.

**AFFECTIVE DYNAMIC SYNTHESES VERSUS
AUTOMATIZED EMOTIONS**

The current work in dynamic, experiential, client-centered, and cognitive/ phenomenological therapies (e.g., Greenberg & Safran, 1989; various chapters in this volume) clearly illustrates that we must recognize two forms of affective processes and emotions. First are those that are already consciously acknowledged by the subject (whether patient, client, or private person), because they are caused by well-learned emotion units or by automatized ego-emotions (perhaps part of the conscious character structures). Second are affects and emotions that actually result from truly novel phenomenal syntheses—*affective dynamic syntheses*—which cause restructuring and reorganization of the subject's construal of experience (cf. Luria, 1973; Sartre, 1939/1960). These truly novel dynamic syntheses may refer to the Other, the world, or the self; but they always constitute affective insights ("Aha experiences") analogous, in the affective domain, to those that were described by classic Gestalt psychologists and others in cognitive problem solving (Pascual-Leone, 1980, 1990a; Piaget, 1971).

Self-recognized affects and automatized emotions are part of the subject's ego-representations—of his/her conscious, explicit knowledge (see Pascual-Leone, 1983, 1984, 1990a,b, for a dialectical constructivist model of the ego/self). In contrast, the dynamic affective syntheses, much more important in psychotherapy, are carried out (as Guidano emphasizes, Chapter 3, this volume) by the subjects' unconscious processes or tacit "knowledge" (but not all unconscious/tacit processes are dynamic syntheses or affective in nature!). The chapters of Rice and Greenberg, McGuire, and Guidano (Chapters 3, 8, and 9, this volume) illustrate these affective dynamic syntheses that emerge spontaneously in clients when prompted by therapists' remarks. As these authors suggest, using different terminology, progress in psychotherapy is marked by fortuitous (albeit induced) sequences of affective dynamic syntheses.[2] These sequences are the drama in the subject's mind that progressively gains for consciousness a valid/realistic representation of the affective problems, and may lead the client to better wisdom in finding remedies (cf. Pascual-Leone, 1990b). That is, paraphrasing a Freudian remark: Where the unconscious was the conscious ego processes shall develop—by virtue of the client's mentation, and without explicit transmission by the therapist of any specialized philosophy or psychology.

Psychoanalytical and cognitive-behavioral therapists nowadays are tacitly using this method of prompting affective dynamic syntheses as a way to therapy (cf. Rachman, 1980; Frijda, 1987). This is well illustrated in the chapter by Butler and Strupp (Chapter 4, this volume). These authors suggest the use of therapists' attitudes and remarks to provide a "corrective emotional experience" (Marmor, 1986) that causes in the client a dialectical contradiction ("mismatch") between his/her old automatized emotional cognitions and expectations (i.e., character structures, scripts— Butler and Strupp's CMPs!—etc.) and the cognitions and emotions that are confirmed by the therapist's attitudes and remarks. This contradiction causes in the client an attentional orienting reaction (Johnson & Lubin, 1967; Sokolov, 1963) toward the mismatching content, which prompts affective dynamic syntheses that bring into consciousness the automatized tacit emotional structures, and eventually corrects them. Alexander, a psychoanalyst who pioneered this sort of therapeutic corrective modeling, may have had some notion of this kind of mechanism (Alexander & French, 1946).

Another common method of therapy that obviously elicits these affective syntheses involves desensitization and *in vivo* experiences, often used with phobics and obsessive-compulsive patients (as illustrated by Foa & Kozak, Chapter 2, this volume). Here the patient's willful and consciously progressive exposure to a situation that is emotionally very disturbing, may cause an affective conflict (a conative contradiction or mismatch) between a growth-oriented partial-self, who seeks healing and wants to face the desensitization situation, and a phobic partial-self (perhaps a set of already automatized character structures) who "wants" to avoid this very experience. Notice that the growth-oriented partial self is here supported and reinforced by affective bonding or "alliance" with the therapist.[3] To prevent misunderstandings it is important to emphasize that a *partial-self*, in my terminology, is nothing more than a collection or subrepertoire (a partial network) of potentially conscious processing units such as schemes or structures (Pascual-Leone, 1990a,b).

Thus conceived, mental conflicts of clients in a desensitization cure may be construed as affective instances of Piaget's *innate equilibration processes* (Pascual-Leone, 1988; Piaget, 1971, 1985; Vuyk, 1981). These mental-attentional processes attempt to resolve the contradiction by enduring the desensitization situation with the emotional support of the therapist/ mentor. This endurance may elicit self-efficacy feelings in the sense of Bandura (1989); but it also leads to re-equilibration in the affective/self-cognitive domain: new dynamic syntheses (emotional experiences) that could eliminate the aversive reactions (cf. Frijda, 1987). All these examples suggest that *a theory of affect and emotion must explicate the difference between affective dynamic syntheses and automatized emotions*.

THE INTENTIONALITY OF AFFECTS AND EMOTIONS

Most psychotherapists, and the authors in this volume, would agree with classic phenomenologists (Scheler, 1973) that affects and emotions are *intentional*. They are intentional in two distinct and equally important senses, which I discuss successively.

In the sense of Husserl (1954/1970), affects and emotions are intentional because they have a referent; that is, they are unconsciously addressed, directed, or ordered to some object or state that is, so to speak, their ultimate goal-object and value/reward.[4] This object or state can be the "loving Other" as in love/attachment, the Other or an inanimate object to be "attacked" as in anger or "avoided" in fear. This referent can also be an internal emotional state coloured by a particular conative quality, such as "sought-after well-being" in joy, "inquisitiveness" in interest (when interpreted as an orienting reaction produced by novelty), or "passive withdrawal" in sadness.

The referent of an affect/emotion has a releasing effect on the affect/emotion in question (this is a *cue-function postulate*). Everyday observations about spontaneous expression of emotions easily confirm this postulate. For instance, it is generally true that willful simulation of a state of affect or emotion tends actually to evoke this emotion (smile and you shall feel happy within!). Thus when the referent can be produced easily in the subject's phenomenal (subjective) experience—as may be the case with joy, interest, or distress—the elicitation of the affect in question may occur shortly after birth (Izard, 1977; Lewis, Sullivan, Stanger, & Weiss, 1989; Malatesta et al., 1989). However when the referent of an emotion cannot be evoked by easily accessible releasing cues, to experience the emotion in question the subject must mentally generate a representation of the referent via his/her active imagination (dynamic syntheses). This representational release of certain affects may be needed before the effects in question can be experienced, even when the affects are innate (cf. Case, 1988; Case et al., 1988; Lewis, 1987; Lewis & Michalson, 1985; Lewis et al., 1989; Sullivan & Lewis, 1989).

To illustrate this point, consider the example of anger discussed by Case et al. (1988). The *releasing situation* of anger is one in which the subject desires and pursues a goal (call its mental representation *M1*) but is prevented by an obstacle or a person from attaining it (call the mental representation of this blocking *M2*). After repeated failures, if the desire grows strong with the failure, the subject might channel into anger this blend of strong desire and repeated emotion of failure. The referent of anger is the possible situation in which the obstacle has been removed; anger itself is a move toward the actual removal via some "aggression." Let us accept that manifest anger is, under these circumstances, an inherited response resulting from the emotional state (which *may* include the referent) of anger (Lewis, 1987; Lewis & Michalson, 1985; Malatesta et al., 1989). Since the emotional state is most highly elicited by the phenomenal (subjective) "awareness" of the referent, and this referent is a mental (but not always "cognitive") pattern constituted by events *M1* and *M2*, the subject must be mentally able to attend simultaneously to these two "events."

Consequently, to be able to generate the anger-releasing pattern in his/her working memory,[5] and thus experience anger, the baby must be able to activate with mental attentional energy (i.e., mental effort or capacity) at least one (M2) and at most two (M1 and M2) affective/cognitive events that are not directly boosted by affect.[6] In a series of studies with babies, my collaborators and I have confirmed a model of mental-attentional growth in infants. According to this model a baby's mental attention can boost two separate mental events or schemes after 4 months of age, and can boost one event (scheme) after 1 month (Alp, 1988; Benson, 1989; Holloway, Blake, Pascual-Leone, & Middaugh, 1987; Pascual-Leone, Johnson, & Benson, 1989).[7] These are the ages at which anger first appears in babies (Malatesta et al., 1989; Lewis et al., 1989; Sternberg, Campos, & Emde, 1983; Sullivan & Lewis, 1989). Even though an affect is innate, its elicitation may necessitate mental attentional capacity (Lewis, 1987).

There is a second sense of intentionality that I must discuss. In this second sense intention is the disposition to act and produce actions ordered to certain results. The classic terms *impulse* and *conation* (i.e., some sort of unconscious will) embody this sense of intentionality. Affects and emotions serve to induce action because of their conative (impulsive) effects that create *affective goals* for the organism. *No cognitive activity occurs without goals, and all goals are ultimately affective; that is, cognition ultimately depends on affect for its direction.* (This postulate is related to Safran and Greenberg's postulate 5, Chapter 1, this volume.) Conative effects of affect are in good part innate. This is shown by the existence across cultures, and even across species, of roughly similar kinds of primary positive and negative affects, and by the recent demonstration that, even in children, positive affects seem to be regulated by the left frontal lobes; however, negative affects are regulated by the right frontal lobes (Davidson & Fox, 1988, 1989; Davidson & Tomarken, 1989; Davidson, Schaffer, & Saron, 1985). *Positive affects* are those that compel the subject to approach the affect's referent, or the object more strongly connected with it. *Negative affects/emotions* are those that lead to a withdrawal from the affect's referent or connected objects. This definition, now being investigated neurophysiologically (Davidson & Tomarken, 1989), is consistent with other more classic definitions (e.g., Miller's [1963] definition of affects as being "go/no go" mechanisms of the brain).

The conative meaning of emotions, even of instinctually based emotions, may be obscure to the subjects, when they first experience them as a
result of affective dynamic syntheses. This lack of conative clarity of the
emergent emotions is recognized by philosophers (e.g., Jaspers, 1970) and
by ordinary subjects in the context of therapy. Psychotherapy can help
subjects in clarifying the hidden, but real, conations of their emotions
(see, e.g., Greenberg & Safran, 1989; Safran & Greenberg, Chapter 2, this
volume).

EQUILIBRATION AND THE DEVELOPMENT OF EMOTIONS

According to Greenberg and Safran the "primary operation" of a therapist
seeking the clients' emotional/existential insight, is to make them "*attend
to their internal experiences.*" And they add: "Affect is being synthesized
in the present from elements that are currently activated" (1989, p. 26).
They are suggesting that therapists must induce clients to work through
sequences of affective dynamic syntheses—mentation (not necessarily
cognition!) that can release and clarify affect. This is *affective equilibration.* But the regulatory mechanism is still obscure in this kind of process.
It might be helpful to relate it to Piaget's theory of equilibration, and to the
"strategies" that Piaget has recognized in subjects engaged in equilibratory
mentation.
    For Piaget (1985) the main releasers of equilibration processes are
contradictions (states of "disequilibrium" created by *disturbances*—i.e.,
by failures to assimilate the present experience, because some of the
activated schemes are mutually incompatible in terms of past learning).
Piaget thought that the process of adapting to new disturbances follows the
path of three successive strategies that Piaget calls, for no good reason,
alpha, beta, and gamma. In *strategy alpha* the subject simply ignores the
disturbances and acts as if they did not exist. In *strategy beta* the disturbances begin to influence the subject's performances by way of accommo-
dation: Schemes are modified to register the fact of the disturbance in
terms of *negations,* schemes that anticipate the failure of important (affectively boosted) expectancies under certain stipulated conditions. (Notice
that Piaget's dialectical negations should elicit negative emotions.) Once
these negations have been registered by the psychological organism, they
become intrinsic motivational agents (*contradictions*) that induce the
search for means of compensating them via *affirmations,* schemes that
can bring about, in the situation, new ways of attaining the purposes that
the original expectations were pursuing. (Notice that Piaget's dialectical
affirmations should elicit positive emotions.) The progressive coupling of
negations with affirmations that compensate them, is the cumulative process that leads to the *strategy gamma.* In gamma all possible disturbances

are represented in the psychological organism by way of negations, and all negations are potentially compensated by corresponding affirmations. When it has reached strategy gamma, the organism is finally well adapted to all expectable variations of his/her environment, without having to experience new disturbances that require problem-solving/learning cycles. Let us consider these strategies within an example representing the emergence and then the extinction of a familiar emotion.

Consider the case of embarrassment, investigated by Lewis and his collaborators (Lewis et al., 1989; Lewis, 1987). Embarrassment occurs when a subject becomes self-conscious of being observed/judged by Others, and is not accustomed to it (the importance of this uniquely human emotion has been emphasized by Sartre, 1966). What is the precise referent (and the releasing situation) of embarrassment? Consider: (1) that the Other (i.e., a person who the subject experiences as another self) and the subject's self are two different causal systems confronting each other; (2) that the subject's, even the child's, "conscious" organization (henceforth to be called the *ego*) has a conscious or subconscious representation of both of them (Pascual-Leone, 1990a, b; Trevarthen, 1986, 1987, 1989; Wallon, 1946, 1954, 1938/1982); and (3) that the child's ego can relate the actions of the self to those of the Other or vice versa.[8]

A canonical situation where embarrassment can be elicited is, as Lewis has shown (Lewis, 1987; Lewis et al., 1989), the "request-to-dance situation".[9] In this situation one person repeatedly asks the subject (a child or unaccustomed adult) to dance by him/herself in front of Others. Conceivably, the subject experiences the Other as being engaged (or about to be engaged) in two functionally related but different mental Acts.[10] The first one is the mental Act (M1) of looking at the subject and, having requested the dance, expecting him or her to dance (in the equilibration model this is a disturbance consciously registered as a negation). The second mental Act (M2) is getting ready to judge how well the child dances (this is an even stronger disturbance registered as a negation). The subject also represents his/her own self as being engaged in two mental Acts. The first one (M3) is the need and feeling/fantasy of obeying the request of Others and dancing well for them (this is a generic affirmation—to satisfy the demands of significant Others—to the negation M1, which the subject has automatized in the past); the second (M4) is the fear of dancing badly and being so judged (this is a second strong disturbance registered as negation). The child, of course, attempts, in a subconscious or self-conscious manner, to coordinate (M5) the affective/cognitive schemes M1, M2, M3, and M4, to reach some sensible decision about what to do. But the contradictory tendencies (M3 versus M4) within him/herself, are so equally strong that no helpful executive plan of action (no good affirmation for M4, i.e., the noncompensated negation) seems to gain control of his/her performance.[11]

Such a constellation of mental events is the *releasing situation* for embarrassment. The *referent of embarrassment* (i.e., the experience of conflict and the tacit goal of solving the conflict created by M2/M3/M4) appears in the subject's consciousness (or in his/her subconscious mind) at this point, and with it embarrassment soon follows. Notice that embarrassment is the affective reaction to a given sort of equilibration strategy beta, and it is also perhaps evolution's attempt to solve the conflict by inducing the Other to change demands (Sartre, 1966, gives a profound phenomenological analysis of this beta-strategy state of shame/embarrassment in face of Others; see part three, Being-For-Others, section The Look). In process-analytical terms, embarrassment results from a complex dynamic synthesis of affects (e.g., dependency, desire/attraction, fear), emotions (e.g., vanity or ambition) and cognitions (expectations about Other, inferred judgmental dispositions of Other). I have described elsewhere (e.g., Pascual-Leone, 1983, 1984, 1987, 1989, 1990b; Pascual-Leone & Goodman, 1979) process mechanisms that might generate these dynamic syntheses.

One observation is pertinent here. To be able to synthesize the referent of embarrassment, and its releasing situation, the child/adult must simultaneously keep in mind (i.e., in the internal "field of activation," or working memory) five different processing units (i.e., mental events or schemes) such as M1 to M5. We have shown in my laboratory that the mental attentional energy or capacity needed to hold simultaneously in working memory five processing units, which are not activated by the situation or by learning factors, does not appear developmentally until the age of 18 to 24 months (Alp, 1988; Benson, 1989; Holloway et al., 1987; Pascual-Leone et al., 1989). Thus, prior to this age babies should not be expected to attain this particular strategy beta and exhibit embarrassment. Children younger than 18 months should only be able to generate strategies alpha in this context. This prediction is born out: Eighteen to 24 months is the age at which embarrassment first appears in performance (e.g., Lewis et al., 1989). The remark just made concerns the developmental emergence (i.e., psychogenetic construction) of equilibration strategies in a particular emotion. But the here-and-now emergence in an adult consciousness (generative construction) of equilibration strategies of affects/emotions follows a similar model and has its own mental-attentional demand. The implication for psychotherapy should be apparent. As Greenberg and Safran (1989) intimate, clients often have not synthesized in consciousness equilibration strategies for some important emotional experiences, since their mental attention was not properly focused on them. The therapist's strategy should then be to arouse maximally the mental attention of the client and to guide, via questioning, the client's focusing on relevant feelings and schemes.

When suitable solutions (*dialectical affirmations*) have thus been developed for all important disturbances (*dialectical negations*), an equilibration strategy gamma begins to emerge. As this happens, stable mental equilibrium appears, and emotions tend to dissipate; the subject's interest (his/her affective goals) shifts to other contents. The same is found in pure cognition: Areas where gamma strategies are still lacking are motivating; but as gamma strategies develop and subjects know solutions for all encountered problems, curiosity and interest decrease and boredom may appear. Gamma strategies, with their operational/coping efficiency, lead to disappearance of strong emotions; thus hot emotion is a marker in psychotherapy. Psychotherapy should seek areas of hot, heightened emotion and move to other domains when emotions mellow (cf. Greenberg & Safran, 1989; Safran & Greenberg, Chapter 1, this volume).

This dialectical constructivist model of affects and emotions accounts for their here-and-now emergence by way of equilibration—restructuring of well-developed schemes via dynamic syntheses and coordinations. But equilibration in turn must be explicated by means of causal organismic mechanisms. In neo-Piagetian theory this is done by means of an explicit processing model (see Pascual-Leone, 1980, 1983, 1984, 1987; Pascual-Leone & Goodman, 1979). I shall only highlight two equilibration factors from this process model:

EF1. An innate *mental-attentional* (mental effort) mechanism that, monitored by currently dominant executive schemes (in turn mobilized by affective goals), can boost with greater activation, or can centrally inhibit ("interruption"), other activated affective or cognitive schemes.

EF2. An organismic *principle of schematic overdetermination of performance/experience*—a reformulation of Freud's "principle of overdetermination"—that ensures the occurrence of a performance, or experience, in such a manner that the following rule applies: The degree to which a particular scheme x contributes to configure the experience/performance in question is a function of the current activation strength (assimilatory weight) of the scheme x, relative to the activation strength of other schemes in working memory. Thus explicated, this Freudian principle prescribes a heuristic method that experiential therapists actually follow: To keep in the client's focus of attention certain experiential content it is important for therapists to ignore (not to react to) client's utterances (schemes) that are unrelated to the content in question (cf. Greenberg & Safran, 1989).

THE PROCESS-ANALYTICAL STRUCTURE
OF AFFECTS AND EMOTIONS

Affects are processes different from cognitions, but with some dynamic properties not unlike those of cognitive units. Both can be cued by releasers (internal and external), can be automatized, can be synthesized by way of the brain's dynamic syntheses (Luria, 1973) in the context of equilibration processes. Both can be intentional, serve to define goals, and seem to be regulated by cortical processes (although affects originate in limbic processes). These and other similarities between affects and cognitions can be explained, without reducing the former to the latter, by accepting that the brain's functional architecture is rather independent from the content—cognitive or affective or mixed—of processes on which it bears. In other words, although constructive processes of affects and emotions are partly similar to those of cognition, the semantics, content, and functional significance of cognition and affects are clearly distinct and separate. In this section, I illustrate this concept of content-independent functional architecture by discussing the concept of scheme and showing how it can be used to clarify the process-analytical structure of affects.

With reference to the psychological processes that it makes possible, we can consider the brain to be constituted by a vast repertoire of structural, mental processing units, each relatively autonomous because it possesses its own set of releasing conditions. These units have been called *schemes* (or schemata), following Kant's creative insight.[12] Nowadays similar processing units are often modeled by means of *productions*, after the computer-simulation theories of Simon and Newell (1972), Anderson (1983) and others, but this representation is not necessary (and connectionist modeling might perhaps be better). Organismic schemes are activated, and tend to apply to produce performance, under minimal conditions of activation—unless they are prevented to do so by other incompatible schemes.

A *scheme* is a functional unit of mental processing that is necessary for praxis (i.e., goal-directed activity, ultimately addressed to the environment so as to satisfy some vital needs). Any scheme, whether conscious or unconscious, cognitive or affective, can be formally demarcated by means of a pair of components: a releasing component and an effecting component (Johnson, Fabian, & Pascual-Leone, 1989; Pascual-Leone, 1969, 1983, 1984; Pascual-Leone & Goodman, 1979; Pascual-Leone, Goodman, Ammon, & Subelman, 1978). The *releasing component* (rc) is constituted by conditions, which can be matched to features of the external or internal state (the input to the scheme in question), creating a cue for the scheme when one such a match has occurred. The *effecting component* (ec) is constituted by effects, which can be applied to constrain the subject's manifest or mental performance. The ordered pair rc:ec suffices to demarcate formally/functionally any scheme. Schemes are recursive units: Any scheme can in turn appear (be copied) as a condition or effect within other schemes. Complex nested structures, serializing or coordinating (chunking) schemes, can be generated in this manner.

But this is the formal/functional demarcation of a scheme. From the perspective of its psychogenetic construction (in terms of its emergence via learning and/or development) an organismic scheme appears as a biological module that embodies the essential characteristics of a segment of goal-directed activity relevant to the organism—that is, the infrastructure of an informational dynamic system or "Act game" that is part of a certain praxis. An *Act game*[13] is a modular pattern of functioning, in tradeoff (i.e., dialectical, accommodation/assimilation) exchange with elements of the situation or context, that "intends" (conation) to produce some result needed for the (tacit or explicit) praxis in question. This result is the goal of the scheme's dynamic system or Act game. The *infrastructure* of an Act game is the conditional set of "perceptions," "operations," "representations," and actions—the constraints on performance and performance patterns—needed for attaining the game's goal. Schemes are organismic units, and they are best demarcated from the perspective of the organism's activity as a whole. Albeit expressed differently, this view is congenial to the epistemology that Guidano intimates (Chapter 3, this volume). From a neuropsychological perspective a scheme is a collection of neurons often distributed over the brain, which are cofunctional, in the sense that they together can bring about certain results (the referent and goals of the scheme in question), and are often coactivated (i.e., activated simultaneously or in a lawful sequence). Schemes are neuronal networks (Greenberg & Safran, 1989), which, albeit defined functionally, have clear neurophysiological representation; and the nature of their content, whether they are cognitive or affective, depends entirely on where in the brain they are located (e.g., sensorial/motor cortical regions versus limbic or associate/prefrontal regions).

Let us use embarrassment again to clarify the notion of an affective scheme. The *releasing component* for the scheme of embarrassment is constituted by the coded relevant aspects (conditions) of the releasing situation: The processing units (schemes) for the events M1, M2, M3, and M4 mentioned above, plus the referent of embarrassment (i.e., the awareness of the conflict and the impulse to resolve it in some way). The *effecting component* is constituted by four different categories of effects that, as Lewis and Michalson (1985) emphasize, are characteristic of all affective schemes. These four categories of effects are:

EC1. A *physiological* or *emotional state* is constituted by all transient physiological changes that accompany, and also serve to reinforce (this is the referent), the affect/emotion. For embarrassment, this is the feeling of blushing, loss of executive control over oneself, the experience of conflict that induces a tacit goal of solving this conflict created by M2/M3/M4, and so on.

EC2. *Conative effects* stipulate tacit goals of the affect in question, whether positive or negative, and tacitly evaluate whether or not the change in the situation approaches these tacit goals. These conative effects also have, at least in part, an innate physiological representation in the brain, as attested by the fact mentioned above that negative affects seem to be regulated by the right prefrontal lobe, whereas positive affects are regulated by the left prefrontal lobe. The conative effect of embarrassment is the tacit goal to avoid the conflict created between the self's own tacit or explicit evaluation and the real or assumed evaluations or demands of the Other. Conative effects are affective-energy boosts (i.e., affective weights) to be applied to cognitive schemes, which are pragmatically relevant for the intentionality (tacit goals) of the affect in question (i.e., escape with fear, attack with anger–hate, approach and/or imitation in attachment, etc.). From this perspective, the application of affective schemes to boost cognitive schemes acts as a multiplier, a mechanism that multiplies by some amount the initial activation weight of the schemes on which it applies. The conative effects of here-and-now dominant affective schemes become the organism's current affective goals, which boost the activation of appropriate executive schemes (Frijda, 1987; Greenberg & Safran, 1989; Pascual-Leone & Goodman, 1979; Pascual-Leone, Goodman, Ammon, & Subelman, 1978).

EC3. *Expressive effects* or *emotional expression*, are potentially observable changes in the face, body, voice, and activity level that usually accompany emotional states (Lewis & Michalson, 1985). They can be innate or acquired, and constitute the signals that enable interpersonal (intersubjective!) dialectical exchanges essential in important Act games of life, which evolution has preserved. The emotional expression of embarrassment I will not describe, for it has been well studied by Lewis et al. (1989) among others.

EC4. The fourth category of effects, found only in emotions but not in primary affects, is a set of *intellective/emotional experiences*. These effects are the self's own conscious or subconscious cognitive elaboration of the affects in question (evaluation, interpretation, goal definition, expressive socialization, referent adaptations, intentional detachment of emotional state from emotional expression, etc.). These intellective effects, as Lewis and Michalson (1985), Frijda (1987), and others have emphasized, are greatly influenced by the person's prior social experiences, and in particular by the relevant models (e.g., mentors) and standards available in the human groups where the subject was formed, and/or to which he/she is adapted.

One might ask whether showing that affects and emotions can be defined in terms of schemes is anything more than an exercise in nomenclature change. It is much more because the theory of organismic schemes, which Piaget pioneered and neo-Piagetians have developed into a process-analytical tool, contains explicit and detailed, experimentally tested, mechanisms that apply on schemes to change them and/or change their manifestation in performance. I refer interested readers to the work of neo-Piagetians in general (e.g., Case et al., 1988; Case, 1985, 1988; Demetriou, 1988) and to the work by me and my associates in particular (e.g., Pascual-Leone, 1980, 1983, 1984, 1987; Pascual-Leone & Goodman, 1979; Johnson et al., 1989; Johnson & Pascual-Leone, 1989).

PRIMARY AFFECTS AND THEIR REPRESENTATION
IN TERMS OF INNATE SCHEMES

Although early ontogenetic emergence of an emotion is an indication of plausible innateness, the age of first appearance can be neither a necessary nor a sufficient indicator (because innate biological characters may have different time schedules). A better indicator of innateness is the irreducibility of an affect/emotion to any combination or adaptation of other affects. This is so because learning or development cannot create something out of nothing: Learning and development are impossible without a sufficient innate basis. This conclusion implies that an epistemological analysis of the informational (i.e., semantic–pragmatic) independence of particular affects/emotions, should be a good basis for a model of primary affects. In this perspective affects/emotions are primary and independent if they are jointly needed to explain the categories of affects intervening in the survival and development of the individual and species. This analysis is the purpose of this section.

Discrete emotions theories, as Malatesta et al. (1989) aptly call them, claim that there is a multiplicity of qualitatively different affects, each with its distinct innate roots. As these authors state, innate emotions "are best conceived as instinct-like behaviors (patterned and organized but flexible) rather than reflex-like behaviors, a distinction that has been emphasized in contemporary ethological theory" (Malatesta et al., 1989, p. 131). This insistence on instinct-like behaviors, as opposed to reflex-like, indicates that they are speaking to innate schemes (as schemes were defined above). But to make them instinct-like presupposes that primary affects are in fact systemic, that is, not isolated affects but dynamic systems of affects, which together can adapt to circumstances (so that "any particular adaptational demand can be met by alternative emotional strategies"; Malatesta et al., 1989, p. 131). Systems of affects, rather than separate affects, are easier to analyze epistemologically, because they are easier to formulate and evaluate in terms of evolution. Also, hypothesizing systems of affects (rather than isolated affects) offers an elegant way of resolving differences between biosocial/nativist theoreticians and constructivist/learning theoreticians: *One can claim a large number of innate and distinct affective systems, while at the same time insisting that each of these innate affective systems is at birth rather undifferentiating (albeit clearly distinct from other systems), becoming differentiated with development and learning.*

Finally, from the point of view of psychotherapy, the assumption of *innate systems* of primary affects may help to explain the amazing easiness with which affects change from one to another in life and during therapy, always maintaining nonetheless their adaptive function and usefulness for coping with experience. This adaptive mobility that cuts across individual affects may be explained by the existence of innate affective systems which, in their interplay, bring about affective/emotional equilibratory regulations. Affective systems such as the ones I propose below may help to capture the complexity of affective processes found in psychotherapy; and may help us to understand the affective change process in therapy. At the center of this proposal is the principle of equilibration (eventually to be explicated by causal neuropsychological mechanisms). This organismic principle regulates the functioning of affective systems, and it gives them, in their coordination, adaptability to the organism's needs.

To illustrate this new concept of *innate affective systems* (Pascual-Leone, 1983, 1990a) it may be useful to contrast two affective systems that in many species, and especially in humans, play a pivotal role in organizing complementary strategies and styles of coping with the world and with Others. I refer to the affective systems of Power and of Love. The leading primary affect of Power is *mastery*; the leading affect of Love is *attachment*. I shall not review the long history of these affective categories (Power/*mastery* versus Love/*attachment*) in literature, philosophy, psychology, psychoanalysis, sociology, and biology/ethology. Instead I will proceed via an epistemological analysis.

It is well known that evolution cares much for the survival of the species but little for the survival of particular individuals. But for a species to survive, its individuals must have a fair chance. A fair chance means to have a second chance, a chance to grow sheltered in dependency and attachment to a mother, but also the chance to be either dominant as an adult and achieve biological survival via the exertion of Power, or be blessed in the ways of Love (and cunning!) and achieve biological survival with the help of protectors and/or the power of a helping group. I am suggesting that Power and Love affects are not only both necessary for survival, but that they maintain a mutual tradeoff or dialectical relationship. To make clear these ideas of dialectical relationships and dialectical analysis, which are important for a proper understanding of affective systems, I must now make a short excursus into epistemology (see also Pascual-Leone, 1983, 1987, 1990a; Pascual-Leone & Sparkman, 1980).

Dialectics studies the tradeoff relations that exist between or among the constituent parts of a dynamic, more or less organized (systemic) totality. It aims at understanding the adaptation (or misadaptation) of a totality *vis-à-vis* its own context, by way of studying the totality's functional constituent parts and their equilibration relations (facilitation, contradiction, etc.) with each other *vis-à-vis* the context. As Lenin (1915/ 1977) wrote: "The splitting of a single whole and the cognition of its contradictory parts . . . is the essence . . . of dialectics" (p. 381). This definition makes clear that in some real sense dialectics is an older and more general (epistemological) approach to the sort of problems studied by system analysis, and by self-organizing system theories (cf. Guidano, Chapter 3, this volume). When a constructivist evolutionary epistemology is added to dialectics, the result, *dialectical constructivism*, yields the developmental-analytical advantages of Piaget's or neo-Piagetian logical constructivism without its inconveniences (e.g., insensitivity to context, lack of process-analytical methods, inadequate causal analysis, etc.).

Power and Love, although independent from each other in terms of processes, are seen related to each other by dialectical functional relations, as soon as we regard them as constituents of the organismic totality—an organism evolved via evolution in continuous interaction with its context. This is the dialectical constructivist perspective I will adopt.

But a closer look at Power or Love quickly shows that they cannot be instruments of environmental survival unless each of them has internal means of adaptation (equilibration) by virtue of its various affective constituents. Epistemological considerations show that the minimal system of dynamic constituents—often called transformations—that could be adaptive (have equilibration capabilities) in a complex environment should consist of a main (or *identity*) *constituent transformation* and three regulating transformations, which I will call *logical negation* (or inverse), *dialectical negation* (or reciprocal), and *supplementary* (or correlative) *transformation*.[14] In the case of Power the *main or identity transformation* would be the affective motive/experience of mastery (the pleasure to achieve and to exercise, the competence-seeking affect). The *logical negation* (*inverse*) of this mastery affect is, of course, the feeling/experience of lack of mastery (incompetence) and vice versa, that is, the undoing of one is the effect of the other affect. The *dialectical negation* (*reciprocal*) of mastery is a qualitatively different affect that can cancel the experience/feeling of mastery via an alternative way, a new affect that *vis-à-vis* its effects on the organism and its performance (its context) is yoked with the main affect into a *relation of contradiction*: growth in the effects of one causes decrement in the effects of the other.[15] Defining dialectical negation (i.e., reciprocal) in this manner, it is apparent that dependency is the dialectical negation of mastery. Finally, the *supplementary* (*or correlative*) of mastery should be an affect that is qualitatively different from mastery, but that *vis-à-vis* its effects on the organism and its performance potentiates mastery, in the sense that growth in one causes growth in the other. It is clear (at least in the Western world) that the supplementary or correlative of mastery is independence.

To see why these four affects constitute an adaptive dynamic system, observe that all four are interrelated in similarly complementary ways: Dependency is the logical negation of independence (and vice versa);

independence is the dialectical negation of incompetence (and vice versa); incompetence is the supplementary or correlative of dependency (and vice versa). Since for each of these affects the other three function either as its supplementary (correlative) or as its negation, the four affects constitute a system which is adaptive (if this argument was not clear, please read again note 13).

Consider now the affective system of Love. The main or identity affect of Love is *attachment,* used here in the technical sense of the word. Its logical negation (inverse) is the absence of (or decrease in) attachment, that is, *unattachment* (nonlove). Its dialectical negation is a qualitatively different affect which is so yoked to attachment in performance that increase in one leads to decrease in the other. This dialectical negation (or reciprocal) is anger/aggression/hate. Finally, the logical negation of anger/aggression/hate and the supplementary or correlative of attachment is friendly indifference (or nonhate).

To see why, in terms of evolution, anger/aggression/hate is the dialectical negation of attachment within the affective system of Love, consider that persons or animals tend to become specialized either in the ways of Power (they are Power-dominated and have weaker Love affects) or in the ways of Love (are Love-dominated and their Power affects are weaker). This becomes so because *Power and Love, as systems, are a dialectical pair.* That is, Power and Love are yoked together by a dialectical relation: The Identity affect of the one is potentiated in performance, respectively, by the logical-negation affect of the other, and vice versa; and the dialectical-negation affect (i.e., the reciprocal) of the one is potentiated by (i.e., connects with), the supplementary/correlative of the other, and vice versa. The reader can easily verify these relations by comparing the effects of Love and Power affects given above. The implication is that increase in the identity of Power tends to cause in performance a decrease in the identity of Love, and vice versa. Due to this dialectical-pair relationship between Love and Power, an individual who is high in Love will tend to become attached to individuals who are high in Power, because their lower Power affects are thus compensated. Since the mastery-drive of the high-Power individuals often tends to impose plans and everyday life choices on their Love-driven partner, without regard to limits, the survival of a high-Love individual should indeed be in jeopardy—were it not for the dialectical negation of attachment, that is, anger/aggression/hate. Indeed, by reacting to abuse with anger/aggression/hate, the Love-driven partner counterbalances and sets limits on the (perhaps unconscious) excessive demands of his/her high-Power partner.

Power and Love constitute jointly the category of primary affective systems dealing with intersubjective relations—social relations within the species. The fact that they constitute a dialectical pair may impose the consequence that Power and Love easily become a typology for classifying people's dominant style, a typology that under innumerous terminologies keeps being reinvented. This fact suggests (see Pascual-Leone, 1990a,b) that the self of a person, that is, his/her self-referring ego-consciousness, is organized around two main complementary pivots: Power and Love affects. These pivots are complementary because their goals are jointly needed, even in pure cognition, for human experience and praxis (e.g., Bakan, 1966; Buber, 1973; Erikson, 1982; Scheler, 1973).

But other affective systems are needed to make superior mammals viable. I shall distinguish two other categories of affective systems. *Another category of innate affective systems deals with the state of the organism as a totality—a holistic affective evaluation. In this category I place the Control, Curiosity, and Joy/Sadness systems.* These systems can be found in Table 13.1.

In all these systems the main affects (symbolized by I, for identity) and their regulatory affects, that is, logical negation (symbolized by N, for negation or inverse), dialectical negation (symbolized by R, for reciprocal), and supplementary affects (symbolized by C, for correlative), maintain with one another, within each system, the kind of functional relations illustrated with Love and with Power.

The Control system corresponds to affects elicited by the appraisal of degree of cognitive control over the here-and-now situation (context). A high degree of control produces a positive affect (which I label with cognitive states that elicit it: certainty/reliable expectation/predictability). A moderate degree of control produces the affects of affective calm and of uncertainty/unpleasant surprise. The absence of control, and more so the appraisal of oncoming catastrophe (i.e., the contrary of control), elicits anxiety, which is the dialectical negation of certainty/reliable expectation/predictability.

The Curiosity system corresponds to affects elicited by the subcortical mechanism of arousal. Its identity affect (i.e., interest/pleasant surprise/orienting reaction) is elicited by a moderate degree of Control (a moderate mismatch with cognitive expectancies; Sokolov, 1963); its reciprocal affect (i.e., boredom/habituation) is elicited by a very high degree of Control (high certainty/reliable expectation/predictability).

Finally, the Joy/Sadness system corresponds to affects elicited by appraisal of a state of well-being in the organism as a dynamic totality. Notice that the Joy/Sadness system is yoked with both the Control system and the Curiosity system into separate logical-pair relations; that is, in both cases the I/N affects of Joy/Sadness are potentiated by (directly relate to) the I/N affects of both Control and Curiosity; and the R/C affects of Joy/Sadness are potentiated by the R/C affects of both Control and Curiosity. The implication is that joy tends to be maximized when, other things being equal, the identity affects of both Control and Curiosity are jointly maximized (which necessitates a moderately high amount of nov-

TABLE 13.1. Primary affect systems

1.   Power system
     [root of ego's "agency"]
I = *mastery*
N = incompetence
R = *dependency*
C = independence

2.   Love system
     [root of ego's "soul"]
I = *attachment*
N = unattachment or nonlove
R = *anger-aggression-hate*
C = friendly indifference

3.   Control system
I = *confidence/reliable expecta-*
    tion/predictability
N = uncertainty/unpleasant surprise
R = *anxiety*
C = affective calm

4.   Curiosity system
I = *interest/pleasant surprise*
N = disinterest
R = *boredom/habituation*
C = motivational indifference

5.   Joy/Sadness system
I = *joy/elation*
N = affective calm
R = *passive sadness/disappoint-*
    ment/depression
C = serenity

6.   Courage/Fear system
I = *courage*
N = cowardice
R = *fear*
C = basic trust/passive acceptance/
    suggestibility

7.   Desire/Disgust system
I = *attraction/appetite/happi-*
    ness/hope
N = unattraction/unhappiness
R = *disgust/rejection/despair*
C = tolerance/active acceptance

elty); and sadness or depression are, other things equal, maximized whenever the reciprocal affects of either Control or Curiosity are maximized
(which generates a range of feelings that, in various degrees and intensi-
ties, mix sadness/depression with "boredom and affective calm" and/or
(versus) "anxiety and motivational indifference."

   The third category of primary affective systems are those oriented
toward definite objects in the here-and-now situation (context): the
Courage/Fear and the Desire/Disgust systems. They are described in
Table 13.1 and should be self-explanatory, after the extended discussion of
Power, Love, and so on.

   A few more general comments about this model of primary affective
systems may be appropriate. Notice that the well-known distinction between positive and negative affects is here preserved, and clarified, by
casting the positive affects as main identity affects (I) and the negative
affects as their dialectical negations (or reciprocals, R). Since their functional role within the system is symmetrical, this choice does not prejudge

their relative importance, which changes both with situations and individual differences.

Two innate linkages regulating dynamic interactions among these primary affective systems are assumed to exist in the workings of this model. One of these systemic regulations (SR1) is that positive-valence (or negative-valence) affects tend to potentiate positive-valence (or negative-valence) affects. The second (SR2) is that the Power-driven disposition tends to increase the sensitivity to positive-valence effects and to decrease that to negative-valence affects. In contrast, the Love-driven disposition has an increased sensitivity towards negative-valence affects, while having a decreased sensitivity toward positive-valence affects. These functional linkages (systemic regulations) among different affects serve to demarcate two styles of emotional coping: the Power style, which leads to development of self structures rich in agency (see Pascual-Leone, 1990a,b), and the Love style of coping—at the origin of self-structures rich in "soul" characteristics (i.e., empathy, feeling for the Other, openness to the Other's needs and demands, etc.; cf. Pascual-Leone, 1990a,b).[16]

It might be useful to illustrate this concept of affective styles (e.g., Power versus Love), and their potential usefulness in psychotherapy, by sketching one example of their possible use in therapy (notice at the outset that the affective strategies and emotions to be explored should not be imposed, but should be reflected from the client's own utterances). Consider a client that is very much within the Power system, of which dominant theme at the start of therapy is mastery. Affective systems, and affective styles in particular, can be truly adaptive in life only if all their affective transformations (e.g., in Power: mastery, incompetence, dependency and independence) are equally flexible, and are able to operate within consciousness. Therefore one initial goal of phenomenological/experiential therapy might be to lead the client to explore in consciousness the (at least four) primary transformations of his/her currently dominant affective system. Thus, with the client mentioned above, the therapist could hope to recognize and reflect manifestations of the dominant affect's reciprocal emotion (dialectical negation), that is, in the case of mastery, dependency. The deeper exploration of this dependency needs, by the client, might lead clients to explore the correlative or supplementary emotion of dependency: incompetence—heretofore a suppressed emotion. Acknowledgment and exploration of his/her areas of incompetence might in turn bring to consciousness his/her previously unconscious overemphasis and overvaluing of mastery/competence. Analysis of concrete life-coping strategies that coordinate these four basic emotional transformations of Power, to foster adaptation, might in turn evoke the system of Love, when limitation of the Power-system strategies become apparent. Exploration of basic transformations of Love might then become the next spontaneous tacit goal of the phenomenological/experiential therapy, and so forth.

In addition to the primary systems described in Table 13.1, there are other secondary affective systems that result from their combination with cognitive schemes in specific sorts of situations (cf. Frijda 1987; Lewis, 1987, in press). Detailed discussion of secondary affects and emotions is of little importance in this model. Table 13.2 gives an implicit definition of two secondary affective systems that are particularly important in psychotherapy: Satisfaction/Sorrow and Pride/Guilt. These two secondary affective systems share an epistemic characteristic that distinguishes them from the primary emotions listed in Table 13.1. *Whereas the primary emotions refer either to the present or the future of experience, Satisfaction/ Sorrow and Pride/Guilt refer instead to the past of experience: They constitute affective evaluations* (value assigning reprocessing) *of experiences that have already taken place, or belong to the subject's history.* As a tentative speculation, I suggest that Satisfaction/Sorrow may have as main constructive core the affects of Love and Joy/Sadness systems, when they are combined in their application to past experience; Pride/Guilt may similarly be generated by the combination of the Power and Desire/ Disgust systems.

Table 13.2 also mentions the Instinctual-Drive systems (sex, hunger, thirst, pain, etc.) and the Cognitive Need/Style systems. The innate instinctual drive systems are analogous in their functioning to, but simpler and more peremptory than, primary affect systems. Cognitive Need/Style systems are developed with learning, as a result of the application of

TABLE 13.2. Four important secondary affective systems

8. Satisfaction/Sorrow system	9. Pride/Guilt system
I = *comfort/satisfaction*	I = *self-esteem/pride*
N = discomfort/dissatisfaction	N = embarrassment/self-dislike
R = *sorrow/regret/distress/active sadness*	R = *guilt/shame/self-alienation*
C = relief/passive acceptance/resignation	C = self-contentment/self-acceptance/passive self-respect
10. Instinctual-Drive systems [sex, hunger, thirst, pain, etc.]	11. Cognitive needs [intrinsic affective motivation for exerting sensorial, motor, and cognitive schemes]
I = *urge/need/pleasure*	
N = satiation	I = *functional need*
R = *aversion/repulsion*	N = saturation
C = tolerance/active acceptance	R = *fatigue/avoidance*
	C = tolerance/active acceptance

primary and secondary affects to the results of exercising cognition. Cognitive needs are emotions and personality styles; they probably develop, along with advanced cognition, by virtue of the same mediational-learning interpersonal processes (communicative praxis) that lead to the emergence of advanced cognition.

It is not possible here to discuss in detail this model of multiple primary affective systems, along with the dynamic organismic assumptions and ego/self model principles that can explain developmental complexities of affective/emotional performance. I will thus conclude this discussion by listing additional systemic regulations of the model that can give more insight into it.

SR3. The primary affective systems suggested in Table 13.1 are postulated to be innate but initially undifferentiated. Their constituent affects may not all be manifested and their interrelations not fully worked out at birth. These affects and interrelations are believed to differentiate with experience and with the growth of self-consciousness. The relative strength of primary affective systems and the affects therein is likely to be different from subject to subject. This innate individual-difference (ID) variation might explain the variability of emotional development as well as the existence of ID that affect considerably the course of cognitive growth (e.g., Kagan, 1989; Marc Lewis, 1989).

SR4. Affects and emotions are cued, via their own releasing conditions, by automatized cognitive schemes (some of which might be innate) or by mental syntheses such as those illustrated above. Often they are initially released by already activated schemes (which may or not be cognitive), and in turn may lead to the activation of new schemes. Thus the field of activation (also called working memory) of the subject can be changed, both in the schemes activated and degree of activation of schemes, by affective schemes (via their multiplier effect on activation weights).

SR5. Not all schemes, whether cognitive or affective, that constitute the current field of activation (working memory) actually apply to generate performance or to create the state of consciousness (cf. Pascual-Leone, 1983, 1984, 1987). Those that are incompatible with the dominant cluster of (compatible) schemes may not be able to apply, unless a change in the field of activation—sometimes brought about by questions or remarks of the psychotherapist—makes them compatible.

SR6. As Freud has emphasized, albeit for different reasons, the actual performance is *overdetermined*. That is, at every moment of the microgenesis of overt or covert performance, performance is determined by the constraints imposed by dominant schemes (which constitute the dominant content, the strongest causal cluster) in the field of activation. If after the application in performance of this first causal cluster of schemes there are "degrees of freedom" left in the to-be-produced performance, the next highest causal cluster of compatible schemes will apply to take some more degrees of freedom in performance; and so on until all the degrees of freedom have been used (Pascual-Leone, 1983; Pascual-Leone & Goodman, 1989).

SR7. In this model of mental processing the basic mental-attentional mechanism is constituted by two general-purpose resources: mental-attentional capacity or *M-capacity*, and mental central inhibition or *Interruption capacity* (I-capacity). In neo-Piagetian theory these two capacities together constitute what William James (1967), Kahneman (1973), and many others have called *mental effort*. Monitored by the subject's *executive schemes* (i.e., by his/her unconscious or conscious plans) the M-capacity can be mobilized and allocated to schemes that are relevant for the executive in question, while the I-capacity is used to inhibit centrally the irrelevant schemes. Thus the field of activation can be changed suddenly, perhaps with the guiding help of a psychotherapist's questions. Whether a lucky change in the field of activation may happen, depends on the totality of schemes available in the subject's field of activation (see Pascual-Leone, 1983, for a "banana republic" analogy that explicates this kind of processing).

I hope that this condensed presentation of a complex model is sufficient to suggest its explanatory potential. Perhaps the reader can by him/herself see how this model might explain defense mechanisms investigated by psychoanalysts, or the dynamic intersubjective processes of nondirective counseling, or the dynamics of self/affect studied by personality-social psychologists (e.g., Higgins, 1987).

CONCLUSIONS

The analyses presented in this chapter were aimed to contribute new ideas to the process-analytical study of affects, emotions, and feelings in psychotherapy; their functional nature and their processing interface with cognition. Three main problematic issues often encountered in the literature have been discussed, and potentially useful new solutions have been proposed for them. The three issues were: (1) the difference between affective "performance" and affective process or, what I believe to be related, the difference between emotions and affects; (2) the problem of the process-analytical psychological unit for affects and emotions, a unit that might become a tool for process and task analysis of affects/emotions in psychotherapy; (3) the problem of reconciling the existence of a multiplicity of innate emotions/affects (for which empirical and rational evidence exists) with the claim, supported by much developmental evidence, that infants' and young children's affects and emotions are undifferentiated, and progressively undergo changes via learning and cognitive growth.

Issue (1) was solved by defining affects as purely affective processes that have differential innate roots, and by defining emotions as affective-cognitive structures resulting from the coordination of affects and cognitions. Since performance is always both cognitive and affective, it is proper to call emotions all manifestations of affects in performance.

Issue (2) was solved by proposing that affects and emotions have as psychological unit the scheme, a well-defined psychological unit that is content-free in its definition, so that cognitive processes and affective processes in fact can and do share the same form of psychological unit. It was emphasized that, although psychological units—schemes—are essential to comprehend emotions, not all emotions can be reduced to schemes: Felt affects/emotions also emerge from dynamic affective syntheses, which are truly novel performance resolutions. These novel dynamic syntheses are a great source of insights for clients.

Issue (3) was solved by positing that there is a multiplicity of innate affective systems, thus upholding the claims of biosocial theoreticians, but claiming that these innate affective systems are not well differentiated at the point of birth; and can only differentiate as a result of developmental and learning processes, which also acknowledges the claim of cognitive-constructivist theoreticians.

A specific detailed model based on these and related principles was presented. Details of the model are tentative. As the Buddhist saying of the second epigraph suggests, the finger pointing to the moon (the model I am here proposing) is not the moon (i.e, the actual processes that I attempt to model). The point of this chapter is to highlight new directions and ways of looking at the "moon," not to claim that this model—my intellectual finger—should be taken as real.

ACKNOWLEDGMENTS

Preparation of this chapter was made easier by an operating research gra.it from Canada's Social Sciences and Humanities Research Council, and by a sabbatical leave from York University. I am grateful to my colleagues Mildred Bakan, David Bakan, Morris Eagle, Les Greenberg, Janice Johnson, and Jeremy Safran for much thoughtful advice. Sandra Locke's assistance made much easier the preparation of the manuscript.

NOTES

1. "L'émotion n'est pas un accident, c'est un mode d'existence de la conscience, une des façons dont elle *comprend* (au sens heideggerien de 'Verstehen') son 'Être-dans-le-Monde'" (translated by J.P.-L.).

2. Notice that to lead to new dynamic syntheses the here-and-now activated (i.e., *present*) affects must be mentally focussed on: This is *mentation*. As Greenberg and Safran (1989) put it: "Affect is being synthesized in the present from elements that are currently activated" (p. 26).

3. I use the term "alliance" here following Greenberg and Safran (1989). Related notions are those of positive "transference/countertransference" and projective "identification" long studied by psychoanalysts; also, the existential/phenomenological notions of empathy and "existential encounter."

4. Values are affective–cognitive structures (i.e., personal schemes; Pascual-Leone, 1983, 1990a), which connect "affect goals" (see below for this construct) with the cognitive schemes of objects, actions, or situations that satisfy the (positive or negative) affective goals in question—thus giving to these cognitive schemes an affective weight (Pascual-Leone, 1990b). Notice that values, albeit related, are distinctly different from motives. A motive (Pascual-Leone, 1990b) is a personal scheme that connects a personal mental operation, or a possible personal act by the person in his/her life (in the "life-world" of Husserl, 1954/1970), to the set of positive/negative affects that will be elicited when the act in question is carried out (cf. McClelland, 1985; Trevarthen, 1986, 1989). One might say that every motive is a personal scheme that gives one or more values as ground-for-choice to the acts (mental operations or overt actions) in the subject's praxis.

5. Notice that when defined as a field of activated processes, working memory can be thought of as either affective or cognitive. This is so because, if it is not due to automatized structures cued by salient perceptual cues, it is produced by mental attentional capacity (a brain hardware resource). This attentional energy or capacity is a content-free, information-free, general-purpose resource, which can be applied onto affective processes to bring them into consciousness (Pascual-Leone, 1983, 1984, 1987).

6. *M1* might be boosted by desire under some circumstances. The verb "boost" is used here as a technical term. It means the functional relation between a causal determinant of scheme activation (such as "mental attentional capacity" or "affect") and a scheme, by virtue of which the former greatly increases the activation level of the latter, thus ensuring that the scheme in question is an important determinant of the to-be-produced performance.

7. Readers familiar with my developmental work might notice that the units of mental capacity we are counting in infancy are those that I and my collaborators (Pascual-Leone, 1987; Pascual-Leone & Goodman, 1979; Johnson, Fabian, & Pascual-Leone, 1989) call e-units. Our behavioral measurement of mental attentional capacity (called M-power) is said to be equal to $e + k$, where both e and k stand for scales of M-power (e-scale is used to boost sensorimotor schemes while k-scale serves to boost the more complex symbolic schemes). The e-units are much smaller than the k-units available to school-aged children.

8. Although this representation (or mentation) of Other and self in their interaction, within the child's ego, is not complete at 20 or 24 months (Case, 1988; Case et al., 1988), what exists at this age suffices to elicit the emotion of embarrassment.

9. Other paradigms of embarrassment studied by Lewis are the "overcomplimentary" and the "mirror" situations. Their task-analytical structure can be shown to be like that of "request-to-dance" situations.

10. I call here Acts, with capitals, mental operative moves coordinated with the figurative schemes on which they apply, and with the figurative schemes that are the result of their application. These coordinated packages of structures are analogous to, but much simpler than, what Piaget has called "operations." They could perhaps be called "proto-operations" (cf. Langer, 1986).

11. Another way of stating the same thing is to say that *no dominant affective goal emerges* and the subject remains disequilibrated (see Pascual-Leone, 1984, 1990b, regarding these tacit processes of "affective choice" that generate *affective goals*).

12. The relative autonomy of schemes postulated here stands in stark contrast with the style of process modeling found in traditional experimental information processing, where psychological units do not, properly speaking, exist, and instead processes are modeled by means of centralized "corporative" modules that are supposed to carry out the various functions needed for the to-be-produced effect. Information-processing models cast in terms of boxes and arrows are customarily of this kind. Recent excellent examples of this style of modeling in the field of emotions are the models of Lewis and Michalson (1985) and of Frijda (1987). In contrast, in the model of organismic schemes proposed here the useful functions of the "corporative modules" are, in part, carried out autonomously by each individual scheme; in part they are carried out not by the affective schemes themselves, but by coactivated cognitive schemes and by a set of organismic "hardware" mechanisms. These mechanisms ensure that all activated schemes together—in "unconscious" collaboration—codetermine performance. In this model, performance is always *overdetermined* by all activated schemes that can apply to produce it, and this is how the effects of "corporative" modular mechanisms are incorporated.

13. I use the expression "Act game" here, inspired by Wittgenstein's notion of "language games" (Wittgenstein, 1958), to refer to a temporally and experientially organized dynamic system of performance patterns that is (are) relevant for the subject's praxis, and functions as a unit in the processing of this performance. Eric Berne's (1964) insightful notion of "games," in transactional therapy, has similar intention and referent in the organism.

14. To see that this is so, consider an operator or functional mechanism capable of an output producing two kinds of transformation. For instance, consider in a car the movements forward and backward. We can call main (identity) transformation one direction of movement, and call the other its logical negation, since one actually reverses the road trajectory of the other. But a single operator or functional mechanism is often maladaptive: Its output is insensitive to circumstances (e.g., imagine a car with no steering wheel; its output under forward or backward transformations would be maladapted to the width and meandering of roads). To make an organization (e.g., the car) more sensitive to circumstances,

the canonical method in engineering is to coordinate the first operator with a second operator (or several others) which is (are each) adaptive to a different relevant variable of the context. This equilibration effect of adding other context-relevant operators is more dramatic when the output of the various operators are dialectically interrelated, in the sense that dynamic tradeoff interactions exist among them. In this case the two transformations of the second operator could serve as dialectical negation (reciprocal) and supplementary (correlative) transformations of the first operator's main transformation. An example is the road effect of forward and backward movement when we endow the car with a steering wheel. On short-range movements, right forward (RF) and right backward (RB) transformations are each the logical negation of the other; left forward (LF) movement is the supplementary (correlative) transformation of RF and left backward (LB) is the dialectical negation (reciprocal) of RF. RB is the logical negation of RF because RB reverses the forward movement by undoing it. LF is the supplementary (correlative) of RF because although preserving the forward movement it reverses the rightward movement of RF—produces a different forward trajectory. LB is the dialectical negation (reciprocal) of RF because it cancels the forward movement by way of a different trajectory, without actually undoing the previous transformation. As any driver knows, these four basic transformations of a car's movement suffice, when cleverly combined, to make the car maneuverable. Thus a dialectical system of two operators, each containing two transformations (a main and its negation), is sufficient for adaptation; and since *two* operators and *two* transformations are minimal in number, this is the minimal system that is adaptable. Some readers may recognize in this system of transformations an analogy to Piaget's well-known model: the so-called INRC group of transformations which is characteristic of formal–operational thinking (Piaget, 1971; Inhelder & Piaget, 1958; Vuyk, 1981). The present model is derived from an epistemological reinterpretation of Piaget's model, but differs markedly from it. For instance, it differs from Piaget's in at least three major ways: (1) It does not form a mathematical group; (2) it is not restricted to conscious, formal-operational thinking; and (3) it is thought to be found in the unconscious affective processes of even young children. In regard to primary affects, this system of transformations might be innately prewired.

15. This is the sort of yoked relation that in a factor analysis would appear as a factor with polarized values, some tests with strong positive factor loadings and others with strong negative ones.

16. Notice the survival value of these systemic regulations with regard to Power and Love styles of emotionality: A person within the Power style must be sensitive to positive affects so as to detect aspects of Others' conduct or achievements that can be used as a means toward Power; on the other hand, an ideal Power-driven person should not be too sensitive to negative affects in order to maximize his/her own endurance. In contrast, a Love-driven person—a person with strong "soul"— should be sensitive to negative affects; he/she should be so in order to signal swiftly his/her negative reaction to Power-driven partners, whenever their demands place the Love person into oppressive situations that might jeopardize survival.

REFERENCES

Alexander, F., & French, T. M. (1946). *Psychoanalytic therapy: Principles and applications.* Ronald Press.

Alp, I. E. (1988). *Mental capacity and working memory in 1 to 3 year olds.* Unpublished doctoral dissertation, York University, Toronto.

Anderson, J. R. (1983). *The architecture of cognition.* Cambridge, MA: Harvard University Press.

Arnold, M. B. (1960). *Emotion and personality* (Vols. I and II). New York: Columbia University Press.

Bakan, D. (1976). *The duality of human existence: An essay on psychology and religion.* Chicago: Rand McNally.

Bandura, A. (1989). Human agency in social cognitive theory. *American Psychologist, 44,* 1175-1184.

Benson, N. (1989). *Mental capacity constraints on early symbolic processing: The origin of language from a cognitive perspective.* Unpublished doctoral dissertation, York University, Toronto.

Berne, E. (1964). *Games people play: The psychology of human relationships.* New York: Grove Press.

Bloom, L., & Capatides, J. (1987). Expression of affect and the emergence of language. *Child Development, 58,* 1513-1522.

Bloom, L., Beckwith, R., Capatides, J., & Hafitz, J. (1988). Expression through affect and words in the transition from infancy to language. In P. Baltes, D. Featherman, & R. Lerner (Eds.), *Life-span development and behavior* (Vol. 8, pp. 99-127). Hillsdale, NJ: Erlbaum.

Buber, M. (1973). *Between man and man.* London: Collins.

Buck, R. (1985). Prime theory: An integrated view of motivation and emotion. *Psychological Review, 92,* 389-413.

Case, R. (1985). *Intellectual development: Birth to adulthood.* New York: Academic Press.

Case, R. (1988). The whole child: Toward an integrated view of young children's cognitive, social, and emotional development. In A. D. Pellegrini (Ed.), *Psychological bases for early education* (pp. 155-184). Toronto: Wiley.

Case, R., Hayward, S., Lewis, M., & Hurst, P. (1988). Toward a neo-Piagetian theory of cognitive and emotional development. *Developmental Review, 8,* 1 -51.

Davidson, R. J., & Fox, N. A. (1988). Cerebral asymmetry and emotion: Developmental and individual differences. In D. L. Molfese & S. J. Segalowitz (Eds.), *Brain lateralization in children* (pp. 191-206). New York: Guilford Press.

Davidson, R. J., & Fox, N. A. (1989). Frontal brain asymmetry predicts infants response to maternal separation. *Journal of Abnormal Psychology, 98,* 127-131.

Davidson, R. J., Schaffer, C. E., & Saron, C. (1985). Effects of lateralized presentations of faces on self-reports of emotion and EEG asymmetry in depressed and non-depressed subjects. *Psychophysiology, 22,* 353-364.

Davidson, R. J., & Tomarken, A. J. (1989). Laterality and emotion: An electrophysiological approach. In F. Boller & J. Grafman (Eds.), *Handbook of neuropsychology* (pp. 419-441). Amsterdam: Elsevier.

Demetriou, A. (1988). *Neo-piagetian theories of cognitive development: An integration.* Amsterdam: North-Holland.

Erikson, E. H. (1982). *The life cycle completed.* New York: Norton.

Frijda, N. H. (1987). *The emotions.* New York: Cambridge University Press.

Greenberg, L. S., & Safran, J. D. (1989). Emotion in psychotherapy. *American Psychologist, 44,* 19-29.

Holloway, R., Blake, J., Pascual-Leone, J., & Middaugh, L. (1987). *Are there common mental capacity constraints in cognitive, communicative and play abilities in infants?* Paper presented at a meeting of the Society for Research in Child Development, Baltimore.

Higgins, E. T. (1987). Self-discrepancy: A theory relating self and affect. *Psychological Review, 94,* 319-340.

Husserl, E. (1970). *The crisis of European sciences and transcendental phenomenology.* Evanston, IL: Northwestern University Press. (Original work published 1954)

Inhelder, B., & Piaget, J. (1958). *The growth of logical thinking: From childhood to adolescence.* New York: Basic Books.

Izard, C. E. (1977). *Human emotions.* New York: Plenum.

Jalley, E. (1981). *Wallon lecteur de Freud et Piaget.* Paris: Editions Sociales.

James, W. (1967). *The writings of William James* (J. J. McDermott, Ed.). Chicago: University of Chicago Press.

Jaspers, K. (1970). *Philosophy* (Vol. 2). Chicago: University of Chicago Press.

Johnson, J., Fabian, V., & Pascual-Leone, J. (1989). Quantitative hardware-stages that constrain language development. *Human Development, 32,* 245-271.

Johnson, J., & Pascual-Leone, J. (1989). Developmental levels of processing in metaphor interpretation. *Journal of Experimental Child Psychology, 48,* 1-31.

Johnson, L. C., & Lubin, A. (1967). The orienting reflex during waking and sleeping. *Electroencephalography and Clinical Neurophysiology, 22,* 11-21.

Kagan, J. (1966). Reflection/impulsivity: The generality and dynamics of conceptual tempo. *Journal of Abnormal Psychology, 71,* 17-24.

Kagan, J. (1989). *Unstable ideas, temperament, cognition and self.* Cambridge, MA: Harvard University Press.

Kahneman, D. (1973). *Attention and effort.* Englewood Cliffs, NJ: Prentice-Hall.

Langer, J. (1986). *The origin of logic: One to two years.* Orlando, FL: Academic Press.

Lenin, V. I. (1977). On the question of dialectics. In K. Marx, F. Engels, & V. I. Lenin, *On dialectical materialism.* Moscow: Progress Publishers. (Original work published 1915)

Lewis, M. (1987). *Thinking and feeling—The elephant's tail.* Paper presented at the Conference on "Thinking and Problem Solving in the Developmental Process: International Perspectives," Graduate School of Applied and Professional Psychology, State University of New Jersey.

Lewis, M. (in press). The development of intentionality and the role of consciousness. *Psychological Inquiry.*

Lewis, M., & Michalson, L. (1985). Faces as signs and symbols. In G. Zivin (Ed.),

The development of expressive behavior: Biology-environment interactions (pp. 153-180). New York: Academic Press.

Lewis, M., Sullivan, M. W., & Michalson, L. (1984). The cognitive-emotional fugue. In C. Izard, J. Kagan, & R. Zajonc (Eds.), *Emotions, cognition and behavior* (pp. 264-288). New York: Cambridge University Press.

Lewis, M., Sullivan, M. W., Stanger, C., & Weiss, M. (1989). Self development and self-conscious emotions. *Child Development, 60,* 146-156.

Lewis, Marc. (1989). Early infant-mother interaction as a prediction of problem solving in toddlers. *International Journal of Early Childhood, 21.*

Luria, A. R. (1973). *The working brain: An introduction to neuropsychology.* New York: Basic Books.

Malatesta, C. Z., Culver, C., Tesman, J. R., & Shepard, B. (1989). The development of emotion expression during the first two years of life. *Monographs of the Society for Research in Child Development, 54*(1-2).

Marmor, J. (1986). The corrective emotional experience revisited. *International Journal of Short-Term Psychotherapy, 1,* 43-47.

McClelland, D. C. (1985). *Human motivation.* Glenview, IL: Scott, Foresman.

Meng, Z. (1989). *The organisational function of emotion on cognitive tasks in infancy.* Invited address at the International Society for the Study of Behavioural Development, Jyväskylä, Finland.

Miller, N. (1963). Reflections on the law of effect produce a new alternative to drive reduction. In M. Jones (Ed.), *Nebraska Symposium on Motivation* (pp. 65-112). Lincoln, NE: University of Nebraska Press.

Pascual-Leone, J. (1969). *Cognitive development and cognitive style: A general psychological integration.* Unpublished doctoral dissertation, University of Geneva.

Pascual-Leone, J. (1980). Constructive problems for constructive theories: The current relevance of Piaget's work and a critique of information-processing simulation psychology. In R. Kluwe & H. Spada (Eds.), *Developmental modes of thinking* (pp. 263-296). New York: Academic Press.

Pascual-Leone, J. (1983). Growing into human maturity: Toward a metasubjective theory of adulthood stages. In P. B. Baltes & O. G. Brim (Eds.), *Life-span development and behavior* (Vol. 5, pp. 117-155). New York: Academic Press.

Pascual-Leone, J. (1984). Attentional dialectic and mental effort: Toward an organismic theory of life stages. In M. L. Commons, F. A. Richards, & C. Armon (Eds.), *Beyond formal operations: Late adolescent and adult cognitive development* (pp. 182-215). New York: Praeger.

Pascual-Leone, J. (1987). Organismic processes for neo-Piagetian theories, a dialectical causal account of cognitive development. *International Journal of Psychology, 22,* 531-570.

Pascual-Leone, J. (1988). Affirmations and negations, disturbances and contradictions in understanding Piaget: Is his later theory causal? *Contemporary Psychology, 33,* 420-421.

Pascual-Leone, J. (1989). An organismic process model of Witkin's field-dependence-independence. In T. Globerson & T. Zelniker (Eds.), *Cognitive style and cognitive development* (pp. 36-70). Norwood, NJ: Ablex.

Pascual-Leone, J. (1990a). Reflections on life-span intelligence, consciousness and ego development. In C. N. Alexander & E. Langer (Eds.), *Higher stages of human development* (pp. 258–285). New York: Oxford University Press.

Pascual-Leone, J. (1990b). An essay on wisdom: Toward organismic processes that make it possible. In R. J. Sternberg (Ed.), *Wisdom: Its nature, origins and development* (pp. 244–278). New York: Cambridge University Press.

Pascual-Leone, J., & Goodman, D. (1979). Intelligence and experience: A neo-Piagetian approach. *Instructional Science, 8,* 301–367.

Pascual-Leone, J., Goodman, D., Ammon, P., & Subelman, I. (1978). Piagetian theory and neo-Piagetian analysis as psychological guides in education. In J. McCarthy & J. A. Easley (Eds.), *Knowledge and development* (Vol. 2, pp. 243–289). New York: Plenum.

Pascual-Leone, J., Johnson, J., & Benson, N. (1989). Mental capacity constraints on symbolic processing: The onset of human language. In J. Johnson (Chair), *Mental capacity constraints on cognition: Studies from the theory of constructive operators.* Symposium conducted at the meeting of the International Society for the Study of Behavioural Development, Jyväskylä, Finland.

Pascual-Leone, J., & Sparkman, E. (1980). The dialectics of empiricism and rationalism: A last methodological reply to Trabasso. *Journal of Experimental Child Psychology, 29,* 88–101.

Piaget, J. (1971). *Structuralism.* New York: Harper & Row.

Piaget, J. (1985). *The equilibration of cognitive structures: The central problem of intellectual development.* Chicago: University of Chicago Press.

Rachman, S. (1980). Emotional processing. *Behaviour Research and Therapy, 18,* 51–60.

Sartre, J.-P. (1960). *Esquisse d'une théorie des émotions.* Paris: Hermann. (Original work published 1939)

Sartre, J.-P. (1966). *Being and nothingness.* New York: Washington Square Press.

Scheler, M. (1973). *Selected philosophical essays.* Evanston, IL: Northwestern University Press.

Shafrir, U., & Pascual-Leone, J. (1990). Post-failure reflectivity/impulsivity and spontaneous attention to errors. *Journal of Educational Psychology, 82,* 378–387.

Simon, H. A., & Newell, A. (1972). *Human problem solving.* Englewood Cliffs, NJ: Prentice-Hall.

Sokolov, J. N. (1963). *Perception and the conditioned reflex.* Oxford, England: Pergamon.

Sroufe, L. A. (1979). Socioemotional development. In J. D. Osofsky (Ed.), *Handbook of infant development* (1st ed., pp. 462–516). New York: Wiley.

Sternberg, C., Campos, J., & Emde, R., (1983). The facial expression of anger in seven-month-old infants. *Child Development, 54,* 170–184.

Sullivan, M. W., & Lewis, M. (1989). Emotion and cognition in infancy: Facial expressions during contingency learning. *International Journal of Behavioral Development, 12,* 221–237.

Thich, N. H. (1974). *Zen keys.* New York: Doubleday.

Trevarthen, C. (1986). Development of intersubjective motor control in infants. In M. G. Wade & T. A. Whiting (Eds.), *Motor development in children: Aspects of coordination and control.* Boston: Martinus Nijhoff.

Trevarthen, C. (1987). Sharing makes sense: Intersubjectivity and the making of an infant's meaning. In R. Steele & T. Threadgold (Eds.), *Language topics: Essays in honour of Michael Halliday* (Vol. 1, pp. 177–199). Philadelphia: John Benjamins.

Trevarthen, C. (1989). Origins and directions for the concept of infant intersubjectivity. *SRCD Newsletter*, pp. 1–7.

Vuyk, R. (1981). *Overview and critique of Piaget's genetic epistemology: 1965–1980.* New York: Academic Press.

Wallon, H. (1946). Le rôle de l'autre dans la conscience du moi. *Journal Egyptien de Psychologie, 2,* i. (Reprinted in *Enfance*, special number, "Henry Wallon, Psychologie et education de l'enfance," 7(3–4), 279–286)

Wallon, H. (1954). *Les origines du caractère chez l'enfant.* Paris: Presses Universitaires de France.

Wallon, H. (1982). *La vie mentale.* Paris: Editions Sociales. (Reprinted from H. Wallon, "La vie mentale," Encyclopédie Française, VIII, Paris: Libraire Larousse, 1938)

Wittgenstein, L. (1958). *Philosophical investigations.* Oxford, England: Blackwell.

PART IV

CONCLUSION

14

Affective Change Processes: A Synthesis and Critical Analysis

JEREMY D. SAFRAN
Adelphi University

LESLIE S. GREENBERG
York University

In this chapter we will summarize and synthesize some of the major themes which have emerged in the previous chapters. We will organize our discussion around a number of different change processes that appear to underlie the various affective change events described by the contributors. While we will treat these processes as distinct in nature, it should be borne in mind that in reality they overlap with one another to varying degrees. Seven different affective processes will be discussed: (1) emotional restructuring, (2) catharsis, (3) experiential symbolization, (4) facilitating cognitive reorganization, (5) motivating adaptive behavior, (6) corrective emotional experience, and (7) affect attunement.[1] A final focus for exploration will be the role of the therapist's emotions in the change process. In our discussion we will attempt to clarify our understanding of the relevant affective processes by integrating the perspectives of the different contributors and by analyzing these processes in terms of the theory summarized in Chapter 1. We will also highlight issues that remain unclear and areas which call for further theoretical refinement.

EMOTIONAL RESTRUCTURING

A number of contributors to this volume make reference to the processes of accessing and modifying cognitive–affective schemata (e.g., Foa &

Kozak, Chapter 2; Engle, Beutler, & Daldrup, Chapter 7; Rice & Greenberg, Chapter 8). These processes are important in their own right and
also as component processes within a number of different affective change
events. The central premise is that people code events not only at a
cognitive level but also at an affective level. For this reason, interventions
that attempt to modify experience at an exclusively cognitive level without
attending to the affective level of representation may fail.

This discrepancy corresponds to the commonly observed split in
therapy between what clients think and feel. In order to be of any theoretical utility, however, it is necessary to go beyond the common language
distinction between thinking and feeling to clarify what we mean by feeling
and what we mean by thinking. Foa and Kozak (Chapter 2, this volume)
adopt Lang's (1984) concept of the fear structure in an attempt to clarify
this issue. In this model, fear is held to be

> . . . represented as a network in memory that includes three kinds of
> information:
> 1. Information about the feared stimulus situations:
> 2. Information about verbal, physiological, and overt behavioral
>   responses; and
> 3. Interpretive information about the meaning of the stimulus and
>   response elements of the structure. (p. 4)

Lang's concept of the fear structure converges in many ways with
Leventhal's (1982, 1984) notion of the emotion schema. Since the emotion schema concept is grounded within a more comprehensive model of
emotion, it may be useful to frame things in these terms. Leventhal's basic
hypothesis is that the individual establishes representations of events that
take place both in terms of the perceived characteristics of the external
events and in terms of his/her own expressive motor and autonomic
reactions to those events. In this model, the individual is seen as continually establishing holistic representations of the self in interaction with the
environment. Emotion is viewed as having a fundamental expressive-
motor component that is based upon neuromotor templates that are wired
into the organism through natural selection.

Since the wired-in expressive motor responses that are evoked by
situations ultimately reflect the goals of the organism (see Safran & Greenberg, Chapter 1, this volume), we represent the meaning of various events
for ourselves in terms of our previous expressive-motor reaction to those
events. Particular classes of situations and our reactions to them thus
become represented in schematic memory as structures in which images
and episodic memories of specific events, and the expressive-motor behaviors and associated autonomic arousals that have been evoked in response
to these events, are tightly linked. Once these schematic structures are
established, encountering either a critical number or configuration of the

relevant schematic components will activate the schema and the contents of the schema will be run off.

Thus, for example, in the case of fear avoidance problems, encountering the phobic stimulus will activate the relevant schematic structure and the individual will experience fear and the associated expressive motor tendencies and action disposition (i.e., escape). Thus as Foa and Kozak (Chapter 2, this volume) point out, these cognitive-affective schemata, or what Lang refers to as fear structures, can be thought of as programs for dealing with feared situations that contain both information about the relevant situation and behavioral responses or dispositions that are automatically elicited when that situation is encountered.

Since it is reasonable to hypothesize that all experiences that are relevant to the basic concerns and goals of the organism are coded in this cognitive-affective format, one might hypothesize that all therapeutic change ultimately involves the modification of memory structures of this type. Foa and Kozak (Chapter 2, this volume) maintain that two conditions are required to modify the fear structure in fear avoidance problems. First, the relevant information must be made available in a fashion that will activate the fear structure. Second, new information must be made available that is incompatible with existing elements in the fear structure in order for a new memory to be formed. They refer to this integration of new memory into the existing fear structure as emotional processing.

While Foa and Kozak restrict their focus to the modification of cognitive-affective structures associated with fear avoidance problems, this type of analysis can be extended to our understanding of the modification of other types of cognitive-affective structures as well. Engle et al. (Chapter 7, this volume), for example, speak about the fashion in which the empty chair approach can be employed to activate and modify an existing cognitive-affective schema in the case of an unfinished business event. Silberschatz and Sampson (Chapter 5, this volume) speak about the modification of pathogenic beliefs about interpersonal relationships. Dahl (Chapter 6, this volume) speaks about the modification of what he terms frames. He argues that therapeutic change involves a modification in affects that function as beliefs about the status of fulfillment of wishes.

When we speak about modifying a specific fear structure in the case of a circumscribed fear avoidance problem, the nature of the schema being modified is reasonably clear. When, however, we extend our analysis to less-circumscribed types of problems, however, the nature of the relevant schema is less clear. One concept which may be useful in discussing emotional restructuring is the construct of the interpersonal schema (Safran, 1986, 1990a,b; Safran & Segal, 1990). An interpersonal schema is a generalized representation of self-other interactions which the individual abstracts on the basis of previous experiences.[2] It is hypothesized that people encode interpersonal events as interactional units rather than as discrete representations of self or other (Main, Kaplan, & Cassidy, 1985).

Interpersonal schemata initially serve the function of allowing the infant to predict interactions with the attachment figure, thereby maintaining proximity to him or her. They are coded, at least partly, in the form of expressive–motor behaviors and images and are more accurately thought of as cognitive–affective structures than purely cognitive structures. Safran (1990a) hypothesizes that these schemata operate at different levels of generality or abstractness and are hierarchically embedded. An interpersonal schema at the highest level of generality would correspond to what Bowlby (1969) refers to as an internal working model. At this level, the interpersonal schema provides an abstract representation of interactions with people in general. This higher-level interpersonal schema is, however, established through the aggregation of lower-level schemata.

At a midlevel of generality the individual establishes interpersonal schemata of interactions with specific types of individuals (e.g., lovers, authority figures). These, in turn, are established through the aggregation of lower-level schemata that represent interactions with specific individuals (e.g., mother, father, brother). These lower-level schemata contain images of prototypical interpersonal events that have transpired as well as expressive motor responses that have been evoked by those events.

Such cognitive–affective schemata can be activated in a number of ways. First, having a new interpersonal encounter that resembles a prototypical interpersonal event may activate the relevant schematic structure. Second, recalling specific images or memories that are coded within the schema may activate the entire schema. Third, contacting and expressing feelings associated with the schema may activate it. The more fully the schema is accessed, the more amenable it will be to restructuring.

Once an interpersonal schema has been accessed, one way of modifying it involves the use of the therapeutic relationship to provide schema-disconfirming experience. Another means involves accessing previously unprocessed emotional experience that is schema-discrepant. We will discuss these processes in a later section of this chapter.

A third process of modification involves operating upon the schema at a more conceptual level. Through articulating the tacit rules and beliefs implicit in the schema (e.g., I must always be strong in order to maintain relatedness) in the form of "hot" or emotionally laden cognitions, the possibility of challenging them at a more conscious level emerges (Safran & Greenberg, 1982, 1986, 1987). Once these rules or core beliefs have been put into words, the client can begin to see the way in which they have been influencing his/her behavior and a process of decentering can take place. These rules, or core beliefs, however, often cannot be accessed unless the relevant schematic structure has been activated.

CATHARSIS

Catharsis is one of the more well-known and controversial affective change processes. It has a history dating back to the very conception of contemporary psychotherapy, with Breuer and Freud's (1895/1955) pioneering of the "talking cure" in psychoanalysis. Although catharsis was subsequently rejected by Freud as a primary change mechanism, it has always retained a role in nonmainstream approaches to psychotherapy, such as Reich's (1942) approach, and neo-Reichian approaches such as bioenergetics (Lowen, 1975). In the 1960s catharsis came to play a central role in emotive therapies such as primal therapy and rebirthing. Despite the long history of cathartic approaches to psychotherapy, the scientific community has always maintained a skeptical attitude toward them. The general public, however, has continued to be fascinated with cathartic approaches. While this fascination may in part be attributable to the dramatic quality of catharsis, repeated testimonials regarding the potency of cathartic experiences suggest the need for careful conceptual and empirical investigation of this phenomenon. One of the problems in conducting research in this area, however, is continuous confusion over the nature of catharsis, and a tendency to group together heterogeneous affective change processes under this general rubric (Greenberg & Safran, 1987).

As McGuire (Chapter 9, this volume) points out, it is important to distinguish between the process of catharsis and the process of experiencing, as described by Gendlin (Chapter 10, this volume) or the type of experiential search described by Rice and Greenberg (Chapter 8, this volume). (We will discuss these processes later in this chapter under the topic of experiential symbolization.) Unlike Gendlin, who appears to deemphasize the importance of catharsis as a change process and who in fact believes that cathartic experiences can interfere with the change process of experiencing, McGuire argues that the catharsis in itself is an important healing process. She maintains that catharsis is "a way in which the client attends in a loving, empathic way to his/her own former hurt and grieves for him/herself."

Our view is that what is typically thought of as catharsis may involve any of a number of component subprocesses. Four such component processes are: (1) experiencing compassion for the self, (2) completing interrupted emotion/action sequences, (3) releasing inhibiting muscular tension, and (4) schematic restructuring.

Experiencing Compassion for the Self

Elaborating on McGuire's (Chapter 9, this volume) suggestion, we hypothesize that catharsis involves a process of experiencing compassion for the self and allowing the spontaneous emergence of previously interrupted emotional experience. This emotional experience, which has, in the past, been interrupted for fear of the interpersonal consequence (see Safran & Greenberg, Chapter 1, this volume), emerges when the client feels sufficiently safe in the therapeutic relationship (see Silberschatz & Sampson, Chapter 5, this volume).

This experience of interpersonal safety facilitates a "letting go," which allows the client to experience a part of the self, previously disowned. This very process of "letting go" entails a change in one's stance toward the self—a softening, which grows as the client's emotional experience emerges and is met with continuing acceptance and validation by the therapist. One form of cathartic experience, focused on by McGuire, involves the expression of sadness and pain that has previously been interrupted. This is a healing process because it allows clients to experience fully nurturance that has previously been unavailable to them and simultaneously facilitates an accepting and nurturing stance toward the self. The emotion of sadness and the act of crying are natural and adaptive responses to being hurt, which elicit nurturant responses in others and allow the individual to feel cared for. Another form of cathartic experience, which we will focus on later, involves the expression of anger.

Completing Interrupted Emotion/Action Sequences

As Engle et al. (Chapter 7, this volume) suggest, Perls's (1973) notion of the Gestalt cycle can be a useful metaphor for understanding one of the processes through which emotional expression in therapy can facilitate change. According to Perls (1973), emotions, once aroused have a natural tendency to push toward completion through the *implementation of action* directed toward the satisfaction of the individual's needs. In this perspective, unexpressed emotions leave one in a state of organismic imbalance until they are expressed in a natural cycle of sensation, awareness, mobilization, contact, and withdrawal. Moreover, as we discussed in Chapter 1, interruption of an emotional experience can interfere with healthy functioning by resulting in a persevering motivational state, which intrudes into working memory and reduces processing capacity. The completion of unfinished business thus involves the completion of an interrupted normal psychophysiological cycle and intense emotional expression in this context can be thought of as a relief from physiological tension.

This notion of emotion as being intrinsically linked to action is also central to the perspective on emotion that Butler and Strupp (Chapter 4, this volume) have adopted from Schafer (1983), and as discussed in Chapter 1, is compatible with contemporary theory, which views emotion as an active disposition. If, as we hypothesized in Chapter 1, the function of emotion is to safeguard and satisfy the goals of the overall system, it may be extrapolated that emotional experience that has not been attended to and dealt with in some way will continue to press for attention.

An important component of what is commonly referred to as catharsis involves the subjective experience, as McGuire (Chapter 9, this volume) illustrates, of release. This experience of release may stem partly from the expression of an action disposition that has been activated but not carried through into action. In the same way that tension builds up in the tip of the tongue phenomenon until the elusive word is finally found, the inhibition of a behavioral system that has been activated may build tension that is only released when the relevant action is implemented.

Releasing Inhibiting Muscular Tension

Another possible component of the subjective experience of release associated with catharsis may be the cessation of muscular tension associated with the interruption of expressive-motor behavior associated with certain emotional experiences. As Reich (1942) theorized, the suppression or interruption of emotional experience may actually involve the suppression of associated expressive-motor behaviors through muscular contraction. If, as contemporary emotion theory suggests, emotional expression involves an expressive motor component, then it is reasonable to hypothesize that the interruption or inhibition of emotional experience is not simply a psychological act. It is also a physical act, in which expressive motor behaviors associated with the relevant emotion are suppressed through muscular contraction. For example, the individual who is angry may clench his/her jaw muscles in order to suppress facial expression associated with anger. As Reich (1942) theorized, over time an individual may develop chronic patterns of muscular tension associated with suppressing particular types of emotional experience. The cathartic experience may thus be associated with a certain sense of release resulting from the relaxing of chronic muscular tension that would be not unlike the release one experiences after relaxing clenched fists.

Schematic Restructuring

As Engle et al. (Chapter 7, this volume) hypothesize, some forms of cathartic experience may operate partly through promoting a type of schematic restructuring. In their chapter, they focus specifically on what Greenberg and Safran (1987) have referred to as the unfinished business event. In this event a process of completing an interrupted emotional sequence is activated by using the Gestalt empty chair procedure to establish an imaginary dialogue with a figure from the client's past.

It may be of some value to speculate about how the chronic interrup-

tion in expression of feelings toward a significant other can lead to pathological functioning. One possibility is that the interruption of feelings
toward another results in the suppression or isolation of the generic
schematic representation of the relevant class of self–other interactions.
As a result of this isolation, the schematic representation is not amenable
to ongoing modification in light of new experiences as the individual
matures. Thus for example, a man who as a child experienced himself as
victimized by a father whom he perceived as powerful and malicious, may
in an attempt to avoid the threatening feelings associated with that experience, also inhibit the activation of the relevant schematic structure. As a
result he will, as he matures, retain a sense of himself as a powerless victim
in interaction with malicious adults. He will not be able to modify his sense
of self or his sense of others in response to new experiences. The activation
of the interrupted feelings and the associated schematic structure may
thus be an important prerequisite in order for him to begin to change his
sense of self in interaction with others. As Engle et al. (Chapter 7, this
volume) suggest, intense emotional expression in the unfinished business
event may unpack emotional schematic memories that can then be subjected to a reinspection, and this process can ultimately lead to a restructuring of schematic memory.

Greater clarification is required, however, regarding how the process of
schematic restructuring takes place. We advance the following hypotheses:

1. By imagining the relevant significant other in the chair and engaging in an emotionally alive dialogue with him/her, the client is able to
activate relevant schematic structures, which include memories of the
relevant individual (e.g., father, mother, lover), memories of the self in
interaction with that individual, and feelings that are associated with those
memories.

2. By expressing previously interrupted feelings toward the imagined
other in the context of an accepting therapeutic relationship, the patient is
able to shift some of the beliefs that inhibit emotional expression.

3. A schematic restructuring may result in part from expressing
intense, previously interrupted feelings toward or in the presence of the
fantasized object of those feelings in the present context and experiencing
this as a valid and acceptable thing to do. This process may be related to a
process described by Rice and Greenberg (Chapter 8, this volume) in
which clients become more accepting of different aspects of the self when
the therapist is able to empathize with his/her emotional experience. In a
similar fashion the client who, for example, expresses previously interrupted feelings of anger toward the imagined figure in the chair and
appraises these feelings as valid and alright in the present context may
begin to restructure a sense of who he/she is. In this situation there may be
a shift in the client's sense of self from one who never got angry at their
mother or father, or one who felt angry and felt bad for feeling angry, to

one who is angry and is acceptable in his/her anger. This type of shift is undoubtedly facilitated by the presence of an empathic therapist who is tacitly validating the experience through his/her presence.

Another important shift that can take place in this context, as Engle et al. (Chapter 7, this volume) illustrate, is a shift from seeing oneself as a victim to seeing oneself as an agent. Thus, for example, in one of the transcript segments provided by them, by directly expressing her resentment at her grandmother for her preoccupation with death and dying, the client shifts from the stance of the powerless child who was subjected to her grandmother's shortcomings, to the stance of an adult who experiences her own feelings, and can take action guided by those feelings. By expressing previously interrupted feelings in an unfinished business event, there can thus be a type of empowerment. This expression of the feelings will not, in itself, empower the client in the real world. Contact with those feelings that have been interrupted, however, can ultimately help to change the patient's sense of who he/she is, thereby leading to mobilization in the real world.

4. As Engle et al. point out, the model of completing unfinished business events presented by Greenberg and Safran (1987) involves an additional component not contained in their model. Specifically, Greenberg and Safran hypothesize that part of the change process involves a modification in the representation of the other through empathy with the other's position. Further efforts to clarify the role of empathy as a change mechanism in this type of context are warranted. Empathy appears to be an important cognitive-affective capacity that allows one to assume another's perspective. For this reason it can be a powerful means of facilitating a disembedding from one's current perceptions and in fact plays an important role in facilitating the decentration process in normal childhood development (Kegan, 1982).

As Greenberg and Safran (1987) point out, however, a prerequisite for this type of empathic process to facilitate change is for the client first to express his/her own interrupted feelings toward the other. Expression of these feelings helps to activate the relevant interpersonal schema, which then becomes amenable to change, through the individual using his or her adult empathic capacity. This prior stage of accessing the relevant schema or the relevant feeling, images, and so on, is vital since without it an attempt to empathize with the other might lead to a type of premature empathy that is self-denying, and which maintains the problem.

EXPERIENTIAL SYMBOLIZATION

McGuire, Gendlin, and Rice and Greenberg (Chapters 8, 9, and 10, this volume) all focus on different aspects of a process we will term *experiential symbolization.* The distinctions made by McGuire (Chapter 9, this volume) between sheer emotion, felt experiencing and catharsis are important ones, and the discussion in this volume between McGuire and Gendlin, we believe, helps to clarify further the difference between these processes. As McGuire suggests, sheer emotion can be thought of as internally generated information associated with basic action dispositions, which are wired into the human organism (e.g., anger, sadness, fear). In contrast, the type of felt experiencing focused on by theorists such as Rogers (1961) and Gendlin (1979), involves the more subtle nuances associated with the tacit meaning of a particular situation for an individual.

When an incident takes place that activates a particular emotional experience, implicit in this emotional experience are learned systemic goals. Through symbolizing one's current emotional experience in conceptualized form, one can derive a more explicit understanding of the personal meanings, values, beliefs, and personal experiences that underlie the current emotional experience. As McGuire (Chapter 9, this volume) states: "While sheer emotion is a narrow, primitive, repetitive response, felt experiencing is a broader bodily sensing of the personal context, past, present, and future intending, as it is functioning in the present moment."

The distinction between sheer emotion and felt-experiencing, initially made by Gendlin (1962), is further clarified by Gendlin's reactions to McGuire's chapter. As Gendlin maintains, the emphasis in experiencing is on the *whole* experience. In other words, not just a specific expressive–motor response to a specific situation, but the expressive–motor response in context of the entire situation. It is this whole configuration then, that provides the individual with information about the meaning of the experience for him/her. The simple emotional response (e.g., anger, sadness) out of context of the relevant situation does not convey the full meaning of the situation for the person.

The transcript presented by McGuire, as well as Gendlin's comments on it, are particularly helpful in terms of clarifying certain aspects of the process of change through experiential symbolization. As McGuire points out, an important part of the change process for this client involves her acquiring a felt-sense of how therapy termination relates to her experience of her loss when her mother died. We are in agreement with McGuire here, that an important part of this change process involves the client's experiencing of the unresolved grief for her mother in context of the nurturing presence of the therapist. This appears to be a multicomponent process that warrants further examination.

One aspect of the change process appears to be what Alexander and French (1946) termed a corrective emotional experience. In other words, the opportunity to resolve her feelings around the separation from her therapist in a constructive fashion helps the client to change her feelings and beliefs about separation in general.

A second component appears to involve an elaboration of the felt meaning of the separation for the client. It appears that in some way the exploration of the meaning of the current separation in terms of her previous experience of loss with the mother appears to be an important part of the change process. Moreover, it appears that a deeper elaboration of the meaning of her original loss of her mother (e.g., when she lost her mother, it felt like she lost her whole family because she was the only female left) appears to be part of the change process as well.

It would be important to clarify in what way the change process involved here is similar to the unfinished business event described by Engle et al. (Chapter 7, this volume) and in what way is it different. Moreover, it would be important to clarify the similarities and differences between the change event described here and the affective change process that would ensue if the therapist had intervened with a transference interpretation. (We will explore this in greater detail later.)

The experiential search event examined by Rice and Greenberg (Chapter 8, this volume) provides further clarification of the process through which experiential symbolization takes place. There appears to be an important similarity between the process described by McGuire and the process described by Rice and Greenberg. Both involve tapping into the tacit meaning provided by bodily felt experience that has not yet been translated into conceptual form. An important difference, however, involves the specific context in which the intervention is applied. McGuire's event involves an exploration of feelings that are evoked in and by the therapeutic relationship. The exploration of these feelings leads back to the exploration of the client's fundamental beliefs and world view as well as critical developmental experiences (as it does in Rice and Greenberg's problematic reaction event). However in the McGuire transcript, the exploration then returns to the context of the therapeutic relationship and an important part of the change process involves the corrective emotional experience of the therapeutic relationship.

Rice and Greenberg's resolution of a problematic reaction begins with the exploration of an out-of-therapy situation. Here again, the exploration leads to the discovery of fundamental client values, beliefs, or system goals that emerge as underlying the problematic reaction. In addition, the process leads to the exploration of formative developmental events.

In this case, however, the process does not lead back to the exploration of the therapeutic relationship, and the ultimate resolution does not directly involve a corrective emotional experience through the therapeutic relationship. It is interesting to note, however, that in both cases relevant historical memories emerge spontaneously. This spontaneous emergence of relevant developmental memories in the context of experiential symbolization, is consistent with the hypothesis that episodic memories, expressive–motor behaviors, images, and autonomic arousal are represented together in a type of prototypical structure or schematic memory and that the activation of critical number or configuration of features of that schematic memory activates other subsidiary components. This spontaneous memory activation parallels certain aspects of a change process that is intentionally activated in psychodynamic therapy through the systematic exploration of historical memories. Is it always necessary to explore and reorganize relevant developmental memories in order to shift the client's current view of themselves in the world? This has been a stance traditionally taken by psychoanalytic theory, although experiential theorists have disagreed. Further investigation of this question is warranted.

The phenomenon of "tasting" described by Rice and Greenberg (Chapter 8, this volume), which involves sampling different and sometimes opposing aspects of a whole emotional experience, provides a further clarification of the distinction made by Gendlin and McGuire between sheer emotion and felt experience. Sheer emotion consists of a specific action disposition and its associated subjective affective experience (e.g., anger, sadness). In contrast, felt experience is a complex constellation of related emotions and thoughts that are often opposing and contradictory in nature. It is also interesting to note that the particular aspects of the feelings that emerge through this tasting process in the change event they describe (i.e. anger and the fear of expressing anger) correspond to what are traditionally referred to in psychodynamic theory as the wish and the defense again the wish.

The ultimate realization experienced by the client in the problematic reaction event described by Rice and Greenberg emerges as quite similar in nature to the type of pathogenic belief described by Silberschatz and Sampson (Chapter 5, this volume). The therapeutic environment offered by the client-centered approach may offer a type of naturalistic laboratory in which affective phenomena that are activated through different intervention strategies in different therapy orientations emerge in a relatively unconstrained form. The relative advantages and disadvantages of different interventions for activating similar affective processes is a topic warranting empirical investigation in the future.

FACILITATING COGNITIVE REORGANIZATION

A number of authors in this volume have explored the role that affective information can play in promoting cognitive reorganization (e.g., Engle et al., Chapter 7; Guidano, Chapter 3; Rice & Greenberg, Chapter 8). Here the central premise is that emotion provides a form of tacit meaning reflecting the overall values and goals of the system. This information may not be represented at an articulated conceptual level. By accessing and processing certain types of emotional information the individual may thus change his/her conscious, articulated sense of who he/she is.

There are a number of ways in which affective information can promote cognitive reorganization. First, affective information that has been previously ignored can facilitate a reorganization of the individual's sense of him/herself by confronting him/her with irrefutable information about previously disowned action dispositions. For example, the individual who has a restricted self-concept in which he/she views him/herself as never being angry will begin to revise this self-concept once he/she begins to allow and access irrefutable affective evidence to the contrary. Acknowledging disowned affects can thus be an important part of what Schafer (1983) refers to as owning disclaimed actions. This process can play an important role in helping to change the client's sense of him/herself from that of a helpless victim of others to that of an active contributor to situations. For example, in the problematic reaction change event presented by Rice and Greenberg (Chapter 8, this volume), the process of beginning to recognize that anger is part of her emotional experience begins to shift the client's self-concept away from that of a puzzled, helpless victim toward the recognition that *she inhibits herself* for fear of hurting others.

As Safran and Segal (1990) point out, the type of cognitive reorganization facilitated by acknowledging previously disowned affects can also contribute to change in another important way. When clients disown certain affective experiences for fear of the interpersonal consequences, they may nevertheless communicate their feelings behaviorally or nonverbally (see Chapter 1). For example, a client may have difficulty conceiving of him/herself as someone who gets angry but may nevertheless communicate his/her anger toward other people through sarcasm or through passive-aggressive acts. This type of communication can contribute to the type of maladaptive transactional cycle described by Butler and Strupp (Chapter 4, this volume), in that others may respond in a negative fashion to the aggressive behavior that is communicated nonverbally, even though the individual is not aware of his/her own hostile feelings. The client may then be bewildered by the situation and see him/herself as a helpless victim because he/she is not aware of his/her own contribution to the cycle. When the client begins to access angry feelings, however, the dilemma becomes less mysterious and he/she begins to gain an understanding of and accept responsibility for his/her own contribution to the cycle.

MOTIVATING ADAPTIVE BEHAVIOR

An important change process touched on by both McGuire (Chapter 9, this volume) and Guidano (Chapter 3, this volume) involves the use of emotional experience as a motivator of adaptive behavior. As we discussed in Chapter 1, emotion not only provides information about the readiness of the system to act in certain ways; it also pushes the system in a certain direction. Thus, for example, the client in McGuire's (Chapter 9, this volume) chapter decides to go back into therapy, after contacting her need for nurturance. Guidano's (Chapter 3, this volume) client, Gordon, contacts feelings of sadness and resentment, which play a role in helping him shift the nature of his marital relationship.

While neither of these chapters elaborate on this phenomenon in detail, our view is that it is of sufficient importance to warrant exploration in future work (Greenberg & Safran, 1987, 1989; Safran & Greenberg, 1986, 1987). Because of the motivational properties of affective experience, accessing previously unintegrated emotions can be an important shift point in the therapeutic process. One can, for example, stay in an abusive relationship indefinitely, despite the fact that one knows at some level that it is not a good relationship. When, however, one begins to access fully previously unintegrated feelings or anger and resentment, one can become motivated to initiate changes that previously seemed too threatening.

A socially isolated client may believe that he/she would be happier if he/she had more friends, and yet continue to fill time with work-related activities. When, however, he/she fully contacts the deep feelings of sadness and loneliness which have previously been only partly integrated, the individual may begin to take the risks involved in rearranging his/her activities.

Pascual-Leone (Chapter 13, this volume) introduces a neo-Piagetian perspective that provides a potentially useful metatheoretical framework for clarifying the organismic–environmental dynamics involved in this type of change process. Using Piaget's concept of equilibration, he suggests that in a well-adapted organism, all possible disturbances are represented by way of negations (i.e., negative emotions), and all negations are potentially compensated by corresponding affirmations (i.e., positive emotions). Thus, for example, a well-adapted organism would experience sadness in response to loss, and sadness would in turn motivate the type of behavior (e.g., recovery of or substitution for the lost object) that would result in positive emotions (e.g., joy).

The ability to process a full range of emotional experience (both positive and negative), would thus in theory be essential in order for an individual to have the type of flexibility necessary to respond adaptively to a wide range of different situations. A corollary and mirror image hypothesis is that confronting new disturbances provides the individual with an opportunity for growth through new equilibration processes, provided he/she is able to attend and process new emotions that may be painful or threatening.

Greenberg and Safran (1987) present a five-stage model of the process through which unintegrated emotions are accessed and ultimately lead to the mobilization of adaptive behaviour. In this model, the client (1) begins attending to an internal state that has previously been avoided, and then gradually proceeds through the processes of (2) accessing the emotional experience; (3) accepting the emotion; (4) symbolizing what the emotion means to them (e.g., "I'm lonely"; "I've been wronged"); and (5) establishing an action intent. Future empirical work will be required to refine this model and to establish its generalizability.

CORRECTIVE EMOTIONAL EXPERIENCE

Both Silberschatz and Sampson (Chapter 5, this volume) and Dahl (Chapter 6, this volume) focus on the process through which the therapist's stance disconfirms what the Mount Zion group refers to as the client's pathogenic beliefs and what Dahl (Chapter 6, this volume) refers to as the client's frame. Butler and Strupp (Chapter 4, this volume) also focus on this process in their examination of the therapeutic "unhooking." By unhooking him/herself from the client's maladaptive transactional cycle, the therapist is able to act in a fashion that provides information discrepant with the client's interpersonal schema, thereby providing new information at an experiential level, which can help restructure the schema.

As discussed earlier, an interpersonal schema will be activated and its components (e.g., images, expressive–motor responses) will be run off, when the features of an interpersonal encounter match a critical configuration of the schematic features. When this occurs in the context of the therapeutic relationship, an ideal opportunity emerges for exploring and restructuring the schematic components. A distinction can be made between the type of corrective emotional experience that takes place as a result of a transference interpretation and the type of corrective emotional experience that takes place when a client gains a felt sense about past relationships in the context of the present therapeutic relationship. This distinction is highlighted by Gendlin's (Chapter 10, this volume) and McGuire's (Chapter 9, this volume) chapters. When a transference interpretation is made, the emphasis is on providing schema-discrepant information through reappraising the situation at a conceptual level (although the interpersonal schema must be activated for this to be more than an intellectual exercise). In the change event examined by McGuire the client subjects the information accessed from the schema to further processing at a cognitive–affective level in order to arrive at a felt sense of the meaning of these old feelings in context with the current relationship. This experiential appraisal plays a parallel role to the conceptual reappraisal that is activated through a transference interpretation.

There is, however, a difference. Affective processing provides an on-going appraisal of current events and experiences for the individual. This affective appraisal reflects and is shaped by tacit values and goals that the individual has developed over a lifetime. Experiential processing thus involves a holistic appraisal of the meaning for the organism of the entire current configuration, that is, the client's current feelings and perceptions, and the therapist's reactions to them. This type of holistic appraisal can thus modify an existing cognitive–affective schema by incorporating new information from the current experience.

One phenomenon described by Silberschatz and Sampson (Chapter 5, this volume), which is particularly interesting from an affective change process perspective, is the emergence of warded-off affect when the thera-pist acts in a fashion that disconfirms the client's pathogenic belief. This observation is consistent with the hypothesis that one of the more impor-tant ways of challenging tacit beliefs or fears that interrupt the experience and expression of emotional experience is through the therapist's behav-ior. The type of dysfunctional beliefs about emotional experience de-scribed by various authors in this volume (e.g., Butler & Strupp, Chapter 4; Engle et al., Chapter 7; Rice & Greenberg, Chapter 8; Silberschatz & Sampson, Chapter 5) are thus an important class of dysfunctional beliefs that have not traditionally been focused on by cognitive therapists but which have been dealt with by psychodynamic therapists as defenses (Safran & Segal, 1990).

These tacit beliefs or dysfunctional beliefs can be explored and chal-lenged at an explicit level by drawing them to the client's attention and interpreting or challenging them in one fashion or another (e.g. Butler & Strupp, Chapter 4, this volume). It is important to emphasize, however, that the content of the intervention may well be overridden by the process of the intervention or the relationship aspect of the intervention. Thus as Rice and Greenberg point out in their discussion of the "prizing event" the therapist's manner in dealing with the client's vulnerability is critical in determining the nature of the subsequent process.

Once warded-off affect has emerged as a result of a passed "transfer-ence test" it can facilitate change in a number of ways. Silberschatz and Sampson (Chapter 5, this volume) suggest that the acknowledgment of warded-off affect can correct a distorted view of one's self and others by leading to the retrieval of memories relevant to understanding the way in which one has developed his/her self-concept.

In an example they cite, a patient, through acknowledging angry feelings toward his parents, retrieves memories of parental humiliation, which help to disconfirm a view of himself as uninteresting, undeserving, and unattractive. It would be important in this type of situation to develop a more-detailed model of the change process. What are the important components of the process and in what sequence do they take place? Does the acknowledgment of anger toward the parents in and of itself contribute to change or is it the reconstruction of the patient's childhood that is important? Is this reconstruction a rational process or a more affectively laden process? In our view, all of the affective processes discussed to this point (i.e., emotional restructuring, catharsis, experiential symbolization, facilitating cognitive reorganization and motivating adaptive behavior) may play a role in this context.

AFFECT ATTUNEMENT

An important area that is touched on by the contributors to this volume (e.g., Gendlin, Chapter 10; McGuire, Chapter 9; Rice & Greenberg, Chapter 8), but is not elaborated on in detail, is the role of affect in the process of empathic communication. A vital aspect of the empathic process involves tuning in to the subtleties of the client's inner world at an affective level. Recent work on affect attunement in developmental psychology is illuminating in this respect. In a series of studies, Stern (1985) and colleagues have demonstrated that infants' mothers automatically attune themselves to the infants' internal affective state and interact in a fashion that demonstrates this attunement.

Consider the following examples taken from Stern (1985). A 9-month-old girl becomes very excited about a toy and lets out an exuberant "AAAH!" as she reaches for it and looks at her mother. The mother responds by looking back, scrunching up her shoulders, and shimmying her upper body. The shimmy lasts approximately the same length as her daughter's "AHHH!" and has the same quality of excitement, joy, and intensity.

A 9-month-old boy is banging his hand on a toy in a rhythmic fashion with pleasure, exuberance, and humor. His mother matches the rhythm and affective quality of the boy's internal experience by saying "KAAA-BAM, KAAAA-BAM, KAAAA-BAM," in rhythm to the boy's banging.

In both these examples, the mother automatically empathizes with the child's internal affective state and communicates her empathic experience, typically by matching the contour and intensity of the child's emotional state in another modality. Affect attunement, then, in Stern's (1985) words "is the performance of behaviors that express the quality of feelings of a shared affect state without imitating the exact behavioral expression of the inner state" (p. 142). Research with mothers who are affectively attuning to their infants indicates that often they do so automatically, but, when asked to reflect on the behavior, will respond that they are simply wanting to "be with the infant" or share in his/her experience.

Further research has demonstrated that mothers who are instructed to misattune their responses to the infant's affective state disrupt the normal interactional sequence and that it remains disrupted until the mother begins to re-attune. Other research demonstrates that some mothers consistently misattune to their child's affective experience.

Accurate affect attunement plays a pivotal role in helping infants become aware of and articulate their affective experience to themselves, and to integrate it into their overall sense of self. Thus, for example, the child who consistently does not have experiences of excitement and exuberance attuned to will not integrate these adaptive feeling states into his/ her sense of self. The child who does not have feelings of sadness or vulnerability attuned to accurately will have difficulty incorporating these more vulnerable feeling states into his/her sense of self.

By the same token, affect attunement by the therapist may play a vital role in helping the client to contact, articulate, and integrate into his/her sense of self, adaptive feeling states that are currently unarticulated. In order for this to take place, however, the therapist must truly be able to attune to the idiosyncratic subtleties, intensity, and contours of the client's emotional experience. An empathic response that captures various cognitive features of the client's internal experience may nevertheless be misattuned to the subtleties of the client's affective experience.

Moreover, another potentially problematic process may take place if the therapist attunes to the client's affective states well enough to in a sense be allowed "inside the client's world" but nevertheless misattunes enough that the nature of the client's experience will be changed when it becomes articulated. In this type of situation what may happen is that, as Stern (1985) puts it, the individual's emotional experience may in a sense be "robbed" or "stolen" from him/her. It is thus critical for the therapist to be able to attune accurately to the subtleties of the client's affective experience.

THE THERAPIST'S EMOTIONS

The focus throughout most of this volume is on the role of the client's emotional experience in the change process. As Izard (Chapter 11, this volume) points out, however, the therapist's emotional experience plays an equally important part in the change process. The client is part of a two-person system, and both members of that system, to paraphrase Sullivan, play an inextricable role in all that takes place. The therapist's emotional experience functions in a number of ways.

First, therapists' emotions provide them with valuable information about the action dispositions that are evoked in them by particular clients. This allows therapists to generate hypotheses about the action dispositions that the clients evoke in other people and about the type of dysfunctional interpersonal patterns that are likely to be characteristic of them. Therapists' emotions thus provide a vital tool in allowing them to clarify the nature of the maladaptive transactional cycle described by Butler and Strupp (Chapter 4, this volume). Moreover, by tuning into and becoming aware of their own emotions, therapists are able to become aware of their own automatic action dispositions. This is vital to the process of unhooking from the client's maladaptive transactional cycle. Therapists who have difficulty processing the full range of emotional experience in themselves will thus have difficulties in unhooking from certain types of maladaptive transactional cycles (Safran & Segal, 1990).

Second, therapists' emotional experience is instrumental in the process of attuning to the client's emotional experience. To the extent that therapists have difficulty fully processing and experiencing certain aspects of their own emotional experience, they will have difficulty attuning to related aspects of the client's experience. Thus, for example, therapists who have difficulty processing feelings of sadness in themselves will have difficulty attuning to such feelings in their clients. Therapists who have difficulty attuning to personal feelings of anger will have difficulty attuning to feelings of anger in clients. Problems in processing the full range of personal emotional experience will thus lead therapists to have systematic biases in attuning to their clients' emotional experience. This will lead to misattunement, which will impede many of the affective change processes that facilitate growth (Safran & Segal, 1990).

A final theme relates to the role of the therapist's emotions in establishing an authentic human encounter. Guidano's intriguing description of the Jessica case (Chapter 3, this volume) raises as many questions as it answers, but it hints at the potentially potent healing impact that an authentic human encounter can have. He suggests that the therapist, in losing his temper, demonstrates to the client that he considers himself to be engaged in a real relationship, and that this in some way shifts the nature of the intervention. While we find it difficult (as does Guidano) to reconstruct, exactly how this interaction may have led to change, it does appear to involve breaking through the barrier to human relatedness resulting from playing the role of the therapist, and allowing an authentic I-Thou encounter to take place.

GENERAL ISSUES

Top-Down versus Bottom-Up Processing

An interesting theme that emerges in reading the different perspectives presented in this book, is what can be framed as the difference between top-down versus bottom-up perspectives on the role of affective processes in psychotherapy. All of the contributors acknowledge that the experience and expression of different kinds of emotion in different contexts can facilitate the change process. In some cases, however, the therapeutic emphasis is on exploring and challenging tacit rules and beliefs that guide the processing of emotional experience (top-down processing), whereas in other cases the therapeutic emphasis is on accessing and intensifying the emotional experience itself (bottom-up). As an example of the first emphasis, consider Chapter 4 by Butler and Strupp (this volume). In their discussion of therapy with the compulsive client, they emphasize the importance of unhooking from the client's deadening interpersonal pull and of analyzing the defenses that interrupt the underlying emotional experience. The emphasis is thus not on facilitating or enhancing the underlying emotional experience itself, but rather on challenging the tacit rules or prohibitions that interrupt that experience. Or consider Guidano's chapter (Chapter 3, this volume). In his analysis of the agoraphobic client, Gordon, the emphasis is on helping the client to develop a conceptual framework that allows him to be open to and make sense of diverse emotional experiences that he has previously interpreted as diffuse anxiety. Here again, the emphasis is on modifying the client's conceptual framework in order to allow him/her to process affective experience in a different way.

   In contrast, consider the unfinished business event described by Engle et al. (Chapter 7, this volume). Here the emphasis is clearly on accessing and intensifying the client's previoulsy interrupted feelings toward the objects of the unfinished business. Little or no emphasis is given to exploring and challenging the fears and beliefs that may be involved in interrupting the expression for the completion of this emotional experience.

   Or, consider the experiencing process described by McGuire (Chapter 9, this volume), or Gendlin (Chapter 10, this volume). Here again, the emphasis is on helping the client to attend to and fully process a current appraisal of the whole situation that is grounded in the client felt-sense or expressive motor reactions. No emphasis is placed on exploring beliefs and tacit rules that may interfere with this type of experiential processing.

   A useful framework for understanding the clinical role played by attending to expressive–motor behavior and emotional memory on the one hand or appraisals and rules and beliefs at the conceptual level on the other, is provided by Leventhal's (1984) model of emotion. As discussed earlier, Leventhal hypothesizes that there are three levels in the emotional processing hierarchy: expressive–motor, schematic, and conceptual. According to him, the expressive–motor level provides the fundamental, wired-in base from which subsequent emotional experience is constructed. The schematic level consists of emotional memories that have developed over time through the encoding of specific events and expressive–motor behaviors and associated autonomic arousal that have been activated by those events. The conceptual level consists of rules and beliefs about emotional processing that guide the way in which the individual synthesizes emotional experience. Thus, for example, an individual who learns that it is dangerous to experience sadness may not attend to expressive-motor behavior consistent with that emotion and may not synthesize it into a conscious experience of sadness. Thus rules and beliefs at the conceptual level play a role in the synthesis or construction of emotional experience.

Since emotional synthesis is both bottom-up and top-down in nature (Greenberg & Safran, 1984), interventions at both levels may be therapeutic. The tendency of contributors in this volume to focus interventions at either the expressive-motor level or the more conceptual level may reflect different theoretical biases. There is no reason, however, for therapists to restrict their focus to one level or the other. Thus, interventions aimed at both the rules governing emotional experience and at the sensory/somatic aspects of feeling may be superior to those focusing on only one aspect of emotional processing.

Core Affective Change Processes

Our review of the affective change events described by the authors in this volume suggests that while some of the events focused on are distinctly different from one another (e.g., completing unfinished business versus focusing), others appear similar in some respects and different in others. For example, spontaneously accessing childhood memories during the focusing event appears similar in some respects to the way in which childhood memories are intentionally worked with when the therapist makes a genetic transference interpretation. The exploration of wishes and fears in the context of the "tasting" procedure described by Rice and Greenberg (Chapter 8, this volume) appears similar in some ways to the exploration of defenses and wishes in psychodynamic therapy and different in other ways.

We hypothesize that there are a number of core affective change processes which can be activated in a variety of different ways. The particular intervention that is employed to activate the change process, however, will ultimately color that change process in a particular way. Thus for example, the use of a transference interpretation to activate a corrective emotional experience will color the ultimate nature of that corrective emotional experience.[3] Similarly, the type of corrective emotional experience resulting from spontaneously recalling memories related to the current therapist–client interaction and then processing this event at an experiential level, will ultimately color the corrective emotional experience another way. The specific change events focused on by the contrib-

utors to this book thus involve underlying affective processes that have
been shaped and colored by the specific therapist interventions that establish the context in which they take place.

In this chapter we have examined a number of processes that apear to
underly the different affective change events. In the future it will be
important to clarify systematically the different interventions that can be
employed to activate these processes as well as subtle differences in the
nature of the ultimate change process that may result from employing
different activating strategies. It will also be important to subject the
specific change events described by the authors to more rigorous empirical
investigation. In addition, it will be important to identify other affective
change events, and evaluate the similarities and differences between those
described here and in other sources (e.g., Greenberg & Safran, 1987).

Although recent years have witnessed a growing interest in the role of
emotion in the therapeutic change process, in many ways work in this area
is still in its infancy. As the different contributions to this book have
demonstrated, the domain of affective change is heterogeneous in nature,
consisting of diverse affective change processes that are similar in some
ways and different in others. Thus, to speak about affective change as a
uniform process such as "emotional insight" or "catharsis" or "emotional
relearning" or "emotional processing" obscures the underlying diversity of
the real phenomena. These contributions can thus be considered the
beginning of an "unpacking" process through which our understanding of
a core dimension of therapeutic change can become progressively more
differentiated over time. This differentiation will involve systematic and
rigorous conceptual and empirical work in which models of important
affective change events are developed and tested. The task that lies ahead is
a substantial one, and it will require the combined efforts of numerous
investigators. The size of this task, however, in no way exceeds its importance.

NOTES

1. This categorization scheme corresponds in some respects the one presented by
Greenberg and Safran (1987, 1989), and diverges in other respects. Our intent is
to provide a scheme that is heuristic in the present context rather than an absolute
or immutable framework.

2. Related concepts have been proposed by Stern (1985), who speaks of representations of interactions that have been generalized, and Horowitz (1979) who speaks
of role relationship schemata.

3. Consistent with a growing number of theorists (e.g., Kohut, 1984; Strupp &
Binder, 1984; Weiss, Sampson, & the Mount Zion Psychotherapy Research Group,

1986), we hypothesize that the impact of the intervention is due to a corrective emotional experience rather than the acquisition of intellectual insight.

REFERENCES

Alexander, F., & French, T. M. (1946). *Psychoanalytic therapy: Principles and applications.* New York: Ronald Press.

Bowlby, J. (1969). *Attachment and loss: Vol. 1. Attachment.* New York: Basic Books.

Breuer, J., & Freud, S. (1955). Studies on hysteria. In J. Strachey (Ed.), *Standard edition of the complete psychological works of Sigmund Freud* (Vol. 2). London: Hogarth Press. (Original work published 1895)

Gendlin, E. T. (1962). *Experiencing and the creation of meaning.* New York: Free Press of Glencoe.

Gendlin, E. T. (1979). Experiential psychotherapy. In R. Corsini (Ed.), *Current psychotherapies* (rev. ed.). Itasca, IL: Peacock.

Greenberg, L. S., & Safran, J. D. (1984). Integrating affect and cognition: A perspective on the process of therapeutic change. *Cognitive Therapy and Research, 8,* 559–578.

Greenberg, L. S., & Safran, J. D. (1987). *Emotion in psychotherapy.* New York: Guilford.

Greenberg, L. S., & Safran, J. D. (1989). Emotion in psychotherapy. *American Psychologist, 44,* 19–29.

Horowitz, M. (1979). *States of mind.* New York: Plenum.

Kegan, R. (1982). *The evolving self: Problem and process in human development.* Cambridge, MA: Harvard University Press.

Kohut, H. (1984). *How does analysis cure?* Chicago: University of Chicago Press.

Lang, P. J. (1984). Cognition in emotion: Concept and action. In C. Izard, J. Kagan, & R. Zajonc (Eds.), *Emotions, cognition and behavior.* London and New York: Cambridge University Press.

Leventhal, H. (1982). The integration of emotion and cognition: A view from the perceptual–motor theory of emotion. In M. S. Clarke & S. T. Fiske (Eds.), *Affect and cognition.* Hillsdale, NJ: Erlbaum.

Leventhal, H. (1984). A perceptual–motor theory of emotion. In L. Berkowitz (Ed.), *Advances in experimental social psychology* (Vol. 17, pp. 117–182). New York: Academic Press.

Lowen, A. (1975). *Pleasure: A creative approach.* Baltimore: Penguin Books.

Main, M., Kaplan, N., & Cassidy, J. (1985). Security in infancy, childhood and adulthood: A move to the level of representation. *Monographs of the Society for Research in Child Development, 50,* (1–2), 66–104.

Perls, F. (1973). *The Gestalt approach and eye witness therapy.* Palo Alto, CA: Science and Behavior Books, Bantam Edition.

Reich, W. (1942). *The function of the orgasm.* New York: Orgone Institute.

Rogers, C. R. (1961). *Client-centered therapy.* Boston: Houghton Mifflin.

Safran, J. D. (1986, June). *A critical evaluation of the schema construct in psychotherapy research.* Paper presented at the Society for Psychotherapy Research Conference, Boston.

Safran, J. D. (1990a). Towards a refinement of cognitive therapy in light of interpersonal theory: I. Theory. *Clinical Psychology Review, 10*, 87-105.

Safran, J. D. (1990b). Towards a refinement of cognitive therapy in light of interpersonal theory: II. Practice. *Clinical Psychology Review, 10*, 107-121.

Safran, J. D., & Greenberg, L. S. (1982). Cognitive appraisal and reappraisal: Implications for clinical practice. *Cognitive Therapy and Research, 6*, 251-258.

Safran, J. D., & Greenberg, L. S. (1986). Hot cognition and psychotherapy process: An information processing/ecological approach. In P. C. Kendall (Ed.), *Advances in cognitive-behavioral research and therapy* (Vol. 5, pp. 143-177). New York: Academic Press.

Safran, J. D., & Greenberg, L. S. (1987). Affect and the unconscious: A cognitive perspective. In R. Stern (Ed.), *Theories of the unconscious* (pp. 191-212). Hillsdale, NJ: Analytic Press.

Safran, J. D., & Segal, Z. S. (1990). *Interpersonal process in cognitive therapy.* New York: Basic Books.

Schafer, R. (1983). *The analytic attitude.* New York: Basic Books.

Stern, D. N. (1985). *The interpersonal world of the infant.* New York: Basic Books.

Strupp, H. H., & Binder, J. L. (1984). *Psychotherapy in a new key: A guide to time-limited dynamic therapy.* New York: Basic Books.

Weiss, J., Sampson, H., & the Mount Zion Psychotherapy Research Group. (1987). *The psychoanalytic process: Theory, clinical observations, and empirical research.* New York: Guilford.

Index